www.harcourt-international.com

Bringing you products from all Harcourt Health Sciences companies including Baillière Tindall, Churchill Livingstone, Mosby and W.B. Saunders

- ▶ **Browse** for latest information on new books, journals and electronic products

- ▶ **Search** for information on over 20 000 published titles with full product information including tables of contents and sample chapters

- ▶ **Keep up to date** with our extensive publishing programme in your field by registering with eAlert or requesting postal updates

- ▶ **Secure online ordering** with prompt delivery, as well as full contact details to order by phone, fax or post

- ▶ **News** of special features and promotions

If you are based in the following countries, please visit the country-specific site to receive full details of product availability and local ordering information

USA: www.harcourthealth.com

Canada: www.harcourtcanada.com

Australia: www.harcourt.com.au

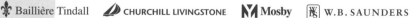
Baillière Tindall   CHURCHILL LIVINGSTONE   Mosby   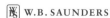 W.B. SAUNDERS

Massage Therapy: The Evidence for Practice

DATE DUE

JUL 22 2002	
JUL 11 2002	
DEC 19 2002 OCT 16 2002	
NOV 20 2003 NOV 17 2003	
AUG 25 2004	
AUG 18 2004	
MAR - 1 2007	
MAY - 7 2007	

For Ashley Montagu,
whose work on touch continues to inspire us

Editor

Grant Jewell Rich PhD LMT
Grant received his PhD in psychology at the University of Chicago. He has been a licensed massage therapist and licensed social worker in both Maine and Ohio. He has served as the 2nd VP for AMTA-Ohio and as the chair of the editorial advisory board for AMTA's *Massage Therapy Journal*. His popular writing has appeared in magazines including *Psychology Today, Massage Magazine, Massage Therapy Journal*, and *Skeptical Inquirer*. Academically, he has edited a number of special issues for such journals as *Anthropology of Consciousness, Journal of Humanistic Psychology*, and (forthcoming) *Journal of Youth and Adolescence*. Having taught at Ohio State University and Antioch College, Grant now serves on the faculty of Bates College, where he teaches courses including research methods and health psychology. He maintains a strong interest in optimal experience, quality of life, and positive psychology.

For Mosby:

Editorial Director: Mary Law
Project Development Manager: Dinah Thom
Project Manager: Gail Wright
Design Direction: Judith Wright

Massage Therapy: The Evidence for Practice

Edited by

Grant Jewell Rich PhD LMT
Bates College, Lewiston, Maine, USA

Foreword by

Janet R. Kahn PhD
Senior Research Scientist, Integrative Consulting, Burlington; Past President of the American Massage Therapy Association Foundation; Member of the NIH National Advisory Council on Complementary and Alternative Medicine; Massage Therapist, USA

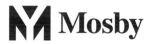 Mosby

EDINBURGH LONDON NEW YORK PHILADELPHIA ST LOUIS SYDNEY TORONTO 2002

MOSBY
An imprint of Harcourt Publishers Limited

© Harcourt Publishers Limited 2002

M is a registered trademark of Harcourt Publishers Limited

The right of Grant Jewell Rich to be identified as editor of this work
has been asserted by him in accordance with the Copyright, Designs
and Patents Act 1988

First published 2002

ISBN 0 7234 3217 1

British Library Cataloguing in Publication Data
A catalogue record for this book is available from the British Library

Library of Congress Cataloging in Publication Data
A catalog record for this book is available from the Library of
Congress

Note
Medical knowledge is constantly changing. As new information
becomes available, changes in treatment, procedures, equipment and
the use of drugs become necessary. The editor, contributors and the
publishers have taken care to ensure that the information given in this
text is accurate and up to date. However, readers are strongly advised
to confirm that the information, especially with regard to drug usage,
complies with the latest legislation and standards of practice.

The
publisher's
policy is to use
paper manufactured
from sustainable forests

Printed in China by RDC Group Limited

Contents

Contributors

Bhakti Arondekar MS is a PhD candidate in the Department of Pharmacy Administration at the University of Illinois at Chicago. She received the UIC-Pharmacia Fellowship in Outcomes Research in the Department of Pharmacy Practice at UIC. The fellowship included one year in the Global Health Outcomes Research Group at Pharmacia in Skokie, Illinois. Bhakti has also served a summer internship at Pharmacia. Her research interests are in pharmacoeconomics and outcomes measurement. She received her MS in Pharmacy and Health Care Administration from the University of Toledo in 1998.

Curtis D. Black BS MS PhD RPh is Interim Chair of the Pharmacy Practice Department and Assistant Dean of Academic Affairs at the University of Toledo College of Pharmacy, and is also Merck Professor of Clinical Pharmacy. His teaching efforts at the undergraduate level focus on pharmaceutics and the development of innovative dosage forms for drug delivery. At the graduate and doctoral level, he focuses on oncology therapeutics and research design. He maintains a teaching practice with a group of medical oncologists and serves as the Chair of the Education and Research Committee of the Stem Cell Transplantation Program at a local medical center. Curtis publishes in the areas of drug delivery, oncology therapeutics and contemporary issues in pharmacy practice. A registered pharmacist, he received his BS degree from the University of Toledo, and his PhD degree from the University of Purdue.

Judie Boehmer MN RN has been a nurse for 13 years at the University of California Davis Medical Center. She is the nurse manager of the University's Birthing Center, Women's Pavilion, and Newborn Nursery. Previously, she has held positions as a staff nurse as well as a nurse educator.

John N. I. Dieter PhD is Senior Research Associate of the Behavioral Perinatology Laboratory at Emory University. He received his doctorate in clinical psychology from Emory University and completed his internship in the Departments of Pediatrics and Psychiatry at the University of Miami School of Medicine. He is a past research associate of the Touch Research

Institute at the University of Miami. John has received a National Research Service Award from the National Institute of Mental Health and is a current recipient of a Young Investigator Award from the National Alliance for Research on Schizophrenia and Depression. He has published research articles and book chapters in the areas of neuropsychology, psychophysiology, chronic pain and early development. His current research focuses on the effects of maternal psychopathology on fetal and newborn development and supplemental stimulation for hospitalized preterm infants.

Eugene K. Emory PhD is Professor of Psychology at Emory University in Atlanta, Georgia. He is the recipient of the NIMH Research Scientist Development Award, and a previous NIH Study Section Member, Cognition, Emotion, & Personality, Human Development & Aging. A Charter Fellow of the American Psychological Society, currently he is a member of the National Academy of Sciences Board on Behavioral, Cognitive, & Sensory Processes, and the National Academy of Sciences Committee on Juvenile Crime, Prevention, and Control. His primary research emphasis is developmental neuropsychology, specifically perinatal behavioral and neural development. He is the author of over 75 published research articles, book chapters and abstracts.

Edzard Ernst MD PhD FRCP(Edin) qualified as a physician in Germany, where he also completed his MD and PhD theses. He was Professor in Physical Medicine and Rehabilitation (PMR) at Hannover Medical School and Head of the PMR Department at the University of Vienna. He came to the University of Exeter in 1993 to establish the first Chair in Complementary Medicine. He is founder/editor-in-chief of two medical journals (*FACT (Focus on Alternative and Complementary Therapies)* and *Perfusion*). His work has been awarded with eight scientific prizes. He sits on the Medicines Commission of the British Medicines Control Agency and on the Scientific Committee on Herbal Medicinal Products of the Irish Medicines Board. In 1999 he took British nationality.

Tiffany M. Field PhD has been conducting massage therapy research at the University of Miami for 25 years and has directed the Touch Research Institute of the Department of Pediatrics for the last 9 years. She received the American Psychological Association Distinguished Young Scientist Award from the NIMH for her research career. She is the author of several series of volumes on high-risk infants, and the author of over 400 journal papers.

Margaret Hodge RN EdD is a Clinical Nurse Scientist at the University of California Davis Medical Center. In addition to her role as a researcher, she is a member of the faculty at California State University, Sacramento, where she teaches a course in Complementary and Alternative Medicine. Her research interests include the role of the nurse in assessing and implementing complementary and alternative therapies.

Monica Holiday-Goodman BS PhD RPh is Coordinator and Associate Professor, Division of Pharmacy and Health Care Administration at the University of Toledo College of Pharmacy. She received her BS and PhD degrees from Northeast Louisiana University, and is also a registered pharmacist. Monica's teaching and research focus on the socio-cultural, educational and administrative aspects of health care provision. She has been an invited speaker to several state and national audiences, and has received state, federal, and corporate funding for her scholarly endeavors. She has numerous publications in peer-reviewed journals, and is also co-editor of the book *Writing Across the Curriculum for Colleges of Pharmacy*.

Sally Klein BSN MSN is a Psychiatric Clinical Nurse Specialist and Assistant Clinical Professor at the University of California Davis Medical Center in Sacramento, California. She received her BSN from the College of Saint Benedict, Minnesota and her MSN from the University of Minnesota. Sally has been in psychiatric–mental health nursing for the past 25 years, with special interests in community mental health and psychiatric consult-liaison nursing.

Silvana Lawvere BA MS LMT has been a licensed massage therapist for the last ten years. She has studied various modalities of massage and has practiced in spas, wellness centers, chiropractic offices, hospitals, and in private practice around the world. Currently, she is a doctoral candidate for a PhD in Epidemiology and Community Health from the State University of New York in Buffalo. She lives in Los Angeles and works at Cedars-Sinai Medical Center as part of a cardiac imaging research group, and is a consultant for alternative medicine research.

Buford T. Lively BS MA RPh EdD HonPharmD is a registered pharmacist, and Professor of Pharmacy and Health Care Administration at the University of Toledo College of Pharmacy. He has also been licensed as a school guidance counselor in West Virginia, as well as earning teaching certification in English and Mathematics. He received his BS degree in Pharmacy and EdD degree in Pharmacy and Health Care Administration from the West Virginia University School of Pharmacy and School of Education and Human Resources, respectively. His other earned degrees are a BS in Mathematics and English and an MA in Guidance and Counseling. He also has an Honorary PharmD from the State of Louisiana. He managed a hospital-based outpatient pharmacy at the West Virginia University Medical Center and a community chain pharmacy before entering academia.

He has served as the Chairman of the Department of Pharmacy Practice at the University of Louisiana at Monroe School of Pharmacy and Health Sciences, Chairman of the Department of Behavioral and Administrative Pharmacy at the West Virginia University School of Pharmacy, Head of the Division of Pharmacy and Health Care Administration at the University of Toledo College of Pharmacy, and Assistant Dean of Administrative and External Affairs at the University of Toledo College of Pharmacy. His general teaching and research areas are in pharmacy and health care administration, outcomes measurements and patient health education. His specific research interests are in patient counseling, communication, writing across the curriculum in pharmacy schools, diversity, and personnel management. He has published over 50 journal articles and has given over 100 presentations at state and national meetings. He is co-editor of the book *Writing Across the Curriculum for Colleges of Pharmacy*, and is also the author of the recently published book *Modern American Pharmacy: An Orientation to Pharmacy Practice*.

Martha Brown Menard PhD CMT received her doctorate in education from the University of Virginia in 1995. She is the author of *Making Sense of Research*, a guide to research literacy for complementary practitioners, and chairs the research grant review committee for the AMTA Foundation. In addition to consulting with individuals and organizations on developing hospital-based massage programs, she maintains a private practice in Charlottesville, Virginia, specializing in massage and bodywork as an adjunct to medical and psychological care.

Ruth Remington PhD RN CS is a nurse practitioner working in central Massachusetts in the ambulatory and nursing home settings. She is also Assistant Professor in Nursing at University of Massachusetts Lowell.

Carol Robinson RN MPA received her Bachelor of Science in Nursing degree from the University of Virginia, Charlottesville in 1973 and her Master in Public Administration from the University of San Francisco, California in 1986. Carol became a Johnson and Johnson Wharton Fellow in 1996. Prior to 1980 she held a variety of nursing positions on the East Coast including staff nurse/charge nurse in ICU/CCU, hospital nursing supervisor, assistant director of nursing and critical care coordinator. She accepted the position of Assistant Director of Hospital and Clinics, Critical Care/Emergency Services at the University of California Davis Medical Center (UCDMC) when she came to Sacramento in 1980. She was in that position until 1991 when she was selected for the Director of Nursing/Associate Director of Hospital and Clinics, Patient Care Services position, also at UCDMC.

Sandra L. Rogers MS PhD OTR is an occupational therapist with 17 years' experience in treating individuals with neurorehabilitation needs, including spinal cord injuries. She has an MS and PhD in Kinesiology from the University of Wisconsin-Madison. Her research interests include utilizing physiological and immunological methods to document outcomes following intervention in individuals who have had neurological trauma. She is currently an assistant professor at the Ohio State University in Columbus, Ohio, teaching in the occupational therapy program and conducting research, and serves as the rehabilitation specialist for the Huntington's Disease Society of America Center of Excellence at Ohio State.

Foreword

Massage Therapy: The Evidence for Practice is an important volume because it deepens and broadens our awareness of the nascent scientific investigation of therapeutic massage. By collecting these papers into one volume, the editor and authors provide a starting point for conversations—conversations within the therapeutic massage community, conversations within the health sciences and research community, and, most importantly, conversations between those two groups. Only good can come from this.

Therapeutic massage is at once one of the oldest of the healing modalities, and simultaneously one of the least studied. In itself this discrepancy is simply an interesting observation likely to prompt speculation. Maybe there has been relatively little research on it because it is so familiar to us. After all, didn't most of our mothers rub our bumps and bruises when we were little? It doesn't take a rocket scientist to know that rubbing helps. Perhaps also because rubbing sore bits and giving backrubs is something we can all do, it is easy to dismiss massage as a household remedy, not 'real medicine' and therefore not likely to be very powerful. Of course it helps, but just a little.

And so, as Kuhn told us (Kuhn, 1970), when ideas or practices are commonly accepted, their investigation is often ignored. Why spend hundreds of thousands of dollars to find out something that we already know? Combine this with the general assumption that at the very least massage, like chicken soup, couldn't hurt you, and you find no pressing sense that investigations are needed to protect public safety. Simply put, there was not much motivation within the health care community to look at massage. This was matched by the lack of interest in research the massage community showed for many years. An all too common attitude seemed to be, 'I see and hear from my clients about the benefits of massage every day. That is proof enough for me.'

There is, however, one very important reason for examining therapeutic massage more closely, and that is that millions of people around the world use it. In 1998, 11% of adults in the USA utilized massage, collectively making an estimated 114 million visits to massage therapists that year (Eisenberg, et al., 1998). In national surveys of Americans' use of complementary and alternative medicine, therapeutic massage is consistently shown to be among the top three modalities used (Eisenberg, et al., 1993).

This usage alone demands that we stop making assumptions about its efficacy or lack thereof, and its safety or lack thereof, and instead conduct systematic inquiry into these issues. We need to know when and why people are using massage. We need to know whether they are in fact deriving any benefit or taking any risk through this behavior; and when massage is shown to have particular effects we need to explore why and how this happens. This volume begins to do that.

To do this in a concerted way will require real change. Consider, for instance, the NIH allocations. Between 1993 and 1997, the Office of Alternative Medicine (OAM) funded 50 studies. This included ten on acupuncture, seven on botanicals or other ingestibles, six on hypnosis or guided imagery, four on massage, three on chiropractic, and one or two each on a total of fourteen other modalities spanning the alphabetical gamut from ayurveda to yoga. In dollar terms, OAM invested $1,881,053 in the study of botanicals, $584,901 in acupuncture research and $115,200 in investigations of therapeutic massage. Funding became even more focused and more discrepant as time went on. By 1999 OAM had become the National Center for Complementary and Alternative Medicine (NCCAM) and in that year it funded eleven studies on botanicals totaling almost five million dollars ($4,902,281), ten studies on acupuncture ($2,703,435), a Center for Chiropractic Research ($650,352), and two studies on meditation ($404,235). There were no studies on massage funded by NCCAM in 1999; one small study ($13,968) on massage had been funded in 1998 (NCCAM).

These numbers do not reflect NCCAM priorities alone. In fact, that is not the main story they tell. The lack of funding for massage research is primarily a product of the small number of proposals on massage submitted to NIH each year. This in turn reflects the relative lack of interest, imagination or preparedness on the part of both the massage and research communities for this enterprise.

Happily, I believe this picture is changing and this book both illustrates and contributes to that change by presenting some of the pioneering work done to date. The volume illustrates something of the span of possible applications of massage that should be investigated. It offers studies exploring the potential of massage to be of benefit to people across the life-span, from Dieter and Emory's solid review of the growing body of literature on kinesthetic and tactile stimulation with premature infants to Remington's work with the elderly. The book offers data exploring the possibility that massage could be of help to people who are coping with serious illness including those with cancer, AIDS, spinal cord injury, and clinical depression. It also offers, in the chapter by Hodge, et al., one of the best of the existing studies examining the potential for massage to ease the stresses of everyday life, in this case the stresses associated with a highly demanding workplace.

This volume represents massage therapy research at its current stage of development. Consonant with the relative lack of funding mentioned earlier, we find here studies with sample sizes that are frustratingly small and cannot really tell us what we want to know. But larger studies will now be done precisely because, as Lawvere so accurately points out in the chapter on massage in ovarian cancer patients, these relatively small studies, at the very least, indicate that it is possible to do research on these topics and with these populations. They are bushwhacking studies, making the path easier for the next folks to travel.

The book also shows us the progress that has been made. The field of therapeutic massage research is more advanced than it was five years ago, the discussions more methodologically sophisticated than they used to be. Gone are the days, for instance, when one could simply label an intervention massage without a solid presentation of the protocol used and the rationale for it.

Grant Rich is to be commended for seeing the need and possibility at this time for a single volume offering a look at the range of research on therapeutic massage. Since there are no peer-reviewed journals devoted specifically to massage research, there is no one place that interested parties can go to stay abreast of it as it emerges. On the contrary, research on therapeutic massage, as the citations in these chapters illustrate, is found in a wide array of journals each with its own substantive focus— adolescence, neuroscience, oncology and the like. This volume, then, offers those new to the field of therapeutic massage a concise look at the range of possible applications. In doing that, it should spark the interest and imaginations of researchers and practitioners in many fields.

In addition, by bringing together the presentation of relatively new data in the same volume with reviews of the literature on areas where it has begun to amass, and discussing the methodological challenges inherent in the field, Rich has offered massage therapy educators an aid in bringing research into our classrooms. This is vital. For massage to mature as a profession, we must produce practitioners who are versed in the basics of research methods and who are capable of and committed to locating and staying abreast of the research. We owe this to our clients. New knowledge is being produced. This book shares some of it and will likely prompt more of it. This information can protect client safety and improve our practice. This is a good contribution.

Janet R. Kahn

REFERENCES

Eisenberg, D. M., Davis, R. B., Ettner, S. L., et al. (1998). Trends in alternative medicine use in the United States, 1990–1997: results of a follow-up national survey. *Journal of the American Medical Association, 280,* 1569–1575.

Eisenberg, D. M., Kessler, R. C., Foster, C., et al. (1993). Unconventional medicine in the United States. Prevalence, costs, and patterns of use. *New England Journal of Medicine, 328,* 246–252.

Kuhn, T. (1970). *The Structure of Scientific Revolutions* (2nd edn). Chicago: The University of Chicago Press.

NCCAM website http://nccam.nih.gov

Acknowledgements

I wish to thank all those who helped me through this long project. Thanks to my fellow members of the former editorial advisory board to the AMTA's *Massage Therapy Journal*: Lisa Mertz, Dawn Jordan, Diane Polseno, Mark Dixon, and Elliot Greene, Past President of the AMTA. Thanks to Janet Kahn PhD, of the AMTA Foundation, for encouragement and support for conference attendance. Thanks to the anonymous reviewers of this book. Thanks to my colleagues in the psychology department at Bates College, especially to Georgia Nigro PhD, Kathy Low PhD, and John Kelsey PhD, who read and commented on parts of the manuscript. Thanks to Clementine Brasier for her humor and patience as I struggled with the copier. Most of all, thanks to Elaine Brewer for her support, counsel, and encouragement throughout this extended process.

Introduction

Grant Rich

The twentieth century has not been kind to touch. In the late 1920s, for example, the renowned psychologist and founder of behaviorism, John Watson, wrote a best-selling child-care book that gave parents the following advice with regard to their children: 'Never hug and kiss them, never let them sit on your lap. If you must, kiss them once on the forehead when they say goodnight. Shake hands with them in the morning' (Hunter & Struve, 1998, p. 50). While early in his career Freud advocated massage in psychotherapy, as he developed his classic psychoanalytic treatment he abandoned touch and favored minimal physical intervention. The ethics of touch in psychotherapy continue to remain a controversial topic, and several recent books are devoted solely to this debate (e.g., Hunter & Struve, 1998; Smith et al., 1998). Outside of the field of psychology, many recent books have explored societal ambivalence towards touch in a variety of cultural, historical, and religious settings (e.g., Johnson, 1993; Montagu, 1986). Touch, depending on the context, may be healing or hurtful. It is certainly always powerful.

Thankfully, one form of healing touch, massage therapy, appears to be making a comeback as we enter the new millennium. While massage has been used for hundreds of years and in numerous cultures, with the rise of biomedicine its use declined in the mid-century United States. Today however, the membership of the American Massage Therapy Association (AMTA) is steadily increasing, and is currently about 47,000. The flagship journal of the AMTA, *Massage Therapy Journal*, has a readership of over 60,000. Even outside the field of massage therapy, professional interest in the field is high; for instance the major journal of the 140,000 member American Psychological Association (*American Psychologist*) recently published a review article on massage therapy effects (Field, 1998). Interest is increasing not only in the consumption of massage therapy, but also in the seeking out of training to become a massage therapist. One recent article notes that 'six hundred and ten state approved and one hundred and forty other massage schools operate in the United States' (Massage and Bodywork, 1999). In addition, more and more public colleges are adding massage therapy programs. One in three US citizens uses some form of alternative medicine (Eisenberg et al., 1993).

In the United States, 28 states and the District of Columbia offer some type of state-wide massage therapy credential, such as a license, certification, or registration. Many other jurisdictions require local licenses for practice in cities, towns, or counties. Twenty-three states use the National Certification Examination for Therapeutic Massage and Bodywork. Most states require a minimum of 500 hours of massage school training, though Texas therapists need only 250 hours plus a 50-hour internship, while New York therapists are required to have a minimum of 1000 hours of training. In Canada, therapists in British Columbia must complete 3000 hours of training and there is speculation that more US states will opt for more stringent requirements in the future (*Massage Magazine*, 2001). Many therapists have additional training in massage and many therapists have college or graduate level education as well. While the pros and cons of mandated licensure are hotly debated, Cohen (2000) notes that some possible advantages of credentialing include better consumer access to alternative health care, increased integration of biomedicine and alternative health, and an improved system for physician referrals and third-party payers. Other potential advantages include reductions in fraud and increases in competence. Readers interested in the legal context of alternative health care are encouraged to read Michael Cohen's books *Complementary and Alternative Health Care* (1998) and *Beyond Complementary Medicine* (2000). Cohen is a Lecturer at Harvard Medical School.

While healing touch has been used for centuries — cave paintings 15,000 years old depict its use (Hunter & Struve, 1998) — *research on massage therapy* is a much more recent development. Massage research tends to be published in a plethora of academic and trade journals aimed at psychologists, nurses, physical therapists, physicians, and other specialists. Researchers may be familiar with research on massage therapy originating in their own discipline, but not with relevant literature originating in other disciplines. Thus, even the research 'experts' are often unaware of pertinent articles on massage therapy (often these articles, if listed at all, are listed in only one specialty's database). Massage therapists and practitioners, and even massage school faculty may be even more at a loss to find a handy 'one stop' source of reliable research on massage. While there are several fine books on massage techniques (e.g., Andrade & Clifford, 2001), currently massage students are often left 'clueless' as to a reliable source for reporting, learning, and understanding research on massage. Thus, I believe that part of the appeal of this book is that it will serve as Grand Central Station for the best of contemporary massage research. Each chapter offers an extensive bibliography of cited sources. The contributors to this volume represent the best of the current massage researchers. Most of the chapter authors hold university or hospital appointments, and several are dually credentialed as doctoral-level researchers and clinical massage therapists. Massage research is an interdisciplinary topic and chapter authors hold advanced degrees in fields including nursing, psychology, pharmacy, medicine, occupational therapy, and epidemiology.

One of my intellectual heroes is the late Ashley Montagu, PhD, anthropologist and author of numerous works on topics ranging from sexism, to racism, to love. He is perhaps best known to the massage world as the author of the seminal work *Touching* (1986). As chair of the editorial advisory board to the AMTA *Massage Therapy Journal* I interviewed Montagu several years ago in his home (Rich, 2000). Throughout our time together I was struck repeatedly by his warmth and wisdom, traits he cultivated throughout his 94 years. None of his comments though, impacted me as greatly as his following words: 'The touching situation is one of communication and connection.' He paused for a moment and let out a long sigh. 'We have been disconnected. Ordinary relationships become extraordinary through the touch situation, really.' My hope is that this volume offers a connecting place where theory may meet practice, and researcher may meet therapist. Such connections are essential, and perhaps extraordinary.

REFERENCES

Andrade, C., & Clifford, P. (2001). *Outcome-based massage*. Philadelphia: Lippincott, Williams, and Wilkins.

Cohen, M. (1998). *Complementary and alternative medicine*. Baltimore: The Johns Hopkins Press.

Cohen, M. (2000). *Beyond complementary medicine*. Ann Arbor: University of Michigan Press.

Eisenberg, D., Kessler, R., Foster, C., et al. (1993). Unconventional medicine in the United States. *New England Journal of Medicine, 328*, 246–252.

Field, T. (1998). Massage therapy effects. *American Psychologist, 53*, 1270–1281.

Hunter, M., & Struve, J. (1998). *The ethical use of touch in psychotherapy*. Thousand Oaks: Sage Publications.

Johnson, D. (1993). *Body*. Berkeley: North Atlantic Books.

Massage and Bodywork. (1999). April–May.

Massage Magazine. (2001). May–June. pp. 182–183.

Montagu, A. (1986). *Touching*. New York: Harper and Row.

Rich, G. (2000). A century of touch. *Massage Therapy Journal, 38*, 6–14.

Smith, E., Clance, P., & Imes, S. (Eds.). (1998). *Touch in psychotherapy*. New York: The Guilford Press.

Methods and massage

SECTION CONTENTS

INTRODUCTION TO SECTION 1

The following two chapters by Edzard Ernst and Martha Brown Menard address important issues concerning research and massage therapy. Ernst's chapter offers an easy to digest introduction to research methods for beginners. Experienced researchers may wish to skip ahead. For those readers who are new to research methodology, the Ernst chapter is a fine place to begin to understand some of the basic issues surrounding choice of research design, including advantages and disadvantages to the designs and special concerns related to conducting research on massage. Martha Brown Menard's chapter focuses on somewhat more difficult research issues and also specifically examines methodological issues relevant to massage. Martha Brown Menard is well suited to author the chapter since she chairs the research grant review committee for the AMTA Foundation.

For those readers who are new to research and who would like pointers to book length treatments of research methods, may I suggest W. Lawrence Newman's *Social Research Methods* (1997), Bordens and Abbott's *Research Design and Methods* (1999), or Shaughnessy, et al.'s (2000) *Research Methods in Psychology*. While these books do not specifically address massage therapy, they do offer standard treatment of social science research design at the undergraduate level. My other suggestions to therapists interested in research are to collaborate with a university or hospital research group and to take a course or two in statistics and research design/methods at a local university or community college.

Quality research in massage therapy is in its infancy and there are many variables which theoretically may play vital roles in the massage experience but which have not yet been systematically studied. One way to analyze the problem is to suggest that the massage experience includes the effects of the therapist, the client, the setting, and the interaction of all of these variables. Specifically, very few studies have examined therapist effects in detail. Therapists vary in amount and type of training, in years and type of experience, in their training in other disciplines relevant to massage, such as nursing, physical therapy, and psychology, and in many other ways. For instance, perhaps part of the effect of the massage derives from positive social interaction between client and therapist, not the physical manipulation of tissue. To examine such an effect, one might envision a study in which therapists spoke with some clients and not others. To date, therapist variables have been neglected in massage research.

The setting in which massage is conducted may also impact the effectiveness of the massage. For instance, is the massage done at the client's home or the therapist's office? What temperature is the room? Is music played? If yes, what kind? What is the lighting like in the room? What is the scent of the room? All of these factors may be operationalized into variables for study by massage researchers. One suspects that data on such variables would be of great interest to schools and practicing therapists seeking to improve their practices. To date, setting variables have been neglected in massage research.

The massage modality employed also may impact the effectiveness of the massage. Are passive joint movements advised? Or is passive touch the technique of choice? Is there a measurable difference between various neuromuscular techniques? Does the use of oil or powder impact the massage experience? Some studies (some of them in this book), do indeed address the efficacy of specific massage techniques and specific massage modalities. More work must be conducted however, to examine the relative efficacy of the component techniques in controlled situations, however. For instance, is the traditional hour-long Swedish massage effective for relaxation due to the stroking component? The petrissage? Or is the whole greater than the sum of the parts?

The client is another basic element in the massage experience and presents numerous possible sources of variation. Aside from the obvious variable of client condition, theoretically one might consider the client's previous experience with 'alternative health' and with massage in particular, the client (and therapist) gender, age, feelings about 'touch' (such as cultural taboos or previous negative experiences with touch or abuse), etc. With the exception of studies focusing on certain clinical conditions, few studies have examined such client variables. Finally, the massage experience includes the interaction of therapist, client, and modality. For instance a given technique may be appropriate in one context with one client but not appropriate with another client in another context. Another example of how interactions may operate is that one therapist may be ideal for client A but terrible for client B. These interactions need to be studied in detail by future researchers.

A final few words about research methods and massage therapy. Traditionally, one important element in the research design of an experiment is to construct a control group that is alike in every way but one to an experimental group and to randomly assign subjects to either condition. Thus one issue frequently raised by massage therapy researchers is the issue of a 'sham' massage group to serve as a control group to an experimental group receiving the genuine massage. Just what might a 'sham massage' be? Some researchers have argued for offering superficial techniques in lieu of deep techniques. Others suggest passive touch instead of the 'real' massage. Still others suggest a treatment group in which subjects do not receive massage, but do receive potentially therapeutic 'nonspecifics' such as attention and conversation with a caring person. Another important issue to bear in mind is the impossibility of the therapist being 'blind' to the treatment. No one has yet devised a convincing way in which the massage practitioner can be naïve as to whether he or she is giving a real treatment or a sham treatment. These two limitations, the issue of blinding the therapist to treatment type, and the issue of inventing a convincing 'sham' massage to serve as a treatment for a control group, have plagued the field of massage research. But what many massage researchers fail to remember is that these issues are also issues in the much larger, much older, and much more established literature on psychotherapy efficacy. While these issues may make research more challenging they do not mean that quality research cannot be conducted on massage.

In an important article in the flagship journal of the American Psychological Association, Past-President Martin Seligman (1995) addresses the state of the evidence for the efficacy of psychotherapy. Every massage researcher should read this article. Let me quote from the study directly. Seligman notes that in the 'ideal efficacy study' all of the following elements should be found (p. 965):

1. The patients are randomly assigned to treatment and control groups.
2. The controls are rigorous: Not only are patients included who receive no treatment at all, but placebos containing potentially therapeutic ingredients credible to both the patient and the therapist are used in order to control for such influences as rapport, expectation of gain, and sympathetic attention.
3. The treatments are manualized, with highly detailed scripting of therapy made explicit. Fidelity to the manual is assessed using videotaped sessions.
4. Patients are seen for a fixed number of sessions.
5. The target outcomes are well-operationalized.
6. Raters and diagnosticians are blind to which group the patient comes from.
7. The patients meet criteria for a single diagnosed disorder, and patients with multiple disorders are typically excluded.
8. The patients are followed for a fixed period after termination of treatment with a thorough assessment battery.

While Seligman was discussing the efficacy of psychotherapy, each of these elements should apply to the ideal study of massage efficacy. Note that Seligman discusses the impossibility of 'double-blind' studies which are common in drug studies but impossible for psychotherapy studies since both therapist and client know what the treatment is. As Seligman puts it, 'Whenever you hear someone demanding the double-blind study of psychotherapy, hold on to your wallet' (p. 965). The same could be said for studies of massage efficacy; double-blind studies are impossible. (How could a massage therapist not know he or she is giving a massage!) Seligman notes that the ideal psychotherapy efficacy study follows patients for a fixed period after the end of treatment. Unfortunately, few massage studies have followed clients for more the 24 hours. Future researchers should certainly aim to examine the long term benefits of massage therapy.

Seligman notes that efficacy studies with the above eight elements have been considered the 'gold standard' (p. 966) for psychotherapy research. However, he then continues to describe 'what efficacy studies leave out' (p. 966). Seligman notes the efficacy studies may 'underestimate or even miss altogether the value of psychotherapy done in the field' (p. 966). Citing Seligman directly (p. 966), these limitations occur since psychotherapy done in the real world (as opposed to in controlled laboratory conditions):

1. is not of fixed duration. It usually keeps going until the patient is markedly improved or until he or she quits.
2. is self-correcting. If one technique is not working, another technique — or even another modality — is usually tried.
3. patients in psychotherapy in the field often get there by active shopping, entering a kind of treatment they actively sought with a therapist they screened and chose.
4. patients in psychotherapy in the field usually have multiple problems.
5. psychotherapy in the field is almost always concerned with improvement in the general functioning of patients, as well as amelioration of a disorder and relief of specific, presenting symptoms.

Seligman notes that to address such issues concerning psychotherapy as it is actually practiced in the real world would require *survey* methods sampling large numbers of users, rather than the type of experimental efficacy study with the eight elements described earlier. Again, Seligman is describing studies of psychotherapy, but the issues are directly relevant to massage researchers as well. For instance, while a controlled efficacy study of massage therapy might require adherence to a manualized protocol, in the real world, therapists often self-correct and change techniques and modalities as they see fit. For example, the therapist might switch from stroking to percussion. Another example might be that in a laboratory experiment the researcher must randomly assign a client to a therapist (one that the client may not necessarily like or feel an emotional connection to), whereas in the real world, clients frequently seek out, screen, and choose therapists of their choice. For instance, a client might seek out a therapist of the same gender. With regard to the fifth item, laboratory studies frequently examine a single condition using specific outcome measures. This technique is very important, but Seligman suggests that perhaps more global measures of life satisfaction, subjective well-being, quality of life, and happiness, may also be important outcome variables to examine in psychotherapy. Theoretically, such variables may indeed be important to the massage experience as well. At any rate, in sum, it appears that both experiments and surveys are useful techniques for massage research as well as for psychotherapy.

A final method of research that may be useful in studying massage therapy are qualitative methods, including interviews and field observations. Such qualitative techniques are commonly used in anthropology, oral history, and some forms of sociology and humanistic psychology. While such methods do not offer quantified results, these methods are excellent exploratory and descriptive tools, especially for topics that have been understudied in the past. Indeed there are now computer programs such as NUD*IST and Ethnograph that assist in the analysis of qualitative data such as interviews or field notes. Perhaps massage researchers of the future will feel comfortable using these methods in conjunctions with experimental and survey methods. One excellent resource on qualitative methods is H. Russell Bernard's (1994) textbook *Research Methods in Anthropology*.

REFERENCES

Bernard, R. (1994). *Research methods in anthropology*. Altamira Press.
Bordens, K., & Abbott, B. (1999). *Research design and methods*. Mountain View, California: Mayfield Publishing Company.
Neuman, W. (1997). *Social research methods*. Boston: Allyn and Bacon.
Seligman, M. (1995). The effectiveness of psychotherapy. *American Psychologist, 50*, 965–974.
Shaughnessy, J., Zechmeister, E., & Zechmeister, J. (2000). *Research methods in psychology*. Boston: Allyn and Bacon.

1

Evidence-based massage therapy: a contradiction in terms?

Edzard Ernst

INTRODUCTION

Massage has a long tradition in several medical cultures. In the USA, it is presently experiencing a most remarkable boost in popularity (Eisenberg et al., 1998). Unfortunately, research has significantly fallen behind this development. This chapter is aimed at discussing issues related to research methodology as they pertain to testing the effectiveness of any form of massage therapy. In tackling some of the most common problems, I will take a pragmatic approach. This chapter is not about dry statistical formulae, it is about simple, common sense aimed at novices to medical research.

AUDIT

Practitioners often confuse audit with research and this has caused much confusion in the area of massage therapy. Clinical audit is the systematic evaluation of clinical activity in its broadest sense (Abbot & Ernst, 1997). It involves the identification of a problem and its resolution through various audit cycles. This can involve examination of the structural aspects of the delivery of care, of the processes involved in delivering care, and of the outcomes of care. The essential quality of clinical audit is that it brings about change, and this aspect is generally under-emphasized. The principal concern of clinical audit, and the outcome indicators integral to it, should be to determine whether treatment, already shown to have a specific effect (efficacy), does so in practice (effectiveness), and whether the resources spent on it are being used to best advantage (efficiency). Thus clinical audit can be usefully applied wherever improvements are to be made in the clinical practice of massage therapy. It is, however, not strictly a research tool, and thus it is excluded from further discussion.

UNCONTROLLED DATA

Traditional use

Massage is amongst the oldest treatment known to mankind (Westhof & Ernst, 1992). Therefore, can anyone doubt that it works? The 'test of time' relies exclusively on experience. While experience is, of course, part of the basis of any clinical medicine, it can be highly deceptive. The history of medicine provides many examples for this to be true. Take blood letting for example; it represented the undisputed panacea for centuries. Its widespread practice must have killed thousands more than it ever benefited (Bauer, 1996). When it was finally discovered to be ineffective, through controlled trials, it was not the intervention but the new (and therefore suspect) method of the controlled trial that was doubted (Lilienfield, 1982). Today we know that blood letting in the form of haemodilution only helps in a few, defined conditions (Ernst et al., 1987).

Traditional use also tells us less about the safety of a therapy than we intuitively assume. But let us assume that a given traditional treatment is *not* burdened with frequent adverse events, which sooner or later make alarm bells ring. It might still be associated with rare or delayed and therefore not immediately obvious yet clinically relevant complications. The 'rule of three' tells us that the number of subjects studied must be three times as high as the frequency of an adverse drug reaction to have a 95% chance that the reaction will actually occur in a studied population (Hanley & Lippman-Hand, 1983). When an adverse drug reaction occurs with a frequency of 1 in 2000, one needs to monitor 6000 users to have a 95% chance that the adverse reaction will be observed at least once. To have a 95% chance that the reaction will occur twice or three times, one has to enroll 9600 and 13,000 patients respectively. The bottom line is that the experience of massage therapists is an unreliable tool to determine either the effectiveness or the safety of their therapy.

Case reports

A clinical research idea often starts with an interesting observation concerning the treatment of a particular patient. A therapist might report: 'I have treated condition X with massage and my patient improved dramatically'.

When put in writing, this initial observation is called a case report (Ernst, 1995). By definition, such case reports are anecdotal evidence; they are essential in clinical medicine as they generate new ideas and constitute experience, but they can never be conclusive. The patient might respond in a different manner or might even have improved without any treatment at all.

Case series

Case series are accumulated case reports evaluated either retrospectively or (more rigorous) prospectively (Ernst, 1998b). They can vary considerably in quality (have better defined inclusion/exclusion criteria, more sensitive endpoints, etc). Case series seem an attractive research tool to many therapists as they do not require informed consent, pose no problem in terms of treatment denial, and fit comfortably into clinical settings. Their most important methodological drawback is the lack of a control group. Thus they have no place in the evaluation of clinical efficacy: their results simply do not tell us whether an observed change was indubitably due to the treatment or to any of the following factors, each of which can influence the clinical results (Ernst, 1998b):

- placebo effect
- natural history of the disease
- regression to the mean
- patient's desire to please the therapist
- therapist's desire for a positive result
- concomitant therapy
- other nonspecific effects.

This, however, is not to say that case series are of no value; the opposite is the case. They are certainly useful, even essential for formulating a hypothesis. In turn, this hypothesis requires testing by other methods, e.g. randomized controlled trials.

Observational studies

Observational studies are very similar to case series. In fact, they are large and well-organized studies without a control group. Because of their size, they may allow comparisons of sub-groups and some inference as to whether or not the observed clinical effect was associated with the therapeutic intervention. For instance, one could conceive a large study of massage therapy where perhaps 1000 consecutive patients with a given condition are treated and the outcome (say pain) is determined. Sub-group analyses could then determine whether patients who were more severely affected or those who received more treatments responded better in terms of pain relief than the rest of the group. The principal drawback does, however, remain: there is no control group that received a different (or no) therapy. Thus observational studies can hardly answer the question whether the perceived effect was caused by the therapy (specific effect) or some other factor (nonspecific effect) (Pocock & Elbourne, 2000).

CONTROLLED CLINICAL TRIALS

The need for controlled studies to evaluate the effectiveness of a treatment is often misunderstood. The 'effectiveness' observed in uncontrolled studies is really the 'perceived effectiveness', which is composed of the specific therapeutic effect plus other, nonspecific factors (see later). Whenever one wants to be certain about the relative importance of these factors and aims at defining the specific effectiveness of the therapy, one has no choice but to conduct controlled trials and compare the results of an intervention group with those of a carefully chosen control group (Fig. 1.1).

When scientifically investigating whether or not a given therapeutic intervention is effective, one essentially asks whether there is a *causal* relationship between the treatment and the outcome. Some may (rightly) argue that most if not all conditions have more than one cause and that therefore this approach is naïve and simplistic. Even though the multi-causality of disease is an indubitable fact, this argument is wrong. By definition, medical treatments are aimed at providing the cause for the clinical benefit quite regardless of multicausal etiologies — a massage therapist treating low back pain treats the patient under the assumption and with

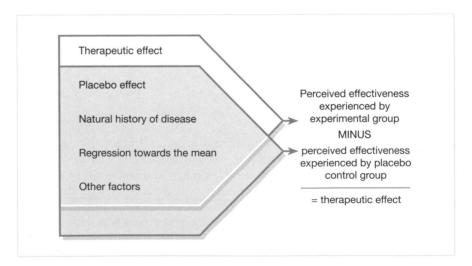

Figure 1.1   Therapeutic effect in relation to other factors determining outcome.

the hope that the massage will ease the pain (which would represent a cause–effect relationship) irrespective of the fact that back pain clearly has many causes. To *not* be interested in the cause–effect relationships in therapeutics means to disregard one of the most essential ingredients in medical therapy (Ernst & Resch, 1996).

Typically, controlled clinical trials are prospective investigations. Yet it is often easier, faster and less expensive to do research retrospectively, for instance, by looking at a number of case notes in an attempt to define which treatment helped best in a given condition. For several reasons this approach is substantially inferior to prospective investigations. There are always several factors that influence the outcome in addition to the treatment given, e.g. the natural history of the disease (Fig. 1.1). Since retrospective investigations are restricted to the data available which, of course, have not been gathered for the purpose of the study, they normally have not been produced under standardized conditions nor do they follow a rigorous predetermined protocol. Inclusion-exclusion criteria (see later) are difficult or impossible to implement on a post-hoc basis because of lack of relevant information, and because randomization (see later) cannot be achieved. Therefore, neither suitability nor validity of the data can be reliably established. Yet, to provide conclusive information on therapeutic effectiveness of a given treatment, all these factors would need accounting for. This can be done reliably *only* with prospective research designs.

Parallel group versus cross-over designs

In trials with parallel groups, participants are split into several (typically two) sub-groups. These receive two different treatments (see later) and the changes that occur in group 1 are compared with those of group 2 (Fig. 1.2). Thus different individuals are compared with each other. This creates numerous confounding factors, and the hope is that, provided both groups are large enough, these will cancel each other out, particularly if the trial was randomized (see later).

In an attempt to reduce confounding, it is tempting to compare one study participant with him/herself. This is the basic concept of cross-over studies (Fig. 1.2). In such trials all participants are treated with two different approaches (e.g. with massage therapy versus drug treatment). To minimize bias, one can randomize the sequence of the two approaches (see later). Essentially the clinical changes in one treatment phase are then compared with those that occur in the other phase.

While cross-over designs have highly attractive features, they are also burdened with numerous problems (Ernst, 1998b). Generally speaking parallel group designs are today considered to be more rigorous.

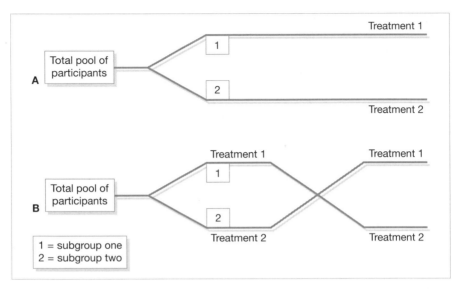

Figure 1.2 Schematic design of parallel group trials (A) and cross-over studies (B).

Placebo controlled trials

The placebo issue is also often misunderstood. No one doubts that the placebo effect can be very powerful indeed (Ernst & Resch, 1994). While in clinical practice we should do everything to make the patient benefit from nonspecific treatment (placebo) effects, we need to exclude them in research aimed at defining specific effectiveness of therapeutic interventions. This is achieved adequately by introducing a parallel group of patients who receive a treatment identical to the treatment under investigation except for the supposed specific treatment effect (i.e. a placebo group). One argument often voiced against this approach is that this neglects the importance of nonspecific treatment effects. This is, of course, not true. The fact that one eliminates a given determinant of a clinical outcome does not mean that one does not appreciate its importance — by eliminating the natural history of the disease in a controlled trial, one by no means disregards its importance. All one attempts is to create a set of circumstances where outcomes and results can be interpreted in a straightforward manner (i.e. 'causality' of the factor under investigation is confounded as little as possible by other factors or circumstances). The trial situation differs critically from the therapeutic situation in this way.

In contrast to what is often said, one can do placebo-controlled trials with *any* form of treatment, even with massage therapy — for instance, one can give sugar pills (placebo) to one group of patients and treat the experimental group with massage therapy. With several therapies (including massage) it is, however, exceedingly difficult or even impossible to find placebos that are *indistinguishable* from the active treatment for the patient and/or therapist, and only such placebos can be used for patient-blinded studies.

In such situations one is often left with the second-best option to an ideal placebo, i.e. an intervention that mimics the active therapy as closely as possible (but not completely), e.g. superficial massage in a trial of Swedish massage of muscular pain. Admittedly these options represent compromises between the feasible and the desirable. Further features can enhance the credibility of such 'imperfect placebos' — for instance, one can make sure that only patients who have no previous experience with the type of massage under investigation are included in a trial. They are therefore less likely to tell the real thing from the imperfect placebo. The development of a credible placebo crucially depends not only on experience but also on creativity and fantasy.

There may be many situations where other controls are adequate or even superior to placebo controls. For instance, whenever a 'gold standard' (accepted form of therapy for a given condition with proven effectiveness) exists, ethical considerations demand to test a given therapy (e.g. massage) against this 'gold standard'. The research question then would be whether massage is as effective as or superior to the standard treatment.

It is also essential that any control treatment (placebo or other) is comparable in terms of factors relating to the clinical setting: identical environment, same team of caretakers, similar length of patient/therapist contact, similar therapeutic relationship, etc.

Blinded versus open studies

Blinding relates to the fact that the two, three or more parties involved in a clinical trial are masked as to the intervention (i.e. active or control). Blinding the evaluator is usually no problem: the assessor (that is, the investigator who quantifies the results, e.g. pain reduction) does not need to know what type of therapy the patient had been submitted to. Blinding patients in trials of massage therapy is probably not achievable. The same obviously applies to the therapist. In essence this means that in clinical massage research only evaluator-blinded trials are feasible.

Randomized versus non-randomized trials

Randomization is the cornerstone of an unbiased assessment of therapeutic effectiveness. A vivid example of how things can go badly wrong is the Bristol Cancer Study (Bagenal et al., 1990), where the lack of randomization was the main reason for flawed results and the confusion that followed. Randomization means that one sample of patients is divided into two or more subgroups through pure coincidence. *Only* this method can achieve that both groups are comparable in terms of known *and unknown* potential determinants of outcome (provided the sample is big enough). Non-randomized trials are wide open to bias. This has several reasons. For instance, investigators might intuitively put the more ill patients into that treatment group for which they hope treatment is more effective, or certain other characteristics render a patient more suitable for one of the two forms of treatment tested. This and the fact that one cannot account for factors that are presently unknown, are crucial reasons why only randomization will guarantee that all treatment groups within a study are comparable and that we are prevented from comparing 'apples with pears' (Schulz et al., 1995).

Inclusion-exclusion criteria

'In view of the differing diagnostic criteria on conventional medicine and complementary therapy, it does not appear possible to define a population which can be randomized for a controlled clinical trial of one form of therapy against another...' (Watt, 1988, p. 151). This quote reflects the notorious problem of inclusion-exclusion criteria and emphasizes the different views held by orthodox and complementary therapists. Yet the problem is not insurmountable. Firstly there is no absolute need to insist on strict inclusion-exclusion criteria (i.e. 'define a population'). They are desirable in order to achieve optimally homogeneous patient samples, which in turn, reduces the 'background noise' in the experiment. Yet they are not mandatory — all we face when relaxing these criteria is the need to increase our sample size. Secondly, one can sometimes use orthodox plus unorthodox criteria in sequence. For instance, one could conceive a trial on patients with rheumatoid arthritis diagnosed by an orthodox physician where the patients are subsequently seen by a therapist who defines the suitability of each patient for the massage therapy under investigation. This 'definition' can be based on anything from reproducible variables to personal intuition. Only if a patient passes both 'filters' will he/she be included in the study. Undoubtedly, this would make any study more tedious, yet it would not render it impossible.

Outcome measures

One often gets the impression that medical research has opted to measure what is measurable instead of what is relevant. Proponents of complementary medicine frequently claim that the known criteria to evaluate success or failure of therapy are not meaningful in their field. Actually this is also true for much of mainstream medicine where surrogate endpoints abound — for instance, blood pressure or serum cholesterol: is it relevant to lower these variables or to prevent a heart attack? The latter is not *a priori* a consequence of the former. What we really want to know is often difficult to measure.

In certain clinical situations encountered by massage therapists there may not be any hard and validated endpoints at all. Yet other meaningful, 'soft' endpoints have been and are being developed — for instance instruments to measure quality of life or well-being (Cella & Tulsky, 1990). Even simple patient preference can be quantified, for instance, in crossover trials. These can be used, depending on the research question, in conjunction with other endpoints like visual analogue scales or 'hard' physiological variables.

SYSTEMATIC REVIEWS

If we accept that the randomized clinical trial is the least biased (yet by no means perfect) method to test for therapeutic effectiveness known today, we still have to admit that one such study is rarely fully convincing. In medical research, one always wants to see independent replications. A single trial could be wrong by chance, through some undetected bias or even through fraud. Where more than one study exists, they often yield different results. For instance, it is conceivable that, for one given indication (say, depression) five studies suggest that massage is effective while five imply that it is not. In such a situation proponents of massage could publish a (apparently evidence-based) review of the positive trials. An opponent could do the same with the negative trials.

This example demonstrates the importance of systematic reviews (and meta-analyses — which are systematic reviews that include statistical pooling of data). Such research projects have to include a detailed explanation where the authors explain what they did and how. They have to demonstrate, for instance, that they included all the data (not just those they liked). This renders a review of this type reproducible and minimizes selection and random biases.

For these reasons, systematic reviews provide, according to the accepted standards of evidence-based medicine (Cook et al., 1997), the most compelling evidence for or against a given therapy (Fig. 1.3). In the realm of massage, several non-systematic (e.g. Callaghan, 1993; Tidius, 1997; Buss et al., 1997) and systematic (e.g. Ernst, 1998a; 1999a,c) reviews have been published.

Systematic reviews are perhaps the best evidence, yet they too are not flawless. Problems can arise when the primary studies are of poor quality (garbage in, garbage out) and when certain (e.g. negative) results never get published (publication bias).

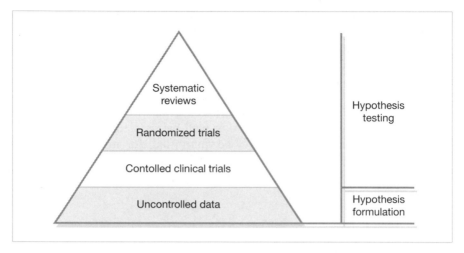

Figure 1.3 Hierarchy of evidence.

THE 'OPTIMAL' TRIAL DESIGN

From the discussion so far it follows that there is no such thing as an 'optimal' trial design. A study can only be optimal in that it answers the question it set out to answer. All types of investigation discussed above can be optimally matched to a research question. In other words, it is the match not primarily the design one should try to get right. Or, to put it bluntly, there are in principle no faulty designs only bad matches (Fig. 1.3).

If, for instance, one wants to generate or strengthen a hypothesis (which would require testing later), case reports or case series are optimal. If one wants to determine whether massage is more effective than no treatment, a randomized, evaluator-blinded study with two parallel groups — one receiving massage and the other no such therapy — is probably ideal. If one requires to know whether massage is superior to another (e.g. gold standard) treatment, the same design but with a different comparison group would be ideal.

It should be re-emphasized that the entire discussion above is directed towards testing the effectiveness of massage therapy. Obviously there are many other areas of research (Table 1.1). It is clear that for all these areas of research, different methods have to be used and the above discussion does not apply.

PRAGMATIC PROBLEMS

In this last section, I would like to give some practical guidance to those who are new to research and would like to give it a try. Many researchers

Table 1.1 Examples of research question matched with adequate research design

Research questions	Examples of possible design
How prevalent is massage therapy?	Surveys
Who uses massage therapies?	Surveys
What are the main indications?	Surveys
What are reasons for using massage therapy?	Personal interviews, postal questionnaires
Are there adverse effects?	Literature review
How frequent are these adverse effects?	Large scale observational study
Does massage offer value for money?	Cost-benefit, cost-utility studies
Which treatment will help a given patient?	Single case study
Which mechanism brings about a given clinical effect?	Investigations using physiological variables
What expectations do patients have?	Personal interviews/qualitative methods
What experiences do patients report?	Personal interviews/qualitative methods
Does massage offer value for money?	Cost evaluation studies

(including myself) have learnt research 'the hard way', e.g. by making all the mistakes themselves. Perhaps the following paragraphs will prevent others from making my mistakes all over again.

Why do research?

There are many reasons to do research, and some are clearly better than others. Enthusiastic novices often want to prove that their therapy works. This is probably one of the worst reasons for doing research. An investigation should *not* set out to *prove* a point but rather to *test* a hypothesis. An investigator with an 'axe to grind' is hardly an objective researcher. Clinical research, in particular, must be patient-centered. Unquestionably, the best reason for doing research is the hope of coming one step closer to the truth and to help (future) patients.

Preconditions

Certain items are essential because, without them, there is no use in even attempting research. It is worth remembering that bad research can be unethical (Emanuel et al., 2000). It can mean not only a waste of resources but also the needless suffering of patients.

An adequate knowledge of research methodology and of the subject area under investigation — for example of treatment modality (e.g. the form of massage therapy to be tested) and disease — are absolute prerequisites. To some degree expertise can be 'bought in' (see later), but the project leader must have at least a minimal understanding of all the issues involved. If you do not have this expertise, acquire it — or do not embark on research.

It almost amounts to a platitude to state that certain infrastructures are also essential. By this I mean things like the time to carry out the work, access to a library, electronic databases and computers as well as the (prospect of) funds to finance all the work and equipment involved. Before you even start planning a research project it might be a good idea to draw up a simple checklist of all the preconditions required in your particular case and go through it one by one.

Background reading

You may want to embark on a subject, say a study of Swedish massage to treat back pain, and not be fully aware of what has been published on this subject already. Yet it is mandatory that you are! Thus it is highly advisable to conduct an in-depth search for all published articles, read all of them thoroughly and make sure you understand all aspects (if you do not, seek help). Failure to do this background research properly might seriously embarrass you and your colleagues later on. You (or someone else) might, for instance, find out that the study you have just done has already been conducted in a more definitive way by someone else. This would obviously render your work redundant and a waste of time, energy and money.

Define your research question

Using the above example, you may have started out with the idea of studying massage for back pain. Now that you have read the published articles on the subject, you will almost certainly have found that the question you are asking is much more complex than originally anticipated. Do you want to formulate or test a hypothesis with your research? What type of patients do you want to study? What type of back pain? What type of massage do you want to test? How do you want to recruit your patients? Do you need to conduct a controlled trial or an observational study? What should the control treatment be (if any) — a 'placebo' or a standard treatment? Can you randomize the treatment groups? Is the treatment under investigation representative for its class? Do you need one therapist or more? What should their qualifications be? Are all conditions optimal for the treatment to work? And so on. Only when you have answered such questions (they will invariably come up when you do your background reading and they will differ according to the nature of your project) will you be able to define the research question. Doing this is essential for deciding which methodology is the best for what you have in mind. It is also a decisive step towards developing a protocol (see 'Recruit a research team').

Check the logistics

This preparatory work will have led you to a more concise idea of what may be coming up. Certain things will have become clear to you and you might, at this stage, what to (re)check whether the logistic preconditions for your research project are fulfilled. For instance, do you have access to the type (and adequate numbers) of patients you need to study? How large should your patient sample be? Is it realistic for you to obtain sufficient funding? Is it likely that you can obtain patient consent for what you plan to do? Is the evolving proposal ethical? Do you have the necessary rooms, help (secretarial back up, research nurses), etc? There will almost certainly be other questions to ask. My advice is, again, to draw up a checklist and tackle one problem at a time.

Recruit a 'research team'

You will probably find that your general research knowledge and experience are not enough to cover all aspects of your project competently. It is therefore usually mandatory to assemble a team for developing a sound protocol of your study and guide you through its experimental phase. Depending on the type of your investigation this team will vary in size and composition. In the example of massage for back pain, it might include a statistician (almost invariably advisable), a clinical expert in back pain (for example, a rheumatologist) and an experienced massage therapist. Make the team as small as possible but as large as necessary.

Within this team you should now organize a series of discussions to evolve a protocol. Subsequently, you might take the lead and draft an outline and circulate it within the team until every team member is satisfied. The team should supervise the entire investigation. Once the protocol is finalized, the planning phase is (almost) finished. All that is needed now is to submit it to the appropriate ethics committee, and secure funding. During this process several (hopefully small) revisions of your protocol may prove necessary.

Obtain funding

Funding is, of course, very often the real obstacle (Ernst, 1999b). Research funds are invariably limited and rejection rates are often high, particularly if you have to compete with applications from mainstream research. Rejections can be extremely disappointing, but you must not be deterred. To succeed you have to try over and over again and learn from the criticisms of those who review your application. Here, too, you should seek expert advice. Establish contact with patient organizations, try all the charities you can think of, use your imagination and leave no stone unturned. If research in massage therapy is ever to get anywhere, I strongly feel that some dramatic changes to the all too miserable present funding situation have to be brought about.

At present there are few funds especially dedicated to such research. Thus we find ourselves competing with mainstream scientists for a more and more limited amount of money. This means that our applications are judged by panels who usually have little understanding of (or sympathy for) complementary medicine. This in turn results in the undeniable fact that very little money is spent on such research (Ernst, 1999c).

I have said and written it before, and I will carry on doing so: in view of the high popularity of complementary medicine (Eisenberg et al., 1998), it is quite simply unethical not to research the subject systematically — and this, of course, requires adequate research budgets.

CONCLUSION

Massage therapy remains grossly under-researched. In particular, clinical trials need to test the effectiveness of defined types of massage for defined conditions. The methodology for doing this is similar to clinical research in other areas. Existing trials of massage therapy are often burdened with significant limitations (Cawley, 1997). Lack of research expertise and research funds are probably the two main reasons for the paucity of reliable evidence in this area. We should find ways of overcoming these obstacles.

REFERENCES

Abbot, N. C., & Ernst, E. (1997). Clinical audit, outcomes and complementary medicine. *Forschende Komplementärmedizin, 4,* 229–234.
Bagenal, F. A., Easton, D. F., Harris, E., & Chilvers, C. E. D. (1990). Survival of patients with breast cancer attending Bristol Cancer Health Care Centre. *Lancet, 336,* 1185–1188.
Bauer, J. (1996). *Die geschichte der aderlässe.* München: Fritsch.
Buss, I. C., Halfens, R. J. G., & Abu-Saad, H. H. (1997). The effectiveness of massage in preventing pressure sores, a literature review. *Rehabilitation Nursing, 22,* 229–234.
Callaghan, M. J. (1993). The role of massage in the management of the athlete, a review. *British Journal of Sports Medicine, 27,* 28–33.
Cawley, N. (1997). A critique of the methodology of research studies evaluating massage. *European Journal of Cancer Care, 6,* 23–31.
Cella, D. F., & Tulsky, D. S. (1990). Measuring quality of life today, methodological aspects. *Oncology, 4,* 29–38.
Cook, D. J., Mulrow, C., & Hayes, R. B. (1997). Systematic reviews, synthesis of best evidence for clinical decisions. *Annals of Internal Medicine, 126,* 376–380.
Eisenberg, D. M., David, R. B., Ettner, S. L., et al. (1998). Trends in alternative medicine use in the United States, 1990–1997. *Journal of the American Medical Association, 280,* 1569–1575.
Emanuel, E. J., Wendler, D., & Grady, C. (2000). What makes clinical research ethical? *Journal of the American Medical Association, 283,* 2701–2711.

Ernst, E. (1995). What is wrong with anecdotal evidence? *European Journal of Physical Medicine and Rehabilitation, 5,* 145–146.

Ernst, E. (1998a). Does post-exercise massage treatment reduce delayed onset muscle soreness? A systematic review. *British Journal of Sports Medicine, 32,* 212–214.

Ernst, E. (1998b). Establishing efficacy in chronic stable conditions, are $n = 1$ study designs or case series useful? *Forschende Komplementärmedizin, 5(suppl 1),* 128–138.

Ernst, E. (1999a). Abdominal massage therapy for chronic constipation, a systematic review of controlled clinical trials. *Forschende Komplementärmedizin, 6,* 149–151.

Ernst, E. (1999b). Funding research into complementary medicine, the situation in Britain. *Complementary Therapies in Medicine, 7,* 250–253.

Ernst, E. (1999c). Massage therapy for low back pain, a systematic review. *Journal of Pain and Symptom Management, 17,* 65–69.

Ernst, E., Matrai, A., & Kollar, L. (1987). Placebo controlled, double-blind study of haemodilution in peripheral arterial disease. *Lancet, 2,* 1449–1451.

Ernst, E., & Resch, K. L. (1996). Evaluating specific effectiveness of complementary therapies — a position paper — Part one, methodological aspects. *Forschende Komplementärmedizin, 3,* 35–38.

Ernst, E., & Resch, K. L. (1994). The science and the art of the placebo. *Update,* 619–622.

Hanley, J. A., & Lippman-Hand, A. (1983). If nothing goes wrong, is everything alright? *Journal of the American Medical Association, 259,* 1743–1745.

Lilienfeld, A. M. (1982). The evolution of the clinical trial. *Bulletin of Historical Medicine, 56,* 1–18.

Pocock, S. J., & Elbourne, D. R. (2000). Randomized trials or observational tribulations? *New England Journal of Medicine, 342,* 1907–1909.

Schulz, K. F., Chalmers, J., Hyes, R. J., & Altman, D. G. (1995). Empirical evidence of bias. *Journal of the American Medical Association, 273,* 408–412.·

Tidius, P. M. (1997). Manual massage and recovery of muscle function following exercise, a literature review. *Journal of Orthopaedic and Sports Physical Therapy, 25,* 107–112.

Watt, J. (1988). *Talking health* (p. 151). London: Royal Society of Medicine.

Westhof, S., & Ernst, E. (1992). Geschichte der massage. *Deutsch Medizinische Wochenschrift, 117,* 150–153.

2

Methodological issues in the design and conduct of massage therapy research

Martha Brown Menard

INTRODUCTION

Much has been written about methodological issues in designing and conducting research on complementary and alternative therapies (Cassileth et al., 1994; Levin et al., 1997; Vickers et al., 1997). Most authors agree that the same methods, both qualitative and quantitative, used to evaluate conventional medicine can and should be applied to complementary and alternative therapies as long as they are applied appropriately. Determining what constitutes appropriate application, however, is where differences of opinion arise (Cassidy, 1994, 1995; Hufford, 1996; Trotter, 2000). Little has been written specifically regarding appropriate methods for investigating massage as a therapeutic intervention. This chapter explores the methodological issues in designing and conducting research on massage therapy from the dual perspective of the research scientist and the clinical practitioner. Some of these arguments have also been made in the book *Making Sense of Research* (Menard, 2002), a guide to research literacy for complementary practitioners.

PROBLEMS IN MASSAGE THERAPY RESEARCH

Despite assurances that existing research methods are sufficiently robust, it is not clear from looking at the bulk of the literature on massage therapy that the application of these methods has produced satisfactory results. Although a number of published studies have found statistically significant results, others have found ambiguous or negative results that are open to interpretation. Relatively few studies have used rigorous methods that can stand up to epidemiological scrutiny. Methodological flaws in many of the studies are obvious and have been noted by others (Cawley, 1997; Ernst & Fialka, 1994;

Field, 1998). Typical criticisms include: small sample size and consequent lack of statistical power; lack of a control or comparison group; lack of random assignment to group; inadequate outcome measure(s); and lack of standardization of the massage protocol used in the study. While there is promising evidence of the effectiveness of massage for certain health conditions (Field, 1998; Vickers, 1996), the small number of systematic reviews conducted on massage therapy have concluded that at present there are too few studies of sufficient quality to definitively say whether or not it works (Ernst, 1999; Furlan et al., 2000). A systematic review of the research on infant and preterm infant massage, one of the few areas where there are a sufficient number of relatively well conducted studies, recently concluded that while the evidence has demonstrated a positive effect, the effect size is too small to warrant its wider use in neonatal care settings (Vickers et al., 2000).

To some extent, these results are not surprising given that serious research on massage therapy is still in its infancy. A related factor is the comparatively small amount of money available to fund studies; thus the large number of pilot studies with small samples. However, other methodological issues in addition to those previously mentioned exist in much of the research conducted and are not always readily apparent to the non-practitioner. These issues include: definitions and theoretical models of massage therapy; lack of involvement of skilled practitioners in the design and conduct of studies; appropriate control interventions and nonspecific effects; and a rush to conduct efficacy studies without a sufficient understanding of massage therapy based on adequate prior research.

DEFINITIONS OF MASSAGE THERAPY

Few studies have explicitly defined just what the term 'massage therapy' means. In the well-known Eisenberg survey on the prevalence and patterns of use of unconventional therapies (Eisenberg et al., 1993), respondents identified more than 100 varieties of massage therapy. Perhaps one reason for this is that the term means different things to different people. I have noticed that within the profession 'massage therapy' tends to be used in a narrower and more technical sense to refer specifically to certain kinds of massage, as distinguished from 'bodywork,' which is separate and different from massage. Adding to this confusion is the fact that the vast majority (96%) of therapists, no matter what their primary discipline, define themselves as eclectic and work in more than one primary discipline (NCBTMB, 1997a,b). Outside of the profession, as the Eisenberg survey shows, 'massage therapy' is used in a broader and more inclusive way to indicate almost any form of touch-based therapy, even some that are energetic in nature and do not involve skin-to-skin physical contact, such as Therapeutic Touch. For the purposes of this chapter, I will use the

---

Box 2.1   Categories of massage and bodywork modalities based on intended therapeutic effect

Promoting structural or physiological change

Swedish massage	Rolfing/connective tissue massage
Myofascial release	Deep tissue/deep muscle massage
Neuromuscular therapy	Craniosacral therapy
Acupressure/shiatsu	Manual lymphatic drainage
Muscle Energy Technique	Counterstrain/Positional Release
Thai massage	Rosen Method
Reflexology	

Promoting comfort

Swedish massage	Craniosacral therapy
Reiki	Therapeutic Touch/Healing Touch

Promoting kinesthetic or neuromuscular education

Trager
Muscle Energy Technique
Alexander Technique
Proprioceptive Neuromuscular Facilitation
Feldenkrais/Awareness Through Movement

Promoting energetic balance or flow

Acupressure/shiatsu	Reiki
Craniosacral therapy	Therapeutic Touch/Healing Touch
Reflexology	

---

term in its broader sense to encompass a range of modalities, that is, both massage and bodywork.

One way to categorize the different kinds of techniques and modalities is on the basis of their intended therapeutic effect, as shown in Box 2.1. Note that a modality can belong to more than one category. The effect of a modality may vary depending upon the application of the technique. For example, Swedish massage can have a stimulating or sedative effect depending upon the rhythm, speed, and pressure with which the massage strokes are applied.

Some guidance regarding this issue may be found in the definitions put forth by two of the major professional organizations. On its website, the most senior professional association of massage therapists, the American Massage Therapy Association (AMTA), defines massage as the application of manual techniques and adjunctive therapies with the intention of positively affecting the health and well-being of the client (AMTA, 2000). The certifying agency for professional therapists, the National Certification Board for Therapeutic Massage and Bodywork (NCBTMB) has a broader practitioner job description supported by a formal job analysis of the field. It defines a practitioner as:

One who employs a conceptual and philosophical framework, and uses knowledge of various systems of anatomy, physiology, and contraindications to facilitate the optimal functioning of individual human beings through the manual application of various modalities. The practitioner assesses the client in order to develop a session strategy, applies relevant techniques to support optimal functioning of the human body, establishes a relationship with the client that is conducive to healing, and adheres to professional standards of practice and a code of ethics (NCBTMB, 1997a).

This is an ambitious definition that clearly states the presence of a theoretical framework supporting the practical application of technique by the practitioner, and it further implies that psychosocial factors are present by virtue of a client–practitioner relationship that is 'conducive to healing.' I do not know of any study to date, that has explicitly defined massage therapy in these terms, that is, as practitioners themselves do.

Definitions are important for several reasons, and the lack of definitions in the majority of studies is troubling. Studies that define massage, by implication or omission, as simply the rubbing of muscle tissue ignore crucial aspects of the therapy under investigation and may be more likely to result in findings that are ambiguous or difficult to interpret. On a more practical level, many studies do not define or describe the specific techniques used in the massage protocol in sufficient detail. As a result, it is impossible for the reader to determine exactly what was done or to evaluate whether or not the protocol was appropriate to the study hypothesis.

STANDARDIZATION OF MASSAGE PROTOCOLS

Related to the issue of definitions is the question of 'standardization.' Massage therapy is not a drug any more than psychotherapy is, and in truth we cannot pretend otherwise, especially for the purpose of research. Those who have taught in a professional training program know that among beginning students, who typically learn a standard routine, qualitative differences are quite readily apparent among the massages they give. As students become proficient practitioners, each develops an individual style. When experienced practitioners are trained in a highly specific protocol, some discernible differences in style and application, such as the amount of pressure used or the timing and rhythm of strokes, will still be present. The implementation of a specific protocol cannot truly be 'standardized'.

An even stronger argument is that in many instances a standardized protocol is not appropriate given the study hypothesis. If the objective of a study is to evaluate the relative effectiveness of various manual approaches for a particular condition, then a more limited protocol specifying the types of techniques used for each approach without any overlapping between approaches would make sense. However, if the question involves evaluating the efficacy of massage generally, a standardized intervention does not represent massage therapy as it is actually practiced because, as the NCBTMB survey showed, practitioners typically combine elements of more than one discipline. Results using a standardized protocol are then limited to that specific protocol and cannot be generalized more widely.

Worse still, standardized approaches do not allow the practitioner to tailor the treatment to the individual client, something that is by definition fundamental to the practice of massage therapy and necessary to make the treatment as effective as possible. The client or patient plays an active role in the therapy and is encouraged to give feedback to the therapist regarding patient preferences for the region(s) of the body to be worked with or to be avoided, the degree of pressure that is pleasant or tolerable, and the amount of time spent on a given region. For example, in one frequently cited study with ambiguous results, massage was tested as an intervention for cancer pain by giving ten minutes of light effleurage on the back, without regard to the patient's diagnosis, the source of pain, or the patient's preference (Weinrich & Weinrich, 1990). While this study has other flaws, a fundamental problem is that the intervention tested bears little resemblance to the way in which an experienced therapist who is familiar with the needs of cancer patients would choose to work with them.

Finally, standardized protocols may present an ethical problem in some situations. For example, participants who are trauma survivors may be uncomfortable with and distressed by having certain areas of their bodies touched. Because their reactions to touch can be highly idiosyncratic, no automatic assumptions can be made about which areas will feel safe to the patient. During 19 years of clinical experience, clients have, at least initially asked me to not touch their hands, feet, legs, arms, lower back, hair, neck, and face during massage. Individualized massage protocols respect the patient's physical and emotional boundaries, which may encourage higher rates of participation and greater adherence to or compliance with the study protocol.

Standardized protocols thus form a rigid straitjacket limiting the effectiveness of the intervention, and are invalid by definition of the therapy as it is practiced. Such studies are likely to avoid Type I error at the expense of promoting Type II error. It is analogous to testing the efficacy of surgery as an intervention by giving every study participant a tonsillectomy no matter what their medical situation requires.

Some may argue that an individualized protocol promotes dilution of treatment and introduces unnecessary variance or error into the study. According to Levin and his colleagues (1997), complex interventions like massage that include individualized treatment can be studied as 'gestalts,' that is, looking at the effects of the whole system of care, rather than breaking it down into its component parts. The virtue of this approach is that it avoids the conventional biomedical model's tendency to reductionism while remaining methodologically sound. In reality, an individualized protocol is more representative of the way massage therapy is practiced and thus has greater ecological or model fit validity (Cassidy, 1995). It also permits greater generalizability of results, allows the therapy to be as effective as possible, and has greater ethical value because it respects the personal boundaries of study participants.

If the study hypothesis does not necessitate one approach or the other, a solution to the standardized versus individualized dilemma is to use a cafeteria style approach, where therapists may choose from a menu of several modalities commonly used or considered useful for a given condition, while other modalities or approaches that are not likely to be particularly effective are excluded. The selected modalities are then applied according to the therapist's judgment and the patient's needs or preferences. It does make sense, however, to standardize some aspects of the treatment such as its duration, time of day given, gender of the therapist relative to the patient, and treatment setting, in order to control these variables. More than one therapist should be used to provide the massage, in order to control for therapist effect as an alternative explanation for results. On a practical level, using more than one therapist anticipates potential scheduling conflicts and prevents therapist burnout. However, because therapeutic relationship between client and practitioner is by definition part of the intervention, the same participant should be treated by the same therapist to the extent that this is logistically possible. Investigating the role of relationship in massage therapy would make an interesting area of study, and one that has general relevance in today's system of health care.

Because we do not know at this point how much variation in individual treatment occurs, it would also be useful to have massage therapists keep detailed notes describing as specifically as possible what they did during each session, along with the rationale for their treatment decisions. These could then be compared among different therapists in a study to see whether significant differences in style exist, and whether or not these are correlated in any meaningful way with the study results.

QUALIFICATIONS OF STUDY PERSONNEL

Where dilution of treatment does surface as an issue, however, is in the qualifications of research study personnel who perform the massage. A number of studies have used personnel with little or no training specifically in massage therapy such as nurses or physical therapists. Nurses and physical therapists typically receive little or no training in the use of specific manual therapy techniques used in massage and bodywork therapy, such as deep tissue work, neuromuscular massage, shiatsu or acupressure, craniosacral therapy, or counterstrain techniques. Although physical therapists do receive some training in rehabilitative manual techniques, schools of nursing no longer routinely teach massage techniques because it is no longer a standard part of evening or PM care, given other demands on nurses' time; massage is now limited to a few simple techniques taught briefly as part of a survey course on complementary and alternative therapies. In contrast, the number of hours required for certification or licensure as a massage therapist in states that regulate massage as a health profession is at least 500 hours. A majority of US therapists (62.4%) report that they have more than 500 hours of entry level training in addition to annual continuing education hours (NCBTMB, 1997a) required to maintain certification and membership in professional associations. It is hardly surprising, then, that studies that fail to use professionally trained therapists to provide the massage treatment have negative or ambiguous results (Richards, 1998; Weinrich & Weinrich, 1990).

In addition, personnel without training or experience in massage cannot provide helpful information to investigators regarding proposed study protocols during the design phase of a study. The lack of such information may pose a potential risk to participants. In my experience, physicians, who are responsible for overseeing participants' medical care and who are often members of the institutional review boards responsible for protecting human subjects, as a group are largely unaware of contraindications and cautions associated with massage under certain health conditions. Many that I have met seem to believe that massage is something that feels pleasant to patients but has no real physiological effects. For example, a physician once asked me to perform Swedish massage on the leg of a patient confined to bed with a diagnosis of a deep vein thrombosis. This condition is one of the few absolute contraindications in Swedish massage because stimulating circulation under these circumstances can dislodge a blood clot, sending it traveling through the bloodstream where it can occlude a vital blood vessel in the heart, lung, or brain. Professionally trained and experienced practitioners can alert investigators to potential problems with protocols, make informed clinical decisions when working with seriously ill patients, and provide a higher standard of care to patients. All of this is not to say that nurses and physical therapists are not qualified, or that they should never provide massage interventions in studies. However, being qualified in one field does not automatically confer proficiency in another. Study personnel should have specific training and experience in the modalities or techniques that will be performed. For example, many physical therapists seek out additional training in modalities not taught in university programs, such as craniosacral therapy. Nurses sometimes complete professional training programs in massage and bodywork, and are eligible for certification or licensure as practitioners.

BLINDING AND CONTROL INTERVENTIONS

It is impossible to use the traditional double blind strategy in studying massage therapy. Obviously, patients know whether or not they are being touched, just as practitioners know whether or not they are touching them. However, study personnel collecting or assessing data can and should be blinded to group assignment whenever possible.

Control interventions pose an interesting challenge. Clearly, the question of what constitutes an appropriate control intervention is always determined by the research hypothesis being tested. In some studies, massage may be compared to an intervention that promotes relaxation but does not involve touch, while other studies may compare social or unskilled touch with the skilled touch that massage provides. The problem is that as a substantial body of research shows, touch in and of itself produces measurable, complex, and sometimes quite dramatic effects (Montagu, 1978), as does relaxation. But the rationale for this strategy assumes that a less active treatment is being compared with one that is more active. How much more active is unknown. If both treatments are active to a similar degree, the null hypothesis can appear to be true when in fact both interventions are effective. Any effects attributed to the intervention tested are wrongly assumed to be due to nonspecific effect, when each intervention may produce effects through other factors that have yet to be identified. However, this strategy is a useful one at present because so little is known regarding the magnitude of the difference, if any, between skilled and unskilled touch.

Sham treatments pose a similar difficulty in that creating a believable sham intervention resembling a true one closely enough runs the risk of eliciting the same effects, and the problem of comparing a less active to a more active intervention still exists. Because there is no such thing as placebo touch, practical difficulties in developing sham treatments are also a consideration. Only one study that I know of has used a credible sham treatment for massage. Evaluating the effectiveness of reflexology for relieving premenstrual syndrome symptoms, Oleson & Flocco (1993) used a sham treatment consisting of pressure applied either too lightly or too roughly to be considered effective on points thought to be ineffective for premenstrual syndrome. Participants in this group reported that they believed they were receiving the true reflexology treatment.

No study of which I am aware has quantitatively examined the possible role of nocebo effects in using sham treatments. Massage therapists usually expect to help people as a consequence of their work. If a practitioner is asked to give a treatment that he or she believes to be ineffective to study participants, the practitioner may unconsciously communicate his or her distress to participants, thus influencing the results. For the same reason, sham treatments are ethically dubious, because practitioners are being asked to knowingly provide an ineffective treatment while withholding a potentially beneficial one. It is also possible that deliberately withholding the intention to help has negative consequences for the practitioner. Janet Quinn (1996), a nurse with experience in designing and conducting research on Therapeutic Touch, has described her own sense of discomfort experienced while giving a placebo Therapeutic Touch treatment as part of a research study, concluding that she would not do it again because it felt too unpleasant.

If the suggestive research on prayer and nonlocal healing compiled by Dossey (1993) is accurate, the practitioner's intention to be of help to the client may influence results in a meaningful way that is statistically measurable. Massage therapists often visualize the anatomical structures and physiological processes they wish to affect during their work with clients, particularly deeper structures that are hard to palpate directly. Perhaps such visualization, along with the desire to help, could be considered a form of focused intention that affects the energetic field of the client. It would be interesting to have data regarding this potential variable in massage research.

NONSPECIFIC EFFECTS

This brings us to the role of nonspecific effects and expectation in massage. Nonspecific response, sometimes referred to as placebo response, has long been misunderstood in health care research. Contrary to the common misinterpretation of the well known study by Beecher (1955), the magnitude of nonspecific effects is not a constant 33% but varies considerably according to Moerman (1983), and can only be determined by measuring it in each study. Another estimate of the magnitude of nonspecific effects is as high as 80%, even when testing drugs and surgical interventions using objective measures (Jonas, 1994). Separating specific from nonspecific effects by the use of a placebo control group is often done in health care research to determine whether or not a given treatment is effective. However, placebo controls are not the only way to determine efficacy.

If a treatment is shown to have no specific effect but reliably induces a positive or desired outcome from nonspecific effects alone, that is no reason to abandon its use. The treatment is effective and may have the advantage of being cheaper or posing less risk of adverse response or side effects. For this reason, the best control may sometimes be a standard treatment group, depending of course on the hypothesis to be tested. It may not always be ethical, practically feasible, or desirable to test massage against a placebo or sham treatment. Also, the additive model, where nonspecific effects plus specific effects are assumed to equal total variance explained, may be much too simplistic. Kleijnen and colleagues (1994) reviewed a series of clinical trials to determine whether interactions between specific and nonspecific effects occurred. They concluded that nonspecific effects can act as a modifying variable, sometimes potentiating the specific effect and in other cases inhibiting it.

Given the difficulties regarding the use of control interventions described previously, it may prove to be impossible to separate the specific from the nonspecific effects of massage therapy. Massage is a highly personal intervention predicated upon touch, one that necessarily involves time and focused attention, and that has a certain amount of face validity, which Jonas (1994) argues is an essential factor in maximizing treatment efficacy. It seems probable that massage is a potent means of engaging nonspecific response. It is interesting that the body systems which have been demonstrated to show the most physiological responsiveness to massage — the integumentary, cardiovascular, autonomic nervous, and neuroimmune systems — are the same ones that are also highly responsive to psychological interventions such as guided imagery, hypnosis, and biofeedback. It is also certainly possible that massage does produce specific effects, such as an increase in the cytotoxicity of natural killer cells (Ironson et al., 1996), through the modulating activity of the higher perceptual centers and the limbic cortex of the brain. Using this line of reasoning, it is also possible that massage produces effects through learned behavior or conditioned response. Many massage therapists have recounted to me instances where clients have said to the therapist that they felt an increased sense of relaxation and well-being upon walking into the office or even knowing that they had an appointment that day. Indeed, as Box 2.1 shows, kinesthetic learning is the stated goal of several modalities, such as Alexander Technique and Feldenkrais. Here again is an argument for viewing research as a collaborative effort on the part of investigator and participant, for studying individual response to treatment, and for studying what factors can maximize treatment effectiveness. From a methodological perspective, it also illustrates the importance of collecting baseline data regarding the extent of previous experience with massage by study participants. In some instances naive participants may be preferable to those with more experience as massage consumers to rule out learning effects.

Because the effects of expectation have been so thoroughly documented in the health care and psychology literature, it is necessary to account for its role in evaluating the effectiveness of massage therapy. Clearly, patients who seek out massage must have some belief that it will help them or else they would not spend time and money to get it. Presumably, patients who choose to participate in research studies of massage must also have some degree of belief or else they would not consent to receive it. By the same token, patients who are averse to massage for whatever reason are likely to refuse it as an intervention. Expectation on the part of patients should be assessed whenever possible so that its role can be measured. Informed consent also raises a related issue: how to provide prospective participants sufficient information with which to make an informed decision without giving away too much information regarding the experimenter's expectations.

One solution is to not label one treatment as active and the other as a sham or placebo, but instead to tell prospective participants that they will receive one of two active treatments, and that each may have benefits.

A novel solution to these problems has been proposed by Cassidy (1994). In her cross-over design, participants are divided into two groups. One group is randomly assigned to receive first treatment A and then treatment B, and vice versa. The other group chooses which treatment they will receive and remains with it unless they become dissatisfied, at which time they are allowed to choose again. In addition, all participants are interviewed. Those who are randomly assigned are asked to respond to their assignment, and those allowed to choose are asked to explain their choice(s). The design is a powerful one because it not only separates the effects of expectation from specific treatment effects but through the use of the interview data examines the ways in which expectation can magnify treatment effects.

TYPES OF RESEARCH STUDIES

A final problem with designing and conducting research on massage therapy has to do with the types of studies that have been conducted. Typically, when little is known about a subject descriptive studies are conducted first, to 'map out the territory' and provide a solid foundation of knowledge to build upon. Analytic studies then follow, and a knowledge base is constructed. Types of studies such as clinical trials or systematic reviews are conducted only when a substantial amount of knowledge has been amassed from previous studies.

With massage therapy, however, this sequence of events has not happened. Massage became popular as a medical intervention in the mid 1800s, thanks to the work of Per Hendrik Ling, Johann Georg Mezger, and their pupils (Kamenetz, 1976). Initial research on the effects of massage was performed by physicians in the Victorian era (Brunton & Tunnicliff, 1894–1895; Edgecombe & Bain, 1899; Jacobi & White, 1880; Mitchell, 1894) and focused on the physiological effects of massage on body functions such as circulation, including blood and lymphatic flow, and muscle function. Research in these and related areas continued until the early 1950s (Carrier, 1922; Drinker, 1939; Elkins et al., 1953; Pemberton, 1945; Wakim et al., 1949). These studies were mostly descriptive in nature, lacking true experimental design and tests of statistical significance. Much of this research has been largely forgotten or dismissed as being out of date, and is seldom referenced outside of massage therapy textbooks, despite its historical and descriptive value. A large percentage of what is currently taught in training programs about the effects of massage is based on these early studies, combined with a healthy dose of clinical observation and belief.

Although the early studies provide some evidence of massage's effects on body systems, evidence as to the usefulness of these effects in treating health care conditions or promoting wellness remains at an early stage. The majority of claims regarding massage's physiological efficacy have not been verified by more recent clinical research (Ernst & Fialka, 1994). Despite this lack of a solid foundation, poorly designed clinical trials of massage and systematic reviews concluding that there is insufficient data continue to proliferate. Proper design and conduct of a clinical trial poses its own challenges, and 'the evidence available to guide many aspects of the design, conduct, and analysis of trials is not always being applied' (Prescott et al., 1999).

While well-designed clinical trials are certainly necessary and help to advance knowledge regarding massage therapy, it also makes sense to focus research funding and efforts on appropriate descriptive and obser-vational studies to create a broader knowledge base. For example, it would be interesting to verify early observed effects of massage on blood and lymphatic flow using modern technology. Because massage has a plausi-ble biological basis, studies that identify and test potential mechanisms by which massage produces its effects are also important. Because mas-sage clearly has significant psychological effects (Field, 1998), it offers a fertile field for investigating mind–body interactions. Studies should routinely collect data on both physiological and emotional variables, as well as the psychological characteristics of participants, all of which may help explain why some people respond more positively to massage than others. At a minimum, studies should collect baseline data concerning psychological factors that are known to affect physiological outcomes, such as anxiety and depression. Studies that examine neuropeptide responses to massage as well as areas of brain activity during and after massage would be valuable and might identify potential mechanisms.

In addition, qualitative studies that focus on patients' experience of massage and its meaning to them are particularly lacking. Qualitative studies are sometimes ignored as an important element of evidence-based medicine, yet they provide information that illuminates impor-tant aspects of the therapist–patient encounter which can also be used to improve the design of quantitative studies. Educational research on massage training is nonexistent and is badly needed as the profession continues to grow exponentially.

RECOMMENDATIONS

Based on these arguments, I make several recommendations to investiga-tors who are designing studies and reporting their results. Some of these recommendations apply to any kind of research, but bear reiteration. Firstly, assumptions about and definitions of massage therapy for the purposes of the study should be clearly articulated. Design decisions should always be determined by the study hypothesis to be tested. Among those particularly relevant for massage research are the choice of an appropriate comparison group and whether to use a standardized or individualized massage protocol. Choices made should be congruent with the hypothesis tested, and their rationale explained. If a sham or placebo treatment is used, investigators should verify that blinding of participants was successful. Dependent variables or outcomes measured should be clinically and socially relevant. As a means to increase validity in research on massage generally, the proper use and implementation of random assignment is especially important.

Secondly, studies should use qualified personnel to provide massage interventions, particularly when individualized protocols are used, in order to maximize treatment effectiveness. Professionally trained and experienced practitioners can provide valuable information to investigators regarding the design of the massage intervention in studies using standardized protocols, again maximizing treatment effectiveness. In studies with individualized protocols, practitioners should keep a detailed record of the treatment provided at each session with an explanation of the rationale for their decisions, which can be analyzed and presented as part of the study results or as a separate paper. More than one therapist should be used to provide treatment, to control for therapist effect, and the same therapist should treat the same patient, to allow the development of a therapeutic relationship. From an ethical standpoint, therapists should also be paid for their time, knowledge, and skill as study collaborators, at a level comparable to other study personnel and commensurate with the work performed, rather than being expected to donate or volunteer their services. Qualifications of massage personnel should be stated in published studies. Such studies should describe the massage protocol used in sufficient detail, so that readers can have a clear understanding of what kind of massage was performed.

Next, study personnel who collect or assess data should be blinded. Data regarding participant expectation and prior experience with massage should be collected and measured whenever possible. Although numerous authors have made the following request before, it bears repeating because it has yet to become standard practice: published results should present estimated effect sizes and confidence intervals, in addition to p values. Statistical tests of significance should be applied appropriately, particularly when multiple outcomes are measured.

It is also important that investigators conducting systematic reviews take some of the methodological issues discussed into account when evaluating or weighting studies for analysis. A systematic review is only as good as the quality of its individual studies will allow. I have yet to see a systematic review that considered the use of professionally trained and experienced practitioners to provide the intervention or that considered whether the massage protocol used was congruent with the study hypothesis as a criterion for evaluating the quality of a study.

Finally, massage schools need to include research literacy as part of the curriculum so that future therapists are conversant with important studies, can distinguish high quality from poor quality research, and have a strong foundation from which therapists can assume roles as active collaborators in helping to design and carry out studies or from which they may pursue further training to design and conduct studies independently.

Having trained in both quantitative and qualitative research methods, I do believe that existing research methods are quite adequate to the task of evaluating massage therapy. However, quantitative methods in particular need to be applied thoughtfully, with attention to the issues discussed here. Health care research has traditionally relied on epidemiological methods and can only benefit from the inclusion of methods drawn from other disciplines such as psychology, anthropology, and education. Clinical trials play an important role but are not the only methodologically sound or rigorous type of study design. Other types of research have value and should be used to inform the design of such trials, and to create a more complete knowledge base in the field of touch-based therapies.

REFERENCES

American Massage Therapy Association (2000). *AMTA Definition of Massage Therapy* [web page]: http://www.amtamassage.org/about/definition.html

Beecher, H. K. (1955). The powerful placebo. *Journal of the American Medical Association, 159,* 1602–1606.

Brunton, T., & Tunnicliff, T. (1894–1895). On the effects of the kneading of the muscles upon the circulation, local and general. *Journal of Physiology, 17,* 364.

Carrier, E. B. (1922). Studies on the physiology of capillaries: Reaction of human skin capillaries to drugs and other stimuli. *American Journal of Physiology, 61,* 528–547.

Cassidy, C. M. (1994). Unraveling the ball of string: Reality, paradigms, and the study of alternative medicine. *Advances, 10*(1), 5–31.

Cassidy, C. M. (1995). Social science theory and methods in the study of alternative and complementary medicine. *Journal of Alternative and Complementary Medicine, 1*(1), 19–41.

Cassileth, B., Jonas, W., & Cassidy, C. (1994). Research methodologies. In *Alternative medicine: expanding medical horizons.* (NIH Publication No. 94-066.) Washington, DC: US Government Printing Office.

Cawley, N. (1997). A critique of the methodology of research studies evaluating massage. *European Journal of Cancer Care, 6*(1), 23–31.

Dossey, L. (1993). *Healing words: The power of prayer and the practice of medicine.* New York: HarperSanFrancisco.

Drinker, C. K. (1939). The formation and movements of lymph. *American Heart Journal, 18,* 389.

Edgecombe, W., & Bain, W. (1899). The effect of baths, massage and exercise on the blood pressure. *Lancet, 1,* 1552–1557.

Elkins, E., Herrick, J., Grindlay, J., et al. (1953). Effect of various procedures on the flow of lymph. *Archives of Physical Medicine, 34,* 31–39.

Eisenberg, D. M., Kessler, R. C., Foster, C., et al. (1993). Unconventional medicine in the United States: Prevalence, costs, and patterns of use. *New England Journal of Medicine, 328*(4), 246–252.

Ernst, E., (1999). Massage therapy for low back pain: A systematic review. *Journal of Pain and Symptom Management, 17*(1), 65–69.

Ernst, E., & Fialka, V. (1994). The clinical effectiveness of massage: A critical review. *Forsch Komplementärmed, 1*, 226–232.

Field, T. (1998). Massage therapy effects. *American Psychologist, 53*(12), 1270–1281.

Furlan, A. D., Brosseau, L., Welch, V., & Wong, J. (2001). Massage for low back pain (Cochrane Review). In: *The Cochrane Library, 4*. Oxford: Update Software.

Hufford, D. J. (1996). Culturally grounded review of research assumptions. *Alternative Therapies in Health and Medicine, 2*(4), 47–53.

Ironson, G., Field, T., Scafidi, F., et al. (1996). Massage therapy is associated with the enhancement of the immune system's cytotoxicity. *International Journal of Neuroscience, 84*(1–4), 205–217.

Jacobi, M., & White, V. (1880). *On the use of the cold pack followed by massage in the treatment of anemia*. New York: G P Putnam's Sons.

Jonas, W. B. (1994). Therapeutic labeling and the 80% rule. *Bridges, 5*(2), 1–6.

Kamenetz, H. (1976). History of massage. In S. Licht (Ed.), *Massage, manipulation and traction* (pp. 3–37). Huntington, New York: Robert E. Krieger Publishing Company.

Kleijnen, J., de Craen, A., van Everdingen, J., & Krol, L. (1994). Placebo effect in double-blind clinical trials: A review of interactions with medications. *Lancet, 344*, 1347–1349.

Levin, J. S., Glass, T. A., Kushi, L. H., et al. (1997). *Medical Care, 35*(11), 1079–1094.

Menard, M. B. (2002). *Making sense of research: A guide to research literacy for complementary practitioners*. Moncton, New Brunswick: Curties-Overzet Publications, Inc.

Mitchell, J. K. (1894). The effect of massage on the number and haemoglobin value of the red blood cells. *American Journal of Medical Science, 107*, 502–515.

Moerman, D. E. (1983). General medical effectiveness and human biology: Placebo effects in the treatment of ulcer disease. *Medical Anthropology Quarterly, 14*(3), 14–16.

Montagu, A. (1978). *Touching* (2nd ed.). New York: Harper and Row.

National Certification Board for Therapeutic Massage and Bodywork (1997a). *1996–1997 NCBTMB job analysis survey findings*. McLean, Virginia: National Certification Board for Therapeutic Massage and Bodywork.

National Certification Board for Therapeutic Massage and Bodywork (1997b). *Background information for NCBTMB's new exam content*. McLean, Virginia: National Certification Board for Therapeutic Massage and Bodywork.

Oleson, T., & Flocco, W. (1993). Randomized controlled study of premenstrual symptoms treated with ear, hand, and foot reflexology. *Obstetrics and Gynecology, 82*(6), 906–911.

Pemberton, R. (1945). Physiology of massage. In *A. M. A. handbook of physical medicine* (p. 141). Chicago: AMA Council of Physical Medicine.

Prescott, R. J., Counsell, C. E., Gillespie, W. J., et al. (1999). Factors that limit the quality, number and progress of randomized controlled trials. *Health Technology Assessment, 3*(20).

Quinn, J. (1996). Therapeutic Touch and a healing way. Interview by Bonnie Harrigan. *Alternative Therapies in Health and Medicine, 2*(4), 69–75.

Richards, K. C. (1998). Effect of a back massage and relaxation intervention on sleep in critically ill patients. *American Journal of Critical Care, 7*(4), 288–299.

Trotter, G. (2000). Culture, ritual and errors of repudiation: Some implications for the assessment of alternative medical traditions. *Alternative Therapies in Health and Medicine, 6*(4), 62–68.

Vickers, A. (1996). Research on massage. In *Massage and aromatherapy: A guide for health professionals*. London: Chapman and Hall.

Vickers, A., Cassileth, B., Ernst, E., et al. (1997). How should we research unconventional therapies? *International Journal of Technology Assessment in Health Care, 13*(1), 111–121.

Vickers, A., Ohlsson, A., Lacy, J. B., & Horsley, A. (2000). Massage for promoting growth and development of preterm and/or low birth-weight infants (Cochrane Review). In: *The Cochrane Library, 2*. Oxford: Update Software.

Wakim, K., Martin, M., Terrier, J., et al. (1949). The effects of massage on the circulation in normal and paralyzed extremities. *Archives of Physical Medicine, 30*, 135–144.

Weinrich, S. P., & Weinrich, M. C. (1990). The effect of massage on pain in cancer patients. *Applied Nursing Research, 3*(4), 140–145.

SECTION 2

Massage research on various conditions

SECTION CONTENTS

INTRODUCTION TO SECTION 2

The following four chapters address the utility of massage therapy for a number of conditions. Tiffany Field summarizes what is known about massage for immune disorders. Her chapter gives special attention to massage for HIV patients, leukemia patients, and for breast cancer patients. For each of these conditions, Field finds that natural killer cell number and cytotoxicity (activity) were increased after massage therapy. Her work with HIV patients includes both studies of adults and adolescents; for adults, Field's protocol included 45-minute massages five days per week for five weeks. In her study of HIV-positive adolescents Field found that after three months of massage treatment, the teenagers reported less depression. Depression is associated with immunosuppression. Field continues to describe her research with pediatric oncology patients. Children with leukemia who received massage therapy showed decreased anxiety and depression and increased immune function.

Field also describes a study she and her colleagues conducted on massage therapy for breast cancer, a cancer which strikes about one in nine women. Her sample of women, who had undergone simple mastectomy, received 30-minute massage sessions twice a week for five weeks. Among her many findings, Field found a reduction in anxiety, depression, and anger. As Field notes, future research should examine potential long-term (over many months) effects of massage therapy and should investigate underlying mechanisms.

In her chapter, Silvana Lawvere, like Tiffany Field, finds decreases in anxiety and depressed mood in a sample of cancer patients. Lawvere studied a small sample of seven ovarian cancer patients undergoing chemotherapy and found decreases in self-reported anxiety and depression and a decrease in self-reported pain. As Lawvere notes, ovarian cancer is the leading cause of death among gynecological cancers, and cancer patients often report anxiety, depression, and pain. Lawvere's study used a licensed massage therapist with over ten years of experience and 30-minute massage therapy sessions. Her study replicates a general finding (Field, 2000) that massage therapy reduces anxiety as measured by the Spielberger State Trait Anxiety Inventory.

In her chapter on immune disorders, Field indicates a need for cost-benefit analyses of massage therapy in the treatment of immune disorders. Buford Lively and colleagues study just this issue in their research on massage therapy for controlling chemotherapy-induced emesis in women undergoing treatment for breast or ovarian cancer. Lively and colleagues remind the reader that the emetic process includes vomiting, nausea, and retching. Anti-emetic drug therapy was given to 14 patients, while 17 patients received massage therapy as an adjunct to anti-emetic drug therapy.

When massage was used as an adjunct, the study found that total days of nausea and vomiting were reduced and that the length of hospital stay was also reduced. The study found that patients who did not receive massage therapy had extra costs averaging $2853.10. Such results are extremely provocative and one hopes to see similar studies for other conditions.

Finally, Sandra Rogers studies massage as a modality to improve health following spinal cord injury. Rogers reminds readers the spinal cord injury is common, and that there are 200,000 people with spinal cord injuries in the United States. Rogers notes that the immune system changes seen in acute spinal cord injury are similar to those found in patients with chronic stress conditions. Her research subjects received 60-minute massages three times weekly for four weeks. Massages were given by licensed massage therapists and advanced students, and subjects were randomly assigned to a therapist, each of whom was blind to the study outcome measures. Rogers reviews a number of immunological and psychological findings for her massage therapy group. Future studies might investigate the necessary duration of treatment as well as its cost-effectiveness.

REFERENCE

Field, T. (2000). *Touch therapy*. Edinburgh: Churchill Livingstone.

3

Massage therapy for immune disorders

Tiffany M. Field

INTRODUCTION

This chapter is a review of a selection of studies on massage therapy for immune disorders including HIV, leukemia and breast cancer. In all of these disorders natural killer (NK) cell number and cytotoxicity (activity) were enhanced following massage treatment. The decrease in stress hormones (for example, cortisol) is thought to mediate the altered NK cell function. Clinical improvement would be expected to follow from less opportunistic infection, inasmuch as NK cells destroy both cancer and viral cells.

Immune disorders involve dysfunction in the immune system — immune cells are destroyed by foreign cells (viral cells). It was expected that massage therapy would attenuate immune disorders such as HIV and cancer because massage therapy has been noted to lower cortisol (stress hormone) in many conditions (see Field, 1998 for review) and cortisol is noted to kill immune cells, for example, NK cells (Ironson et al., 1996), that in turn kill viral and cancer cells (Whiteside & Herberman, 1989). In this chapter a selection of massage therapy studies on HIV and cancer are reviewed. The data from these studies combined suggest that massage therapy positively affects immune function in immune disorders.

HIV-POSITIVE PATIENTS

Although the effects of massage have rarely been studied in the context of immune disorders, the data from relaxation studies are suggestive. Progressive muscle relaxation has contributed to increased NK cell activity and decreased antibody titers in elderly adults (Kiecolt-Glaser et al., 1985). Helper T lymphocyte cells have also increased in medical students who practiced relaxation more frequently (when they were undergoing exams), (Kiecolt-Glaser et al., 1986). Further, relaxation therapy has been associated with increased NK cell cytotoxicity (activity) and NK cell number in melanoma patients (Fawzy et al., 1990). Finally, HIV positive subjects who practiced relaxation more frequently had better immune functioning one year after their diagnosis, and slower disease progression two years later in at least two studies (Antoni et al., 1991; Ironson et al., 1996).

HIV-positive adults

A study on massage therapy with HIV adults, assessed changes in anxiety and depression, in cortisol levels and immune function following five weeks of massage therapy treatment (Ironson et al., 1996). Twenty-three HIV-positive and ten HIV-negative men were recruited for the study. Over half the sample (14 of 23) had CD4 counts below 500. Most of the subjects were asymptomatic and only two subjects were on antiretrovirals (both on AZT). The 45-minute massage protocol, provided five days per week for five weeks, was a combination of stretching, rocking, squeezing, and holding applied to the head, neck, arms, torso, legs and back.

The massage therapy had no effects on the immune measures related to disease progression in HIV including CD4, CD4/CD8 ratio, beta 2 microglobulin, and neopterin. However, NK cell number and cytotoxicity (activity) increased for the massage therapy group. These changes may have related to the decreased cortisol noted during the massage period. Decreases in cortisol (and anxiety) were significantly correlated with enhanced NK cell number and cytotoxicity.

The importance of NK cell number and cytotoxicity (activity) in HIV positive persons is twofold. First, since the virus itself infects and destroys CD4 cells, the NK cells represent another type of immune cell that may still afford some protection. In later stages of HIV infection, persons with low CD4 counts, who remain asymptomatic may have greater NK cell function (Solomon et al., 1993). Second, NK cells repeatedly provide protection against both viruses and tumors (Whiteside & Herberman, 1989). Viruses (opportunistic infections like pneumonia) are often seen in AIDS patients, as are several malignant diseases (Epstein & Scully, 1992). Lower NK activity is associated with the development of metastases and shorter survival time in patients with cancer (see Whiteside & Herberman, 1989 for a review).

Inasmuch as elevated stress hormones (catecholamines and cortisol) negatively affect immune function, the increase in NK activity probably related to the decrease in these stress hormones following massage therapy. Because NK cells are the front line of defense in the immune system, combating the growth and proliferation of viral cells, the HIV patients who received the massage therapy would probably experience fewer opportunistic infections such as pneumonia and other viruses that often kill them. Inasmuch as NK cells are also effective in combating cancer cells, cancer patients might also benefit from massage therapy.

HIV-positive adolescents

The lack of change in the disease markers, the CD4 cells and the CD4/CD8 ratio, may have related to the patients being immune compromised (over half having CD4 counts below 500). Thus, our next study sampled less immune compromised adolescents. HIV-positive adolescents with a mean CD4 count of 466 were recruited from a large urban university hospital's outpatient clinic and randomly assigned to receive massage therapy ($n = 12$) or progressive muscle relaxation ($n = 12$) twice per week for 12 weeks (Diego et al., 2001). To evaluate the effects of treatment, participants were assessed for depression, anxiety and immune changes before and after the 12-week treatment period. The adolescents who received massage therapy reported feeling less anxious and were less depressed than those who experienced relaxation therapy. They also showed enhanced immune function by the end of the 12-week study. Immune changes included increased NK cell number (CD56 and CD56+CD3−). In addition, the HIV disease progression markers including CD4 number and the CD4/CD8 ratio increased for the massage therapy group only.

Following three months of treatment, the HIV-positive adolescents who received massage therapy reported feeling less depressed than the adolescents who participated in progressive muscle relaxation sessions. In addition, those in the massage therapy group showed improved immune function supporting previous research on decreased depression (Field et al., 1992; Ironson et al., 1996) and improved immune function (Hernandez-Reif et al., 2001; Ironson et al., 1996) following massage therapy.

HIV infection is commonly accompanied by psychological distress, often manifested as depression and anxiety, which may increase HIV symptomology (Jewett & Hecht, 1993). Stress and anxiety might overactivate the hypothalamic-pituitary-adrenal axis (HPA) resulting in the production of cortisol and neuropeptides that may further suppress the immune system, NK cells in particular (Lutgendorf et al., 1996; Zorilla et al., 1996; Madhavan et al., 1995). Although this study did not assess cortisol, the positive massage therapy effects on NK cell number and cytotoxicity might be explained by this treatment's ability to reduce stress and anxiety, which in turn might trigger a reduction of HPA activity, lowering cortisol levels and resulting in improved immune function. Increased NK cell number and activity signifies an important gain in HIV infection as NK cells have been shown to provide protection against common AIDS opportunistic diseases such as tumors and viruses (Whiteside & Herberman, 1989). In addition, it is believed that in advanced HIV cases characterized by low CD4 counts, persons who remain asymptomatic may have greater NK cell functioning (Solomon et al., 1993).

The effect on the HIV disease marker (CD4/CD8 ratio) shown in this study but not in the study conducted by Ironson and colleagues (1996) might be explained by the high incidence of depression in our sample. Depression has been linked to immunosuppression through the effects that adrenaline (epinephrine) and noradrenaline (norepinephrine) have on immune function, including decreased CD4 number and CD4/CD8 ratio (Ravindran et al., 1995). Massage therapy then by reducing depression might also help to improve T-lymphocyte activity, including CD4/CD8 ratio and CD4 number, in HIV-infected adolescents.

BREAST CANCER

Breast cancer is one of the most common cancers among women (one in every nine) (National Cancer Institute, 1999). Although breast cancer treatment depends on many factors, most particularly the stage of the disease, the most common treatments are surgery followed by chemotherapy or radiation therapy.

Because NK cells increased in our HIV studies and because they are thought to ward off cancer cells as well as viral cells, as already mentioned, massage therapy was explored as a potentially effective intervention for breast cancer patients.

The breast cancer study examined the effects of massage therapy on boosting the immune system by increasing NK cell number and cytotoxicity, and enhancing psychological status by reducing depression and anxiety. Because massage therapy has been effective with numerous physical and psychological conditions associated with breast cancer (anxiety, depression, elevated stress and stress hormones, compromised immune system, and pain), massage therapy was also expected to reduce these problems in breast cancer patients. Thirty-six women diagnosed with Stage I or II breast cancer who had undergone simple mastectomy (the removal of a breast) within the past 18 months were included in the study. The mean age of the group was 52 years. Because radiation therapy affects immune measures, the women were not entered into the study until completion of their radiation and chemotherapy treatment, which lasted for six to seven weeks following surgery.

The 30-minute therapy sessions were conducted by volunteer massage therapists three times a week for five consecutive weeks. The therapy was comprised of moderate pressure, smooth strokes, covering the head/neck, shoulder, chest, arms, legs and back.

The data analyses suggested the following: anxiety was reduced for the massage therapy group after the first and the last sessions; depressed mood was also reduced for the massage therapy group after the first and last sessions and from the first to the last day of the study; and anger decreased for the massage therapy group from the first to the last massage day. Also, depressive and hostility symptoms decreased for the massage therapy group from the first to the last day. Biochemical changes included increased dopamine and serotonin levels from the first to the last day.

Analysis of the immune measures

Paired sample t-tests, conducted separately for each group, revealed significant increases for the massage therapy group in NK cell numbers and lymphocytes.

Correlations

A positive correlation was noted between avoidant coping and NK cell numbers and a negative correlation between intrusive coping style and urinary dopamine values. A negative correlation was also noted between anxiety scores and lymphocytes, suggesting that the lower the anxiety level the higher the lymphocyte numbers.

The immediate effects of massage therapy for women with breast cancer were decreases in anxiety, depressed mood and anger. Depressed mood on the Profile of Mood States (POMS) also decreased across the study period, as did depression and hostility on the Symptom Checklist 90R. Similar massage therapy effects have been reported for other chronic illnesses including HIV (Ironson et al., 1996), multiple sclerosis (Hernandez-Reif et al., 1998), fibromyalgia (Sunshine et al., 1996), and chronic fatigue syndrome (Field et al., 1997).

Surprisingly, the women in the massage therapy group did not show a decrease in cortisol stress hormone, noradrenaline (norepinephrine) or adrenaline (epinephrine) values, as has been shown in other massage therapy studies (Field et al., 1996, 1997; Ironson et al., 1996). In relation to the HIV men's study data, the women with breast cancer had higher catecholamine and cortisol values. That the women in the control group showed an increase in the stress hormone noradrenaline (norepinephrine) over the five weeks suggests that the women who did not receive massage were more stressed by the end of the five-week control period. The men in the HIV men's study received daily massage whereas the women in the present study were massaged three times a week. Perhaps more frequent massages or a longer intervention period is required to decrease catecholamine levels for breast cancer patients. The findings also suggest that massage therapy three times a week may be sufficient to keep stress hormone levels from rising.

The women in the massage therapy group showed increased dopamine and serotonin levels on the last day of the study. This increase may reflect the massaged group's improved mood and decreased depression as both serotonin and dopamine have been noted to increase in depressed individuals following massage therapy (see Field, 1998).

Of greatest interest in the current study was that women who received massage therapy showed an increase in NK cell number and lymphocytes. The increase in NK cell number supports an earlier HIV men's massage therapy finding (Ironson et al., 1996) and a recent HIV adolescent massage therapy study (see Diego et al., 2001 for review). That massage therapy increased NK cells and that NK cells specialize in destroying virus-infected cells and tumor cells (Brittenden et al., 1996) has important implications for massage as an intervention for immune compromised illnesses. The increase in lymphocytes following three times weekly massage therapy sessions had not been previously reported. Lymphocytes are precursor cells of immunologic function as well as regulators and effectors of immunity and play an important role in the activation of helper T cells (Hyde, 1992).

Also of interest in the study were the associations between coping style, biochemistry and immune response. Avoidant coping was associated with increased NK cell numbers and intrusive coping was associated with decreased dopamine levels. Women who avoid thinking about cancer may be less depressed or stressed and this may explain their better immune response, inasmuch as stress has been shown to impair immune function (Zorilla et al., 1994). Women who have intrusive thoughts or are preoccupied with their cancer diagnosis may be more prone to depression and lower dopamine (Rogeness et al., 1992). Higher anxiety scores were also correlated with lower lymphocytes, suggesting that greater anxiety negatively impacted the immune system. However, one unexplained finding was the negative correlation between anxiety scores and cortisol levels since typically higher anxiety is correlated with higher cortisol values.

The present study is limited with respect to assessing longer-term effects of massage therapy on breast cancer. Further research is required to examine whether extended massage therapy treatments (e.g., over six months) can keep the cancer in remission. Moreover, whether similar massage therapy benefits would be gained for other types of cancer or immune compromised conditions requires further study.

In summary, the self-reports of reduced stress, anxiety, anger/hostility and improved mood and the corroborating findings of improved immune function suggest that massage therapy has positive applications for breast cancer survivors. That elevated anxiety levels and coping style correlated with immune and biochemistry measures suggest the need for interventions, like massage therapy, that offer psychoneuro/immunological benefits for breast cancer patients.

PEDIATRIC ONCOLOGY PATIENTS

Cancer treatment can cause distress in children related to the anxiety and pain associated with medical procedures (such as bone marrow aspirations, lumbar and venous punctures and chemotherapy) and nausea and vomiting (resulting from chemotherapy and from anticipatory anxiety associated with treatment). These repeated procedures may lead to anxiety and depression.

The potential benefits of relaxation therapy have been explored for stress management and pain reduction in leukemic patients (Pederson, 1996) and for reducing feelings of nausea and anxiety induced by chemotherapy in cancer patients (Arakawa, 1997). Distress levels in children with leukemia have been notably lower following a combination of pharmacological and psychological interventions (Kazak et al., 1996). One study reported the use of cognitive behavioral techniques from both parent and child as instruments to improve positive mood during painful procedures (Broome et al., 1998). Imagery using visualization has also resulted in fewer distress behaviors during painful procedures such as children undergoing cardiac catheterization (Pederson, 1995).

As noted above in the HIV and breast cancer studies, a significant reduction in anxiety levels and enhanced immune function (increased NK cell number and cytotoxicity) in HIV-positive men suggest that massage therapy positively affects the immune system. Thus, massage therapy was used with children being treated for leukemia to reduce the children's anxiety and depressed mood and enhance their immune function. Massage was the preferred therapy because other relaxation therapy techniques require more active participation and understanding by the participant. The parents were taught to give the massage therapy so that it could be given on a daily basis, could be cost effective and might reduce the parents' stress. For example, anxiety and cortisol levels have been reduced in elderly volunteers from giving children massage (Field et al., 1998). Teaching the parents to massage their child was expected to give the parents a more active role in their child's treatment, thereby reducing their own anxiety levels and sense of helplessness. Having the parents massage the children at home was also less likely to cause an association between massage and any painful, uncomfortable medical procedures at the hospital. In addition, having the parents as therapists was considered more cost effective and potentially helpful for the parent–child relationship.

Twenty children (mean age 7.2 years) with leukemia participated in this study. The children were randomly assigned to the massage or control group. The massage therapy training sessions were conducted by two massage therapists who guided the parents through the 20-minute massage by having them practice it on their child under the direction of the therapist. Once they felt comfortable doing the massage, the parents were instructed to give the massage before bedtime every day for 30 days. The 20-minute massage consisted of applying moderate pressure for 30-second periods on the face, neck, shoulders, back, stomach, legs, feet, arms and hands.

Analyses of the data on the parents' and child's anxiety and depressed mood measures suggested that the massage therapy group parents had lower anxiety and depressed mood levels after the massage therapy sessions on the first day of the study. Similarly, the massage therapy group children had lower anxiety and depressed mood levels after the massage therapy sessions on the first day of the study.

The massage therapy group parents' depression also decreased across the course of the study. Most importantly, the massage group children's white blood count and neutrophil count increased significantly across the one month treatment period. The reduction of anxiety in the parents may have resulted from their having a more active role in their children's treatment. The children's lower anxiety following massage may have in turn contributed to their improved immune function.

CONCLUSION

These then are the improved functions noted following massage therapy. In addition to the immune changes noted in each study — most commonly increased NK cell number and activity — anxiety, depression, stress hormones (cortisol) and catecholamines significantly decreased. Increased parasympathetic activity may be the underlying mechanism for these changes. The pressure stimulation associated with touch increases vagal activity which in turn lowers physiological arousal and stress hormones (cortisol levels). The pressure is critical because light stroking is generally aversive (much like a tickle stimulus) and does not produce these effects. Decreased cortisol in turn leads to enhanced immune function.

Further research is needed, however, not only to replicate these empirical findings but also to study underlying mechanisms. Until underlying mechanisms are known, the medical community is unlikely to incorporate these therapies into practice. In addition to mechanism studies, treatment comparison studies are important not only to determine the relative effects and combined effects of different therapies such as the massage therapy combined with aromatherapy, but also the within-therapy variations such as the best massage techniques for different conditions and the arousing versus the calming effects of different types of treatment, for example, the arousing effects of rosemary and the calming effects of lavender (Diego et al., 1998). Further, cost benefit analyses need to be conducted to establish the cost effectiveness of massage therapy for the treatment of immune disorders.

ACKNOWLEDGEMENTS

I would like to thank those individuals who participated in these studies. This research was supported by an NIMH Senior Research Scientist Award (MH#00331) to Tiffany Field and funding by Johnson and Johnson.

REFERENCES

Antoni, M. H., Baggett, L., Ironson, G., et al. (1991). Cognitive-behavioral stress management intervention buffers distress responses and immunologic changes notification of HIV-1 seropositivity. *Journal of Consulting and Clinical Psychology, 59*, 906–915.

Arakawa, S. (1997). Relaxation to reduce nausea, vomiting, and anxiety induced by chemotherapy in Japanese patients. *Cancer Nursing, 20*, 342–349.

Brittenden, J., Heys, S., Ross, J., & Eremin, O. (1996). Natural killer cells and cancer. *Cancer, 77*, 1226–1243.

Broome, M. E., Rehwaldt, M., & Fogg, L. (1998). Relationships between cognitive behavioral techniques, temperament, observed and pain reports in children and adolescents during lumbar puncture. *Journal of Pediatric Nursing, 13*, 48–54.

Diego, M. A., Field, T., Hernandez-Reif, M., et al. (2001). HIV adolescents show improved immune function following massage therapy. *International Journal of Neuroscience, 106*, 35–45.

Diego, M., Jones, N., Field, T., et al. (1998). Aromatherapy positively affects mood, EEG patterns of alertness and math computations. *International Journal of Neuroscience, 96*, 217–224.

Epstein, J. B., & Scully, C. (1992). Neoplastic disease in the head and neck of patients with AIDS. *International Journal of Oral Maxillofacial Surgery, 21*, 219–226.

Fawzy, F. I., Kemeny, M. E., Fawzy, N. W., et al. (1990). A structured psychiatric intervention for cancer patients. II. Changes over time in immunological measures. *Archives of General Psychiatry, 47*, 729–735.

Field, T. (1998). Massage therapy effects. *American Psychologist, 53*, 1270–1281.

Field, T., Grizzle, N., Scafidi, F., & Schanberg, S. (1996). Massage and relaxation therapies' effects on depressed adolescent mothers. *Adolescence, 31*, 903–911.

Field, T., Hernandez-Reif, M., Quintino, O., et al. (1998). Elder retired volunteers benefit from giving massage therapy to infants. *The Journal of Applied Gerontology, 17*, 229–239.

Field, T., Morrow, C., Valdeon, C., et al. (1992). Massage reduces anxiety in child and adolescent psychiatric patients. *Journal of the American Academy of Child and Adolescent Psychiatry, 31*, 124–131.

Field, T., Sunshine, W., Hernandez-Reif, M., et al. (1997). Massage therapy effects on depression and somatic symptoms in chronic fatigue syndrome. *Journal of Chronic Fatigue Syndrome, 3*, 43–51.

Hernandez-Reif, M., Field, T., & Theakston, H. (1998). Multiple sclerosis patients benefit from massage therapy. *Journal of Bodywork and Movement Therapies, 2*, 168–174.

Hernandez-Reif, M., Ironson, G., Field, T., et al. (2001). Breast cancer patients have improved immune functions following massage therapy.

Hyde, R. (1992). *Immunology*, 2nd Edition. Pennsylvania: Harwal Publishing Co.

Ironson, G., Field, T., Scafidi, F., et al. (1996). Massage therapy is associated with enhancement of the immune system's cytoxic capacity. *Journal of Consulting and Clinical Psychology, 84*, 205–218.

Jewett, J., & Hecht, F. (1993). Preventive health care for adults with HIV infection. *JAMA, 269*, 1144–1153.

Kazak, A. E., Penati, B., Boyer, B. A., et al. (1996). A randomized controlled prospective outcome study of a psychological and pharmacological intervention protocol for procedural distress in pediatric leukemia. *Journal of Pediatric Psychology, 21*, 615–631.

Kiecolt-Glaser, J. K., Glaser, R., Williger, D., et al. (1985). Psychosocial enhancement of immunocompetence in a geriatric population. *Health Psychology, 4*, 25–41.

Kiecolt-Glaser, J. K., Glaser, R., Strain, E., et al. (1986). Modulation of cellular immunity in medical students. *Journal of Behavioral Medicine, 9,* 5–21.

Lutgendorf, S., Antoni, M. H., Shneiderman, N., & Fletcher, M. A. (1996). Psychosocial counseling to improve quality of life in HIV infection. *Patient Education and Counseling, 24,* 217–235.

Madhavan, P. N., Shwartz, N., & Shwartz, S. (1995). Synergistic effect of cortisol and HIV-1 envelope peptide on the NK activities of normal lymphocytes. *Brain and Behavior, 9,* 20–30.

National Cancer Institute. Office of Cancer Information, Communication, and Education (OCICE) 1999.

Pederson, C. (1995). Effect of imagery on children's pain and anxiety during cardiac catheterization. *Journal of Pediatric Nursing, 10,* 365–374.

Pederson, C. (1996). Promoting parental use of nonpharmacologic techniques with children during lumbar punctures. *Pediatric Oncology Nursing, 13,* 21–30.

Ravindran, A. V., Griffiths, L., Merali, Z., & Anisman, H. (1995). Lymphocyte subsets associated with major depression and dysthymia: Modification by antidepressant treatment. *Psychosomatic Medicine, 57,* 555–563.

Rogeness, G. A., Javors, M. A., & Pliszka, S. R. (1992). Neurochemistry and child and adolescent psychiatry. *Journal of the American Academy of Child and Adolescent Psychiatry, 31,* 765–781.

Solomon, G. F., Benton, D., Harker, J., et al. (1993). Prolonged asymptomatic states in HIV-Seropositive persons with CD4 positive T-cells/mm^3: Preliminary psychoimmunologic findings. *Journal of Acquired Immunodeficiency Syndromes, 6,* 1173.

Sunshine, W., Field, T., Quintino, O., et al. (1996). Fibromyalgia benefits from massage therapy and transcutaneous electrical stimulation. *Journal of Clinical Rheumatology, 2,* 18–22.

Whiteside, T. L., & Herberman, R. B. (1989). The role of natural killer cells in human disease. *Clinical Immunology and Immunopathology, 53,* 1–23.

Zorrilla, E., McKay, J., Luborsky, L., & Shmidt, K. (1996). Relation of stressors and depressive symptoms to clinical progression of viral illness. *American Journal of Psychiatry, 153,* 626–635.

Zorrilla, E., Redei, E., & DeRubeis, R. (1994). Reduced cytokine levels and T-cell function in healthy males: Relation to individual differences in subclinical anxiety. *Brain Behavior and Immunity, 8,* 293–312.

4

The effect of massage therapy in ovarian cancer patients

Silvana Lawvere

INTRODUCTION

Despite the increasing use of alternative medicine and specifically massage therapy (MT) among cancer patients, the efficacy of MT has not been evaluated in a clinical sample of ovarian cancer patients. Previous studies of MT in other samples have demonstrated a reduction in cancer-related symptoms. This randomized cross-over trial evaluated the effect of MT on self-reported anxiety (Spielberger State Anxiety Inventory), depressive mood (Visual Analogue Mood Scale), and pain (Memorial Pain Assessment Card) among seven hospitalized, white, aged 44 to 75, ovarian cancer patients undergoing chemotherapy at the Roswell Park Cancer Institute, Buffalo, NY. Six of the seven women (85.7%) self-reported using some form of alternative medicine.

Patients were randomized to one of the following sequence groups: first a 30-minute MT treatment followed the next day by a 30-minute rest period, ($n = 3$) or, first the rest period followed the next day by the MT treatment ($n = 4$). The mean percent change in scores from pre to post MT were: anxiety (33% reduction), depressive mood (38% reduction), and pain (9% reduction). These reductions were compared, using a paired *t*-test, to the corresponding percent changes for the rest period: anxiety (6% reduction), depressive mood (13% reduction), and pain (5% increase). The reduction in anxiety was statistically significant ($p = 0.002$). These initial findings, though drawn from a select sample, contribute to a growing body of research that suggests that MT may improve quality of life within a biopsychosocial approach to cancer care.

Many patients remain dissatisfied with management of anxiety, pain and/or depressive mood, despite the medical advancements that have been made in the diagnosis and treatment of cancer (Burke et al., 1994). This study was designed to examine the efficacy of massage therapy (MT) in alleviating anxiety, depressive symptoms, and pain in ovarian cancer patients undergoing chemotherapy.

A study published in the *New England Journal of Medicine* found that 34% of their representative sample had used unconventional forms of medical treatment in the previous year (Eisenberg et al., 1993). MT was found to be the third most frequently used alternative treatment. Alternative medicine is also being explored by cancer patients, and by ovarian cancer patients, who account for 4% of all cancer patients (Tortolero-Luna & Mitchell, 1995). With the growing use of MT in the US it is crucial to undertake scientific investigation regarding its effectiveness.

The purpose of this study was to demonstrate the possibility of conducting a randomized controlled clinical trial that would evaluate the efficacy of MT compared with usual care among ovarian cancer patients undergoing chemotherapy. Instrumentation was developed and tested to assess depressive mood, pain, and anxiety, as well as to collect background information. No past MT studies have investigated the efficacy of massage on anxiety, depressive mood and pain in this sample. The information derived from this study is crucial for both patients and clinicians alike.

The hypothesis of this study is that MT treatments will produce a short-term, less than 24-hour, 20% reduction of anxiety, depressive mood, and pain symptoms among ovarian cancer patients undergoing chemotherapy, when compared with the same patients receiving usual care in the form of a rest period.

LITERATURE REVIEW

Ovarian cancer is the second most common cancer of the reproductive system in women (Tortolero-Luna & Mitchell, 1995). It is the leading cause of death for all gynecological malignancies (Tortolero-Luna & Mitchell, 1995). The US incidence rate between 1986–1990 of ovarian cancer was 14.3/100,000 women, the mortality rate for the same period was 7.8/100,000 women (Tortolero-Luna & Mitchell, 1995). These incidence rates have remained somewhat stable for the past 30 years. The five-year relative survival rate is still 39–46% (Tortolero-Luna & Mitchell, 1995; American Cancer Society, 1997). Ovarian cancer is more common among white women than among African American women and it increases dramatically after age 40 (Tortolero-Luna & Mitchell, 1995). Although age and race are known risk factors, the etiology is not well understood.

Portenoy et al. (1994) found the prevalent symptoms in the 151 ovarian cancer patients studied were: worrying (71.7%), lack of energy (68.8%), feeling sad (63.8%), pain (61.8%), feeling nervous (61.5%), having difficulty sleeping (57.3%). Another study showed that 85% of women experienced at least some anxiety during treatment of gynecologic cancers (Rollison & Strang, 1995). This may be associated with uncertainty about the outcome of the illness, fear of death, being in the hospital setting, as well as with the various invasive tests and treatments involved.

Depression and depressive mood are major problems among cancer patients, with prevalence estimates ranging from 40% to 64% (Portenoy et al., 1994; Spiegel, 1996; Middleboe et al., 1994). Though there is a high prevalence of depressive mood among cancer patients, it is often not diagnosed. The symptoms of depression may be attributed to the disease or to the treatment of the disease.

It is estimated that 30–40% of patients in the intermediate stages of cancer and 60–80% in the more advanced stages experience pain (Ferrel-Torry & Glick, 1993). Dorrepaal et al. (1998) found that 83% of the cancer patients they studied said that tension and nervousness increased the pain they were experiencing. Although cancer patients are treated with analgesics, Bonica (1990) reports that 20–40% of cancer patients are not successfully treated for pain. Montazeri et al. (1996) include pain relief as one of the most important areas for improving the quality of life for ovarian cancer patients.

The majority of the research on cancer pain reduction has looked at treatments that revolve around analgesics. Increased tolerance to analgesics can present several problems (Brucra & Lawlor, 1997). Patients are often in need of progressively higher doses, but the risk of side effects increases the higher the dose. As opioid exposure increases, many patients develop toxicities, like delirium, myoclonus, grand mal seizures and hyperalgesia (Bruera & Lawlor, 1997).

MT simultaneously acts in multiple ways. Soft tissue manipulation can improve circulation (Tappan, 1988) and can reduce pain caused by the accumulation of irritants, which are flushed away with increased blood flow between muscle fibers caused by the repeated motion of massage (Zerinsky, 1987). MT can stimulate large diameter sensory nerves that inhibit pain transmission (Melzack & Wall, 1965). One mechanism may relate to increased parasympathetic activity: 'The pressure stimulation associated with touch increases vagal activity, which in turn lowers psychological arousal and stress hormones' (Field, 1996). Touch is believed to stimulate the release of endorphins and enkephalins, which can increase a sense of subjective well-being (Tappan, 1988). Massage reduces muscle tension and spasm, and hence relaxes the patient (Tappan, 1988). It been shown to significantly reduce heart rate (McKechie et al., 1983), it can have a positive psychological effect (Field et al., 1996a), and may be associated with feelings of being nurtured and cared for (Tappan, 1988).

Much of the research on MT has had methodological problems including small sample size, lack of adequate control groups, varied treatment length, treatments which are too short, and massages which are of poor quality due to inadequate training and lack of standardization. The data from several studies has shown that MT can have an immediate effect on reducing both physiological and psychological symptoms (Ferrel-Torrey & Glick, 1993; Field et al., 1996a,b; Ahles, 1995; Fishman et al., 1995; Meek,

1993; Nixon et al., 1997; Weinrich & Weinrich, 1990). These outcomes have been measured both by established indices and through physiologic measurements. The research generated at the Touch Research Institute International in Miami, (Field et al., 1996a, b; Field, 1995) and at the Dartmouth Medical Center (Ahles, 1995) has been the exception. It has been able to overcome these methodological obstacles with larger sample sizes, standardized treatment lengths, appropriate control groups, and well-trained massage therapists.

Research on the effectiveness of MT has been completed with a range of samples, including cancer patients. A clinical trial by Weinrich & Weinrich (1990) on a sample of cancer patients investigated the effectiveness of MT, looking specifically at the effects of MT on cancer pain. Patients were randomly assigned to a MT and to a control group. The MT group received 10 minutes of massage to the back while the patients in the control group were visited for 10 minutes. A pain index was administered before, immediately after, one hour after, and two hours after, the massage treatment or visit.

Potential methodological problems in this study include: participants were undergoing various types of treatments for various types of cancer; and the time since receiving medication for pain within the control and treatment groups was variable. Such factors may produce inter-group variability as well as intra-group variability. The MT treatments were only 10 minutes long, and the instruments were administered immediately following the treatment. It has been shown that a therapeutic effect is not fully manifested immediately following the massage and at least a 10-minute period should be allowed between the end of the massage and the administration of indices and/or physiologic measurements (Ferrell-Torrey & Glick, 1993). Moreover, seven nursing students that had received only a one-hour training session had given the treatments. Another possible limitation of this study is that the treatment and control groups were not demonstrating equal pain levels prior to the intervention, and the initial baseline pain measures were quite low. A study strength appeared to be the use of a 10-minute visit with a nurse as the control treatment for the MT treatments. This strategy may address both the possible placebo effect as well as the potential effect of human contact alone.

Ferrell-Torrey and Glick (1993) found a statistically significant ($p = 0.05$) reduction in pain (as measured by visual analogue scales) and anxiety (as measured by the Spielberger State Trait Anxiety Inventory) in nine male cancer patients who received back massages. This study suggests a possible short-term benefit from just one 30-minute massage. However, this study was exploratory, had no control group, and used cancer patients at various stages and sites.

Corner et al. (1995) also evaluated MT in a cancer population. This study examined the interaction effect of MT and aromatherapy on 52 people. Participants were randomized to three groups. Group 1 received 30-minute massages once a week for eight weeks with almond oil, while Group 2 received the same massage schedule with essential oils (a blend of lavender, rosewood, lemon, rose and valerian). Group 3 received usual care. Study measures, the Holmes and Dickerson Distress Scale and the Zigmond Hospital anxiety and depression scale, were administered prior to, and 24-hours after, the massage treatments. Since the measurements were taken after 24 hours and not immediately after the MT sessions, this study was specifically looking at the longer-term cumulative effects. There was a peak reduction in anxiety after three or four sessions ($p = 0.05$) in both of the MT groups. However, the patients were not matched according to cancer site or stage of disease.

Wilkinson (1995) examined quality of life in 28 cancer patients and investigated MT and the interaction effect of MT and aromatherapy oil (i.e., chamomile oil). Fifty-one cancer patients (3 males and 48 females) were randomized into one of three groups. Patients had various cancer sites and stages of cancer. Both massage groups demonstrated a reduction in anxiety ($p < 0.001$), as measured by the State Trait Anxiety Inventory, and higher quality of life readings ($p < 0.05$), as measured by the Rotterdam checklist. The MT plus aromatherapy group had larger reductions on the above indices. This study also used a perception questionnaire that consisted of open-ended questions about patient satisfaction and perceptions about the benefits of massage. Although an open-ended questionnaire collecting information about perceptions may be helpful in a pre-study investigation, it is possible that these open-ended questions may have biased the participant when reading the other two standardized instruments.

One of the earlier studies was done by Sims (1986), who investigated the use of MT with six breast cancer patients. The McCorkle Symptom Distress Scale and Likert mood scales measured the outcomes of interest. The author indicated that there was a 15.4% improvement in distress scores ($p = 0.05$). This study was the only one to use a cross-over design. The design would have been appropriate, except for the extremely small sample size of six women and for the fact that there was no attempt to randomize volunteers. Having only volunteers may introduce bias, since these people may believe MT to be beneficial to them.

To summarize the state of the field, several studies examined cancer patients. Sims (1986) was the only investigator who looked at the effects of MT on a cancer population that included patients with only one cancer site (breast cancer) and the only one who used a cross-over design, but with only six participants. Ahles (1995) performed the only study on cancer patients with the use of licensed massage therapists. The findings from all these studies suggested that MT did produce positive results. Most of these studies however did not have a large enough sample size to achieve sufficient statistical power and were preliminary or pilot studies. More research needs to be done in this area to investigate the efficacy of MT in a sample of cancer patients all experiencing the same type of cancer.

One problematic premise of most MT studies was that massage was performed as a nursing intervention. This poses many problems. The quality of the MT treatments is questionable. These nurses would need the time, energy, extensive training and physical and emotional space to achieve maximum success with MT. In many of these studies the nurses who performed the massage had only short training, and only for that particular study. The practitioner must feel at ease with his/her work, to be effective at calming the patient. The therapist's experience and familiarity with issues of inhibitions concerning touch is crucial. With a growing body of research that supports the effectiveness of MT, issues of the implementation of MT must be thought out.

The majority of the studies that utilized massage therapists were done at the Touch Research Institute International at the University of Miami Medical school (Field et al., 1996a, b; Field, 1995) and at the Dartmouth-Hitchcock Hospital (Ahles, 1995). These studies were among the most methodologically sound studies and all produced positive results.

MEASURES USED

The State Trait Anxiety Inventory (STAI) (Box 4.1) was first developed by Spielberger in the 1960s when all available scales measured trait, rather than state anxiety, and was revised in 1983 (Spielberger et al., 1983). The STAI consists of two 20-item questionnaires that measure current anxiety (state) as well as the tendency to experience anxiety (trait). Only the State portion of the inventory was utilized, because the inventory was given to each patient four times in two days and change in current anxiety was the primary outcome of interest. Reliability and validity have been repeatedly demonstrated (Murphy, 1994; Thompson, 1989). This test has been sensitive to changes in anxiety levels after massage treatments in a cancer population (Ferrell-Torrey & Glick, 1993). Its advantages are: low cost, minimal time (5–10 minutes), and it is self-administered. No interviewer qualifications or training are needed to administer the STAI. Drawbacks include: the anxiety items are not specified for clinical morbid anxiety which is a drawback in clinical research, the test is most likely measuring perceived anxiety, and the scale has a number of somatic questions that can cause difficulties when used in a hospital setting.

First developed by Aitken (1969), the Visual Analogue Mood Scale (VAMS) (Box 4.2) has the advantage that the patient does not have to review his emotional status under numerous, and often painful, headings. A mark on the line toward the left represents 'as depressed as you have ever been',

Box 4.1   Spielberger State Anxiety Inventory for adults scoring key

To use this, line up with test. Simply total the scoring weights shown on the stencil for each response category. For example if the respondent marked 3, then the weight would be 2. Refer to the manual for appropriate normative data. A decrease in score represents a decrease in anxiety.

	NOT AT ALL	SOME- WHAT	MODER- ATELY SO	VERY MUCH SO
I feel calm	4	3	2	1
I feel secure	4	3	2	1
I am tense	1	2	3	4
I feel strained	1	2	3	4
I feel at ease	4	3	2	1
I feel upset	1	2	3	4
I am presently worrying over possible misfortunes	1	2	3	4
I feel satisfied	4	3	2	1
I feel frightened	1	2	3	4
I feel comfortable	4	3	2	1
I feel self-confident	4	3	2	1
I feel nervous	1	2	3	4
I am jittery	1	2	3	4
I feel indecisive	1	2	3	4
I am relaxed	4	3	2	1
I feel content	4	3	2	1
I am worried	1	2	3	4
I feel confused	1	2	3	4
I feel steady	4	3	2	1
I feel pleasant	4	3	2	1

Box 4.2   The Visual Analogue Mood Scale scoring key

The Visual analogue scale, question 21, will be scored on a ordinal basis from 1 to 10. An increase in score represents a decrease in self-reported depression. The line was divided equally in to ten parts and scored accordingly. One end has the value 10 stating 'Not at all depressed' and at the other end has a value of 1 stating 'As depressed as you've ever been'.

toward the right represents, 'not at all depressed'. In this study the scale was presented on an 8.5 by 11 inch piece of paper along with the other instruments. This scale is useful when measuring the change in depressive mood during the course of an illness rather than determining an absolute level (Little & McPhail, 1973). This scale can be used multiple times in a day, and has been used when repeated measures were needed. When this instrument was correlated to similar scales in hospital patients with various conditions, the results were between 0.61–0.8 (Aitken, 1969; Little & McPhail, 1973). However, after discharge the validity was extremely low.

Luria (1975) reported test-retest mean levels in the range 0.56–0.8. The medium r range was 0.52–0.84 ($p < 0.001$). The across-patient test-retest reliability coefficients were significant in all diagnostic groups. The 2-hour reliabilities were 0.73–0.91, the 24-hour reliabilities 0.52–0.72 (Luria, 1975; Folstein & Luria, 1973).

The advantage of the VAMS is its simplicity and the low cost of administration, since untrained personnel can administer it. It can be self-administered or read aloud to the patient who must put the mark on the line. It will take only approximately 15 seconds to answer the question. Note, however, that the definition of depression is nonspecific, since this instrument cannot provide a diagnosis of depression per se.

The Memorial Pain Assessment Card (Box 4.3) used in this study was first developed by the Analgesic Studies Section of the Memorial Sloan-Kettering Cancer Center to assess the relative potency of new analgesic drugs (Fishman et al., 1987). The card was an 8.5 by 11 inch card with eight pain intensity descriptors and three visual analogue scales (Fishman et al., 1987). It has been found to be valid, reliable, efficient and sensitive when used with cancer patients (Fishman et al., 1987; Kornblith et al., 1995), is inexpensive to administer, and can be self-administered in about 20 seconds.

This study was a pilot study for an eventual full-scale randomized clinical trial that utilized a two-period cross-over design. A randomized clinical trial (RCT) is an epidemiological experiment such that the participants in a study are randomly allocated into groups, usually called study

---

Box 4.3   The Memorial Pain Assessment Card scoring key

An increase in score represents a decrease in self-reported pain.

Question 23 will be scored as follows:
  8 No pain
  7 Just noticeable
  6 Weak
  5 Mild
  4 Moderate
  3 Strong
  2 Severe
  1 Excruciating

The Visual Analogue Scales will be scored on a ordinal basis from 1 to 10. The lines were divided equally in to ten parts and scored accordingly.

Question 22
  One end has the value 10 stating 'Least possible pain' and the other end has a value of 1 stating 'Worst possible pain'.

Question 24
  One end has the value 10 stating 'Complete relief of pain' and the other end has a value of 1 stating 'No relief of pain'.

Question 25
  One end has the value 10 stating 'Best mood ever' and the other end has a value of 1 stating 'Worst mood ever'.

The scores for the Visual Analogue Scales and question 23 will be added for one final score.

and control groups, to receive or not receive an experimental treatment or drug. The results are assessed by rigorous comparison of rates of disease, death, recovery, or any other outcome of interest. These trials are regarded as the most scientifically rigorous methods for hypothesis testing available (Fletcher & Fletcher, 1988; Last, 1995). The advantage of a clinical trial is that it can cut down on extraneous factors, and systematic error. Clinical trials, when done correctly, produce the strongest evidence for cause and effect (Hulley & Cummings, 1988). The information gained in a clinical trial cannot always be generalized to groups, except to the population from which the sample of the clinical trial was drawn. Interventions tend to be ideal in a clinical trial but are not ideal in common practice, hence clinical trials can only measure efficacy and not effectiveness.

A two-period cross-over study is a method of comparing two or more treatments or interventions such that when the patients complete the course of one treatment they are later switched to the another treatment. When investigating two treatments, A and B, half the study participants will be randomly allocated to undergo treatment A, followed by treatment B, while the other half will be randomized to undergo treatment B, followed by treatment A. An appropriate length of time separates these two treatments and is known as the wash-out period. Fleiss (1981) states that a cross-over design should be used only when the treatment under study is short-acting. If the treatments may be long-acting, a cross-over design should be avoided, because a long wash-out period may not preserve the homogeneity of various variables — most notably, stage of disease. The major advantage is that the number of patients needed for a two-period cross-over study with a specified power is one-fourth of the number needed with a parallel groups study with the same power (Fleiss, 1981). A disadvantage of this AB/BA design is the possibility that the effect of the first treatment will carry over and bias the data on the effects of the second treatment (Fletcher & Fletcher, 1988; Last, 1995).

METHODS

The sample consisted of seven, white, ovarian cancer patients who were undergoing chemotherapy treatments. Patients were from the Roswell Park Cancer Institute, which is the first cancer research treatment and education center in the USA and is now the third largest in the country. Recruitment stopped at seven participants because there was a change in the clinic's protocol regarding which patients would receive their chemotherapy as outpatients and which would be inpatients. Effectively only the 'sicker' patients would have become inpatients under the new protocol.

All the patients included in this study had been diagnosed as having ovarian cancer. All were still under the original guidelines, which had the ovarian cancer patients remain in the hospital for two to three days after each course of chemotherapy. They were in various stages of cancer and in various stages of treatment.

The exclusion criteria were as follows: (1) patients with visible skin problems or open sores; (2) patients who cannot read or write; (3) patients who had surgery in the last six weeks; (4) patients taking anticoagulants; (5) patients with broken bones or other acute musculoskeletal injuries; and (6) patients with known spinal cord metastasis. [Patients were previously excluded from chemotherapy if they had low platelet count (thrombocytopenia) or low white blood cell count (neutropenia).]

Information was collected by chart review by the clinic's research nurse prior to the chemotherapy treatment, to establish which patients were ovarian cancer patients, and which patients were eligible for the study. The investigator verbally reviewed the inclusion and exclusion criteria with each patient. She read aloud the consent form to the patients that both agreed to participate and met the inclusion criteria.

This study was a preliminary pilot study for an eventual randomized clinical trial that utilized a two-period cross-over design. This method has been described in detail in the literature review. The duration of the study was approximately one month. The first patient was recruited in June, 1998 and the last patient was seen in July, 1998. Each participant was followed for two consecutive days.

Patients who agreed to participate and who qualified were randomly allocated (block randomization) using a random numbers table to one of the following two sequence groups: MT treatment followed by a rest period treatment (M/R) versus a rest period followed by a MT treatment (R/M) (Fig. 4.1). One day separated the two treatments. This small time between intervals ensured that the patients were in the same stage of cancer and treatment, and under the care of the same physician.

A New York State licensed massage therapist gave one 30-minute MT treatment to every participant. The control treatment consisted of a 30-minute rest period. The sequence in group 1 was the MT treatment followed by the rest period (M/R), while in group 2 the rest period was first,

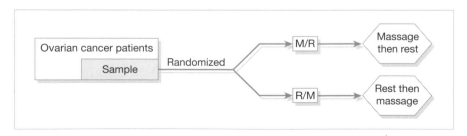

Figure 4.1 Randomization of the sample into two treatment sequence groups.

followed by the MT treatment (R/M). There was a 20–26-hour wash-out period between sessions.

The volunteer New York State licensed massage therapist was a white, 43-year-old female with 13 years of experience giving MT treatments. She had been trained in a variety of bodywork and behavioral therapies. The massage therapist was trained for the study to ensure consistency. The training protocol involved learning the standardized MT (Lawvere, 1999) procedure mentioned later and administering this treatment several times to the investigator to ensure that the treatment was done consistently. A checklist made sure that each aspect of the massage was included in the treatment. In addition, procedures that had not been included in the protocol were systematically eliminated.

The massage therapist and study coordinator determined the operational definition of the standardized MT treatment used for the study. This treatment was an integrative approach that utilized both Swedish and connective tissue modalities of MT. Biotone dual-purpose massage lotion was used for all of the massage treatments. The massage therapist did not engage the patient in conversation, except to respond to the patient's inquiries or to address physical or psychological comfort levels. The pressure of the massage was adjusted to the patient's pain tolerance.

For the first 15 minutes the patient was prone. After coaching the patient in deep breathing the therapist began the massage using the following standardized procedure. The therapist first utilized the Swedish massage stroke effleurage on the back. Effleurage strokes are smooth, long, rhythmical strokes which glide over the skin without attempting to move the deep muscle masses (Tappan, 1988). These effleurage strokes on the back moved first from the neck down the sides of the spine over the erector spinae muscles. Then the stroke moved out over the hips, returned over the quadratus lamborum and trapezius muscles, and ended by moving around the shoulders and back over the suboccipitals of the neck. Approximately five of these strokes were performed. Connective tissue techniques were then used on the rhomboids, trapezius, erector spinae and on the attachments of the quadratus lumborum. Connective tissue massage is a slower, deeper massage and works on a more concentrated area. The goal of this technique is to break up adhered connective tissue in between muscle fibers.

The therapist utilized effleurage on the legs. Several strokes were done, beginning at the ankle and moving over the Achilles tendon, the calf, and the hamstrings. Friction (a Swedish technique) was then used on the Achilles tendon and on the insertions of the gastrocnemius, the biceps femoris, and the semitendinosous muscles. Friction strokes are small circular movements that are done with the tips of the fingers, the thumb, or the heel of the hand (Tappan, 1988). Like connective tissue massage, friction works the deep muscle masses. It differs from connective tissue massage in that the small circular strokes remain in one location, while connective tissue strokes move more slowly and cover larger areas. Both these techniques are believed to break down the minor adhesions between the skin and the underlying tissue.

The patients then turned over and received the next 15 minutes of the treatment in the supine position. First, effleurage was used on the dorsal surface of the foot. Friction with the thumbs and knuckles was then used on the full plantar surface of the foot. Repeated effleurage and petrissage strokes were done on each of the legs. Petrissage is another Swedish massage stroke which works by milking and kneading the belly of the muscle (Tappan, 1988).

Next, the hands and arms were massaged. First the arm was put in an assisted stretch position. Then the hand was massaged using thumb friction. The forearm and upper arm were massaged using effleurage and petrissage, and this procedure was repeated on the other hand and arm.

The neck was massaged using effleurage strokes which originated at the rhomboids, with the massage therapist's hands under the patient and then moved over the upper trapezius muscles. Friction was used on the attachments of the muscles from the occiput to the ears. Light petrissage was then done on the upper trapezius muscles. Next, gentle friction was used on the scalp. Light effleurage and petrissage was also used on the face. After the massage therapist was finished with the standardized procedure, she instructed the patient to rest for a few minutes. After 5–10 minutes the study coordinator administered the post treatment indices. The study coordinator was instructed not to discuss the MT treatment with the patient.

All the participants of this study acted as their own controls. During the usual care portion of the study, data was collected with the same schedule as the MT treatment. Patients were instructed to 'rest and have quiet time' during the 30-minute 'treatment' and the staff was instructed not to interrupt patients unless medically necessary. To ensure quiet and no disturbances, the study coordinator closed the patients' doors. During this period patients were instructed not to watch television and not to have visitors. This procedure was followed in order to keep the patients in bed. These patients were not supposed to receive medical interventions during this treatment time. Although there was a standardized procedure for the control sessions, there was no significant deviation from usual care.

The dependent variables were symptoms of anxiety, depressive mood and pain, as measured by the following instruments: the Spielberger State Anxiety Inventory (a decrease in score represents a decrease in self-reported anxiety); the Visual Analogue Mood Scale (an increase in score represents a decrease in self-reported depressive mood); the Memorial Pain Assessment Card (an increase in score represents a decrease in self-reported pain).

A self-administered questionnaire collected background information prior to randomization and prior to any interventions. It provided information on potential covariates; continuous data on age; and categorical data on education, income levels, race/ethnicity, marital status, zip code and employment status. Dichotomous information about past experiences with massage and other alternative medicine treatments was also collected. Each participant filled out a short health history including questions concerning past mental disorders. Before the interventions, the investigator collected information regarding primary site of cancer and the time since initial diagnosis.

The schedule for the administration of the background questionnaire, for randomization and for each of the three instruments which were each administered four times per participant is shown in Fig. 4.2. After it was established that patients had met the inclusion criteria, and had signed the consent form, the investigator then gave all patients the self-administered background questionnaire. The background questionnaire was administered prior to any experimental treatment. After the patients had completed the background questionnaire, they were allocated to one of the two sequence groups by the randomization scheme.

The above indices were administered both prior to, and again 5–10 minutes after, the massage treatment or control treatment was completed. The investigator presented the self-administered outcome instruments to the study participants. The instruments were presented in the following order: (1) State Anxiety Inventory, (2) Visual Analogue Mood Scale, (3) Memorial Pain Assessment Card.

All participants completed both treatment and control portions of the study. The Statistical Package for the Social Sciences (SPSS) was used to

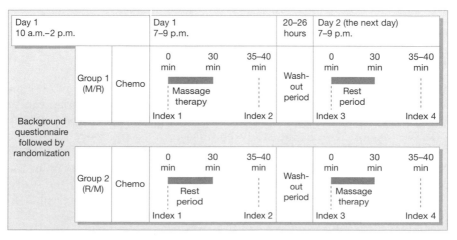

Figure 4.2 Protocol schedule.

analyze the data. Each participant filled out each index four times, one each before the treatment or control period and one each after the treatment and control period. A paired t-test was used to compare the differences from the baseline of the treatment or control session to 35–40 minutes later. The primary outcome measured was the change between the pre- and post-treatment indices. This makes the assumptions that there are no period effects, no residual carry-over effect and no treatment period interaction. The t-tests were done again using the ratio of this above difference over the baseline measure (the percent change from baseline). This was done for each of the three instruments.

In order to combine the data from each of the sequence groups, an ANOVA was done to evaluate the variance of the percent change following the MT sessions during the M/R sequence and the R/M sequence. An ANOVA was also done to compare the rest periods of each sequence group. In order to access the possibility that there could be a residual carry-over effect resulting from the sequence of treatments, t-tests were used to compare the last index score from day one with the first index score in day two. In the M/R group this meant comparing the post MT index with the pre rest index. In the R/M group the post rest index was compared with the pre massage index. P-values and confidence intervals were then calculated for each of these paired t-tests.

After looking at the t-tests for the entire sample, the participants were stratified by sequence group (M/R versus R/M), and also by past experience with MT (yes versus no). The paired t-tests were done for both the absolute change in score and for the percent change of score on each of the three indices for the stratified samples. This was done in order to rule out the possibility that there could have been a residual carry-over effect resulting from the sequence of the treatments or a different response to treatment with different history of receiving massage.

RESULTS

During the study period, seven eligible women were recruited and underwent a MT treatment and a rest period treatment. Of the ovarian cancer patients seen by the gynecology clinic during the study period only one was excluded from the study because of a past surgery within the six weeks prior to the intervention. All (100%) of the patients who met the inclusion criteria and were asked to participate agreed to be in the study and completed both the MT and rest period portions of the study. Sociodemographic characteristics of study participants are presented in Table 4.1.

Table 4.2 lists the type and number of alternative medicine practices used by the study participants. Six of the seven participants (85.7%)

Table 4.1 Sociodemographic characteristics of study participants

Characteristic	M/R[a] sequence group (n = 4)		R/M[b] sequence group (n = 3)		All patients (n = 7)	
	n	%	n	%	n	%
Age (years)						
44	1	25.0	0	–	1	14.3
51	1	25.0	0	–	1	14.3
52	1	25.0	0	–	1	14.3
56	0	–	1	33.3	1	14.3
58	1	25.0	0	–	1	14.3
70	0	–	1	33.3	1	14.3
75	0	–	1	33.3	1	14.3
mean	51.3		67.0		58.0	
SD[c]	5.7		9.8		10.9	
Race						
White	4	100.0	3	100.0	7	100.0
Marital status						
Married	1	25.0	0	–	1	14.3
Not married/single	2	50.0	0	–	2	28.6
Divorced	0	–	3	100.0	3	42.9
Widowed	1	25.0	0	–	1	14.3
Household income (U.S. dollars)[d]						
< 5,000	0	–	1	33.3	1	16.7
5,000 ≤ 10,000	1	33.3	0	–	1	16.7
10,000 ≤ 15,000	1	33.3	0	–	1	16.7
15,000 ≤ 20,000	0	–	2	66.6	2	33.2
30,000 ≤ 35,000	1	33.3	0	–	1	16.7
Education (years completed)						
12	1	25.0	2	66.6	3	42.9
13	1	25.0	1	33.3	2	28.6
14	1	25.0	0	–	1	14.3
16	1	25.0	0	–	1	14.3

[a]M/R is the group receiving the massage therapy treatment followed by the rest period.
[b]R/M is the group receiving the rest period followed by the massage therapy treatment.
[c]SD = standard deviation.
[d]One participant had missing data regarding income.

reported having used some form of alternative medicine in the past. One participant (14.3%) reported using six different forms of alternative medicine. Three participants (42.9%) reported using MT in the last year, although none had received MT more than a year before the intervention.

Table 4.3 displays the characteristics of the distributions of scores on the Spielberger State Anxiety Inventory for the MT treatments and rest periods for all participants, regardless of sequence group assignment (n = 7). Note that the Spielberger State Anxiety Inventory has a possible range of score from 20 to 80 points. A decrease in score indicates a decrease in self-reported anxiety.

Table 4.2 Type and number of alternative medicine practices used by study participants

Type of practices[a]	In the last year		More than a year ago		Ever	
	n	%	n	%	n	%
Vitamins	4	57.2	4	57.2	4	57.2
Chiropractic	2	28.6	2	28.6	4	57.2
Massage therapy	3	42.9	0	0	3	42.9
Dietary changes	1	14.3	1	14.3	2	28.6
Exercise	0	0	2	28.6	1	14.3
Herbs	1	14.3	1	14.3	1	14.3
Acupuncture	0	0	0	0	1	14.3
Relaxation	0	0	0	0	1	14.3
Yoga	0	0	0	0	1	14.3
Spiritual healing/prayer	1	14.3	1	1	1	14.3
Meditation	0	0	0	0	0	0
Folk doctor	0	0	0	0	0	0
Number of practices						
0					1	14.3
1					2	28.6
3					1	14.3
4					2	28.6
6					1	14.3
ever					6	85.7

[a]Not mutually exclusive.

Table 4.3 Characteristics of the distributions of scores on the Spielberger State Anxiety Inventory for massage and rest among all participants[a]

	n	Minimum	Maximum	Mean	Standard deviation
Massage					
Before	7	27	57	43.43	11.87
After	7	20	34	28.14	4.95
Raw change	7	−4	−25	−15.29	7.45
Percent change	7	−0.15	−0.44	**−0.33**	0.10
Rest					
Before	7	27	54	40.57	10.91
After	7	28	55	37.71	10.06
Raw change	7	7	−11	−2.86	6.04
Percent change	7	0.15	−0.20	−0.06	0.13

[a]The possible range of scores is from 20 to 80 points. A decrease in score indicates a decrease in self-reported anxiety.

The scores before and after the rest period ranged from 27 to 54 points and from 28 to 55 points, respectively. This resulted in a raw change in scores that ranged from −7 to 11 points (mean reduction ± SD = 2.86 ± 6.04). A 6% reduction in anxiety scores was noted following the rest period (mean reduction ± SD = −0.06 ± 0.13).

The range of scores before, and after, the MT treatment were from 27 to 57 points and from 20 to 34 points, respectively. The raw change in scores ranged from 4 to 25 points (mean reduction ± SD = 15.29 ± 7.45). A 33% reduction in anxiety scores was observed following the MT session (mean reduction ± SD = −0.33 ± 0.10).

Table 4.4 presents the data for the comparisons of overall and stratified scores on the Spielberger State Anxiety Inventory. Combining the anxiety scores following treatment from the two sequence groups allowed for the overall comparison of the MT and rest treatments. This was done because there was no observable residual carry-over effect and the variances did not have statistically significant differences.

The t-tests comparing the last anxiety score from day one with the first anxiety score of day two were not statistically significant. Specifically, the t-test for the M/R group compared the anxiety score post massage with the anxiety score pre rest ($t = -0.930$, $p = 0.421$) and the t-test for the R/M group compared the anxiety score post rest with the anxiety score pre massage ($t = -1.567$, $p = 0.258$). Although a paired t-test has little power with

Table 4.4 Comparisons of scores on the Spielberger State Anxiety Inventory: overall and stratified by sequence group and past experience with massage therapy[a]

	n	Mean	Standard deviation	Confidence interval	t[b]	p[c]
Overall						
Raw change	7	−12.43	7.85	5.17–19.69	4.19	0.006
Percent change	7	−0.27	0.14	0.14–0.40	5.20	0.002
Sequence group						
M/R[d]						
Raw change	4	−14.75	9.91	−1.02–30.52	2.98	0.059
Percent change	4	−0.31	0.18	0.02–0.59	3.45	0.041
R/M[e]						
Raw change	3	−9.33	3.51	0.61–18.06	4.60	0.004
Percent change	3	−0.22	0.05	0.09–0.35	7.34	0.018
Past experience with massage therapy						
No						
Raw change	4	−10.00	4.55	2.77–17.23	4.40	0.022
Percent change	4	−0.21	0.05	0.13–0.29	8.40	0.004
Yes						
Raw change	3	−15.67	11.24	−12.25–43.59	2.41	0.137
Percent change	3	−0.35	0.19	−0.11–0.81	3.31	0.080

[a]The possible range of scores is from 20 to 80 points. A decrease in score indicates a decrease in self-reported anxiety.
[b]Two paired t-tests were performed (raw change and percent change) on scores for each participant comparing the massage therapy and rest treatments.
[c]p-values are 2-tailed.
[d]M/R is the group receiving the massage therapy treatment followed by the rest period.
[e]R/M is the group receiving the rest period followed by the massage therapy treatment.

this limited sample size, there does not appear to be residual carry-over from day one to day two of the study in either sequence group.

ANOVA was used to compare the variances of the percent change in anxiety scores following the MT treatment ($F = 1.944$, $p = 0.222$) in each of the two sequence groups. This was also done for the rest period ($F = 0.019$, $p = 0.896$). Since the differences in the variances were not statistically significant, the data was combined, despite the limitations of an ANOVA with this limited sample size. This lack of difference in the variances may indicate that there is no period effect, but again it is difficult to interpret with this limited sample size.

The data was stratified by sequence group and by past experience with MT. Changes in anxiety during the MT and rest period sessions for all participants ($n = 7$) were compared using a paired t-test, a statistically significant difference was observed for both the raw change ($t = 4.19$, $p = 0.006$) and percent change ($t = 5.20$, $p = 0.002$).

Table 4.4 also presents data with patients stratified by sequence group (M/R or R/M). For the M/R group ($n = 4$), the percent change ($t = 3.45$, $p = 0.041$) demonstrated statistical significance, while the raw change ($t = 2.98$, $p = 0.059$) did not. In the R/M sequence group ($n = 3$), the percent change ($t = 7.34$, $p = 0.018$) and the raw change ($t = 4.60$, $p = 0.004$) remained significant.

Anxiety scores were also evaluated by past history of experience with MT (yes/no). Both the raw change ($t = 4.39$, $p = 0.022$) and the percent change ($t = 8.40$, $p = 0.004$) demonstrated statistical significance for participants with no past experience with MT ($n = 3$). No systematic differences were observed for participants with past experience with MT: raw change ($t = 2.41$, $p = 0.137$), percent change ($t = 3.31$, $p = 0.080$).

Table 4.5 displays the characteristics of the distributions of scores on the Visual Analogue Mood Scale for the MT treatments and rest periods for all participants, regardless of sequence group assignment ($n = 7$). The Visual Analogue Mood Scale has a possible range of score from 1 to 10 points. An increase in score indicates a decrease in self-reported depressive mood.

The range of scores before, and after, the MT treatment were from 1 to 10 points and from 5 to 10 points, respectively. The raw change in scores ranged from 0 to 10 points (mean reduction $\pm$ SD $= 2.29 \pm 1.80$). A 38% reduction in depressive mood was observed following the MT session (mean reduction $\pm$ SD $= 0.38 \pm 0.43$).

The scores before, and after the rest period ranged from 2 to 10 points and from 4 to 10 points, respectively. This resulted in a raw change in scores that ranged from -2 to 2 points (mean reduction $\pm$ SD $= 0.14 \pm 1.35$). A 13% reduction in depressive mood was found following the rest period (mean reduction $\pm$ SD $= 0.13 \pm 0.41$).

Table 4.6 presents the data for the comparisons of overall and stratified scores on the Visual Analogue Mood Scale. Combining the depressive mood

Table 4.5   Characteristics of the distribution of scores on the Visual Analogue Mood Scale for massage and rest among all participants[a]

	n	Minimum	Maximum	Mean	Standard deviation
Massage					
Before	7	1	10	6.00	3.16
After	7	5	10	8.29	2.06
Raw change	7	0	5	2.29	1.80
Percent change	7	0.00	1.25	**0.38**	0.43
Rest					
Before	7	2	10	7.00	2.71
After	7	4	10	7.14	2.12
Raw change	7	−2	2	0.14	1.35
Percent change	7	−0.29	1.00	0.13	0.41

[a]The possible range of scores is from 0 to 10 points. An increase in score represents a decrease in self-reported depression.

Table 4.6   Comparisons of scores on the Visual Analogue Mood Scale: overall and stratified by sequence group and past experience with massage therapy[a]

	n	Mean	Standard deviation	Confidence interval	t[b]	p[c]
Overall						
Raw change	7	2.14	1.07	1.15–3.13	5.30	0.002
Percent change	7	0.25	0.55	−0.26–0.76	1.18	0.282
Sequence group						
M/R[d]						
Raw change	4	2.25	1.26	0.25–4.25	3.58	0.037
Percent change	4	0.22	0.76	−0.99–1.43	0.58	0.605
R/M[e]						
Raw change	3	2.00	1.00	−0.48–4.48	3.46	0.074
Percent change	3	0.28	0.19	−0.19–0.75	2.58	0.123
Past experience with massage therapy						
No						
Raw change	4	2.50	1.29	0.45–4.55	3.87	0.030
Percent change	4	0.53	0.41	−0.12–1.17	2.61	0.080
Yes						
Raw change	3	1.67	0.58	0.23–3.10	5.00	0.038
Percent change	3	−0.13	0.54	−1.48–1.22	−0.41	0.719

[a]The possible range of scores is from 0 to 10 points. An increase in score represents a decrease in self-reported depression.
[b]Two paired t-tests were performed (raw change and percent change) on scores for each participant comparing the massage therapy and rest treatments.
[c]p-values are 2-tailed.
[d]M/R is the group receiving the massage therapy treatment followed by the rest period.
[e]R/M is the group receiving the rest period followed by the massage therapy treatment.

scores following treatment from the two sequence groups allowed for the overall comparison of the MT and rest treatments. This was done because there was no observable residual carry-over effect and the variances did not have statistically significant differences.

The t-tests comparing the last depressive mood score from day one with the first depressive mood score of day two were not statistically significant. Specifically, the t-test for the M/R group compared the depressive mood score post massage with the depressive mood score pre rest ($t = 1.260$, $p = 0.297$) and the t-test for the R/M group compared the depressive mood score post rest with the depressive mood score pre massage ($t = -2.000$, $p = 0.184$). Although a paired t-test has little power with this limited sample size, there does not appear to be residual carry-over from day one to day two of the study in either sequence group.

ANOVA was used to compare the variances of the percent change in depressive mood scores following the MT treatment ($F = 1.097$, $p = 0.343$) in each of the two sequence groups. This was also done for the rest period ($F = 1.839$, $p = 0.233$). Since the differences in the variances were not statistically significant, the data was combined, despite the limitations of an ANOVA with this limited sample size. This lack of difference in the variances may indicate that there is no period effect, but again it is difficult to interpret with this limited sample size.

The data was stratified by sequence group and by past experience with MT. Changes in depressive mood during the MT and rest period sessions for all participants ($n = 7$) were compared using a paired t-test, a statistically significant difference was observed for the raw change ($t = 5.30$, $p = 0.002$), but not for the percent change ($t = 1.18$, $p = 0.282$).

Table 4.6 also presents data with patients stratified by sequence group (M/R or R/M). For the M/R group ($n = 4$), the percent change ($t = 0.58$, $p = 0.605$) did not demonstrate statistical significance while the raw change ($t = 3.58$, $p = 0.037$) was significant. In the R/M sequence group ($n = 3$), the percent change ($t = 7.34$, $p = 0.018$) and the raw change ($t = 4.60$, $p = 0.004$) remained significant.

Depressive mood was also evaluated by past history of experience with MT (yes/no). The raw change ($t = 3.87$, $p = 0.038$) was statistically significant while the percent change ($t = 2.31$, $p = 0.080$) did not demonstrate statistical significance for participants with no past experience with MT ($n = 3$). A systematic difference was observed for participants with past experience with MT in regards to raw change ($t = 5.00$, $p = 0.038$), but not for the percent change ($t = 0.41$, $p = 0.719$).

Table 4.7 displays the characteristics of the distributions of scores on the Memorial Pain Assessment Card for the MT treatments and rest periods for all participants regardless of sequence group assignment ($n = 7$). The Memorial Pain Assessment Card has a possible range of score from 1 to 37 points. An increase in score indicates a decrease in self-reported pain.

Table 4.7 Characteristics of the distributions of scores on the Memorial Pain Assessment Card for massage and rest among all participants[a]

	n	Minimum	Maximum	Mean	Standard deviation
Massage					
Before	7	14	31	21.57	5.32
After	7	21	24	22.14	1.07
Raw change	7	−10	9	0.57	6.86
Percent change	7	−0.32	0.64	**0.09**	0.30
Rest					
Before	7	18	29	23.14	3.44
After	7	21	32	23.14	4.72
Raw change	7	−3	1	−1.00	1.73
Percent change	7	−0.17	0.04	−0.05	0.08

[a]The possible range of scores is from 1 to 37 points. An increase in score represents a decrease in self-reported pain.

The range of scores before, and after, the MT treatment were from 14 to 31 points and from 21 to 24 points, respectively. The raw change in scores ranged from −10 to 9 points (mean reduction ± SD = 0.57 ± 6.86). A 9% reduction in pain was observed following the MT session (mean reduction ± SD = 0.09 ± 0.30).

The scores before, and after, the rest period ranged from 18 to 29 points and from 21 to 32 points, respectively. This resulted in a raw change in scores that ranged from −3 to 1 point (mean reduction ± SD = −1.00 ± 1.73). A 5% reduction in pain was found following the rest period (mean reduction ± SD = 0.05 ± 0.08).

Table 4.8 presents the data for the comparisons of overall and stratified scores on the Memorial Pain Assessment Card. Combining the pain scores following treatment from the two sequence groups allowed for the overall comparison of the MT and rest treatments. This was done because there was no observable residual carry-over effect and the variances did not have statistically significant differences.

The t-tests comparing the last pain score from day one with the first pain score of day two were not statistically significant. Specifically, the t-test for the M/R group compared the pain score post massage with the pain score pre rest ($t = 1.093$, $p = 0.354$) and the t-test for the R/M group compared the pain score post rest with the pain score pre massage ($t = 1.375$, $p = 0.303$). Although a paired t-test has little power with this limited sample size, there does not appear to be residual carry-over from day one to day two of the study in either sequence group.

An ANOVA was used to compare the variances of the percent change in pain scores following the MT treatment ($F = 0.153$, $p = 0.712$) in each of the two sequence groups. This was also done for the rest period ($F = 0.713$,

Table 4.8 Comparisons of scores on the Memorial Pain Assessment Card: overall and stratified by sequence group and past experience with massage therapy[a]

	n	Mean	Standard deviation	Confidence interval	t^b	p^c
Overall						
Raw change	7	1.57	43.86	−2.92–6.07	0.86	0.425
Percent change	7	0.13	0.26	−0.11–0.37	1.34	0.228
Sequence group						
M/R[d]						
Raw change	4	1.25	2.21	−2.28–4.78	1.13	0.342
Percent change	4	0.07	0.10	−0.08–0.22	1.43	0.249
R/M[e]						
Raw change	3	2.00	7.64	−17.72–21.72	0.44	0.705
Percent change	3	0.22	0.41	−0.81–1.24	0.91	0.460
Past experience with massage therapy						
No						
Raw change	4	0.00	4.69	−7.46–7.46	0.00	1.00
Percent change	4	0.03	0.17	−0.24–0.30	0.38	0.731
Yes						
Raw change	3	3.67	5.13	−9.08–16.41	1.24	0.341
Percent change	3	0.27	0.34	−0.57–1.10	1.36	0.306

[a]The possible range of scores is from 1 to 37 points. A decrease in score indicates a decrease in self-reported pain.
[b]Two paired t-tests were performed (raw change and percent change) on scores for each participant comparing the massage therapy and rest treatments.
[c]p-values are 2-tailed.
[d]M/R is the group receiving the massage therapy treatment followed by the rest period.
[e]R/M is the group receiving the rest period followed by the massage therapy treatment.

$p = 0.437$). Since the differences in the variances were not statistically significant, the data was combined, despite the limitations of an ANOVA with this limited sample size. This lack of difference in the variances may indicate that there is no period effect, but again it is difficult to interpret with this limited sample size.

The data was stratified by sequence group and by past experience with MT. Changes in pain during the MT and rest period sessions for all participants ($n = 7$) were compared using a paired t-test; No statistically significant differences were observed; raw change ($t = 0.86$, $p = 0.425$) and the percent change ($t = 1.34$, $p = 0.228$).

Table 4.8 also presents data with patients stratified by sequence group (M/R or R/M). The differences in the raw change and the percent change did not demonstrate statistical significance for either sequence group.

Pain was evaluated by past history of experience with MT (yes/no). No systematic differences were observed for participants with or without a past MT history.

The massage therapist filled out a questionnaire regarding adherence to the MT protocol upon completion of each MT session. A visual analogue scale with at one end the value 10 stating 'did not adhere to the protocol at all' and at the other end a value of 1 stating 'completely adhered to the protocol'. The therapist reported a score of 1 on six patients and a 6 on the seventh patient. Although there was an attempt to keep interruptions during the MT treatments and rest period sessions to a minimum, one diabetic patient was interrupted during the massage for a blood draw and a hospital priest visited another patient during the rest period in order to schedule an appointment.

DISCUSSION

Preliminary findings from this clinical trial provide evidence to support that MT may produce a short-term (less than 24-hour), 20% reduction in anxiety and depressive mood among ovarian cancer patients undergoing chemotherapy, when compared with the same patients receiving usual care in the form of a rest period. In fact, there was a 33% reduction in anxiety and a 38% reduction in depressive mood. We also observed a 9% reduction in pain. If this level of reduction in pain can be repeated in a full-fledged clinical trial it will have clinical significance, regardless of statistical significance. These reductions were compared, using a paired t-test, with the following corresponding percent changes for the rest period: anxiety (6% reduction), depressive mood (13% reduction), and pain (5% increase). Only the reduction in anxiety was statistically significant ($p = 0.002$). These results support previous findings which have shown a reduction in anxiety (Ferrell-Torrey & Glick, 1993; Field, 1995, 1996; Field et al., 1996a,b, 1998a,b,c; Ahles, 1995; Corner et al., 1995; Wilkinson, 1995), depressive mood (Field et al., 1996a, 1998a,b; Corner et al., 1995; Sims, 1986), and pain (Ferrell-Torrey & Glick, 1993; Field, 1996; Weinrich & Weinrich, 1990; Field et al., 1998a) in relation to MT treatments. Although these other studies investigated various MT protocols (i.e. different MT techniques, lengths of treatments, numbers of treatments and varying samples) findings in terms of the direction of effect (i.e. reduction in symptoms) have been consistent. Only one study to date showed no effect when investigating MT (Dunn et al., 1996).

This study is one of the few known studies evaluating the efficacy of MT among cancer patients receiving the same chemotherapy treatment for the same cancer site. Use of a cross-over design dramatically increases the homogeneity of the covariates, when comparing the mean differences of the treatment and rest period indices, and theoretically produces less biased results (Senn, 1994). Moreover, this study has four times the power of a parallel designed study with seven participants, since the number of patients that are needed for a two-period cross-over study with a specified power is one-fourth of the number needed with a parallel group study design with the same power (Fleiss, 1986).

This study did not experience problems with non-compliance and attrition that frequently are a problem in the conduct of clinical trials. Perhaps due to the brevity of the time-frame of the study, this study had a 100% response rate and complete compliance with no drop-outs. Although the massage therapist reported only 60% completion of the standardized MT protocol with one patient, this patient's data was included in the analysis based on the intent-to-treat policy. All of the other treatments complied 100% with the protocol. No adverse side effects were evident in the use of MT. Contrary to what would appear to be the case, the patients' past experience with massage did not appear to produce a positive bias. Those patients who had a past experience with MT appeared to have less reduction in symptoms.

The main study limitation is the small sample size, but this sample may serve as a basis to establish an effect size to be used in a future, larger trial. Results are not generalizeable to patients other than white females with ovarian cancer that are undergoing chemotherapy. Patients were not all in the same stage of cancer or treatment. It is important to note, however, that since each patient acted as her own control, there were equal numbers of each stage of cancer in the treatment and control group means. In addition, the control group most likely did not adequately control the placebo effect, and the difference between a MT session and a control session was clear to patients, so they were subsequently not blinded. In addition, knowing the order of the sequence of treatments may have introduced bias.

Another possible limitation is the length of the wash-out period. Although this period, of 20 to 26 hours, has been shown to be sufficient in some studies, other studies have indicated that it may not be long enough. The t-test indicates that there is no residual carry-over effect after the wash-out period, however with this limited sample size, only a large residual carry-over effect would be able to be detected. This length was chosen so that the treatments could be given at the same time of day and because of the practical restrictions. In order to ensure a high completion rate, we had the patients complete both treatments during one stay in the hospital.

An additional potential bias is the fact that the floor nurses may have been introducing bias by saying things like 'you are so lucky to be getting a massage today', along with other positive remarks referring to MT.

Only self-reported subjective outcome measures were used in this study. It would be advantageous for a future study of this kind to incorporate objective physiologic measures (i.e. serum cortisol levels as a marker for anxiety).

Finally, bias may have been introduced due to the use of repeat measures. Each patient completed each of the indices four times. Patients may have remembered the answer they gave on a previous index, and it might have affected their answer on subsequent indices.

This preliminary pilot study provided us with an initial understanding of the efficacy of MT in the treatment of anxiety, depressive mood and pain in ovarian cancer patients undergoing chemotherapy. It demonstrated that it is feasible to use a cross-over study design. Although this pilot study did not have sufficient statistical power, it established an effect size which will be needed when calculating sample size and power for a future, full-fledged clinical trial. This study has been an important first step in investigating this specific clinical sub-group of women in relation to MT. Obviously, continued research will be needed to clearly define the efficacy, effectiveness and duration of effect of MT.

This study has clarified the specific direction future studies might take, both in regards to which endpoints to pursue (anxiety, depressive mood, and/or pain) and in regards to study design. Self-reported subjective measures will need to be supplemented with physiologic measures in future studies.

Future studies will also need to analyze the cost effectiveness related to the use of massage therapists in oncology settings. It is important for future research to include clinical trials with sufficient sample size that reach statistical power levels in the 80% and above range. This will enable future researchers to begin to stratify data to evaluate age, sex and other possible covariates. In addition, if at all possible, the methodological drawbacks that were outlined above in past studies and in this pilot study will need to be avoided. It is crucial that various applications of MT be rigorously tested and evaluated to assess the benefits, potential hazards and costs. Furthermore, prescriptive information needs to be established about duration of optimal individual treatment lengths, as well as about the differing effects of singular, versus multiple treatments. Since MT is a behavior utilized by a growing number of patients, and in particular cancer patients, this information is needed for both the patients and the clinicians.

In summary, preliminary findings from this study replicate and expand upon previous studies demonstrating, in other samples, the use of MT treatments for temporary reductions in anxiety, depressive mood, and pain. MT can improve the quality of life and subjective well-being of ovarian cancer patients enduring caustic cancer treatments and may be a welcome addition to oncology units and a useful adjunct to existing treatments.

REFERENCES

Ahles, T. (1995). Massage therapy for bone marrow transplant patients (personal communication).
Aitken, R. (1969). A growing edge of measurement of feelings. *Proceedings of the Royal Society of Medicine, 62*, 989–996.
American Cancer Society. (1997). *Facts and figures.* New York: ACS.

Bonica, J. (1990). *The management of pain*. Philadelphia: Lea & Febiger.

Bruera, E., & Lawlor, B. (1997). Cancer pain management. *Acta Anaesthesiologica Scandinavica, 41*, 146–153.

Burke, C., Macnish, J., Saunders, A., et al. (1994). The development of a massage service for cancer patients. *Clinical Oncology, 6*, 381–385.

Corner, J., Cawley, N., & Hildebrand, S. (1995). An evaluation of the use of massage and essential oils on the well-being of cancer patients. *International Journal of Palliative Nursing, 1*, 67–73.

Dorrepaal, K., Aaronson, N., & VanDam, F. (1998). Pain experience and pain management among hospitalized cancer patients: a clinical study. *Cancer, 63*, 593–598.

Dunn, C., Sleep, J., & Collett, D. (1996). Sensing an improvement: an experimental study to evaluate the use of aromatherapy, massage and periods of rest in an intensive care unit. *Journal of Advanced Nursing, 21*, 34–40.

Eisenberg, D., Kessler, R., Foster, C., et al. (1993). Uncon-ventional medicine in the United States. *New England Journal of Medicine, 328*, 246–252.

Ferrell-Torrey, A., & Glick, O. (1993). The use of therapeutic massage as a nursing intervention to modify anxiety and the perception of cancer pain. *Cancer Nursing, 16*, 93–101.

Field, T. (1996). Touch therapies for pain management and stress reduction. In R. Rozensky (Ed.), *Health psychology through the life span: practice and research opportunities*. Washington: American Psychological Association.

Field, T. (1995). Therapy for infants and children. *Journal of Developmental and Behavioral Pediatrics, 16*, 105–111.

Field, T., Grizzle, N., Scaffidi, F., & Schanberg, S. (1996a). Massage and relaxation therapies' effects on depressed adolescent mothers. *Adolescence, 31*, 904–911.

Field, T., Henteleff, T., Hernandez-Reif, M., et al. (1998c). Children with asthma have improved pulmonary functions after massage therapy. *Journal of Pediatrics, 132*, 854–858.

Field, T., Ironson, G., Scafidi, F., et al. (1996b). Massage therapy reduces anxiety and enhances EEG pattern of alertness and math computations. *International Journal of Neuroscience, 86*, 197–205.

Field, T., Scanberg, S., & Kuhn, C. (1998b). Bulimic adolescents benefit from massage thrapy. *Adolescence, 33*, 555–563.

Field, T., Peck, M., & Krugman, S. (1998a). Burn injuries benefit from massage therapy. *Journal of Burn Care and Rehabilitation, 19*, 241–244.

Fishman, B., Pasterniak, S., Wallenstein, S., et al. (1987). The Memorial Pain Assessment Card. *Cancer, 60*, 1151–1158.

Fishman, E., Turkheimer, E., & DeGood, D. E. (1995). Touch relieves stress and pain. *Journal of Behavioral Medicine, 18*(1), 69–79.

Fleiss, J. (1981). *The design and analysis of clinical experiments*. New York: John Wiley & Sons.

Fletcher, R., & Fletcher, S. (1988). *Clinical epidemiology*. Baltimore: Williams & Wilkins.

Folstein, M., & Luria, R. (1973). Reliability, validity, and clinical application of the visual analogue scale. *Psychological Medicine, 3*, 479–486.

Hulley, S., & Cummings, S. (1988). *Designing clinical research*. Baltimore: Williams & Wilkins.

Kornblith, A., Thaler, H., & Wong, G. (1995). Quality of life of women with ovarian cancer. *Proceedings Annual Meeting Society Clinical Oncology, 14*.

Last, J. (1995). *A dictionary of epidemiology*. New York: Oxford University Press.

Lawvere, S. (1999). *The effect of massage therapy on self-reported anxiety, depressive mood, and pain in ovarian cancer patients: a pilot study*. Buffalo: State University of New York.

Little, J., & McPhail, N. (1973). Measures of depressive mood at monthly intervals. *British Journal of Psychiatry, 122*, 447–452.

Luria, R. (1975). The validity and reliability of the Visual Analogue Scale. *Journal of Psychiatric Research, 12*, 51–57.

McKechie, A., Wilson, F., Watson, N., & Scott, D. (1983). A preliminary report on the value of connective tissue massage. *Journal of Psychosomatic Research, 27*, 125–129.

Meek, S. (1993). Effects of slow stroke back massage on relaxation in hospice clients. *Journal of Nursing Scholarship, 25*, 7–21.

Melzack, R., & Wall, P. (1965). Pain mechanisms: a new theory. *Science, 150*, 971–979.

Middelboe, T., Ovensen, L., Mortensen, E., & Bech, P. (1994). Depressive symptoms in cancer patients undergoing chemotherapy: a psychometric analysis. *Psychotherapy and Psychosomatics, 61*, 171–177.

Montazeri, A., McEwen, J., & Gillis, C. (1996). Quality of life with ovarian cancer: current state of research. *Supportive Care in Cancer, 4*, 169–179.

Murphy, L. (1994). *Tests in print IV*. Lincoln: The University of Nebraska Press.

Nixon, M., Teschendorff, J., Finney, J., & Karnilowicz, W. (1997). Expanding the nursing repertoire: the effect of massage on post-operative pain. *Australian Journal of Advanced Nursing, 14*, 21–26.

Portenoy, R., Kornblith, A., & Wong, G. (1994). Pain in ovarian cancer, prevalence, characteristics, and associated symptoms. *Cancer, 74*, 907–915.

Rollison, R., & Strang, P. (1995). Pain, nausea and anxiety during intra-uterine brachytherapy of cervical carcinomas. *Supportive Care in Cancer, 3*, 205–207.

Senn, S. (1994). The AB/BA crossover: past, present and future? *Statistical Methods in Medical Research, 3*, 303–324.

Sims, S. (1986). Slow back massage for cancer patients. *Nursing Times, 82*, 47–50.

Spielberger, C., Gorsuch, R., & Lushene, R. (1983). *Manual for the State Trait Anxiety Inventory*. Palo Alto: Consulting Psychologist Press.

Spiegel, D. (1996). Cancer and depression. *British Journal of Psychiatry, 30*, 109–116.

Tappan, F. (1988). *Healing massage techniques*. Norwalk: Appleton and Lange.

Thompson, C. (1989). *The instruments of psychiatric research*. New York: Wiley.

Tortolero-Luna, G., & Mitchell, M. (1995). The epidemiology of ovarian cancer. *Journal of Cellular Biochemistry, 23*, 200–207.

Weinrich, M., & Weinrich, S. (1990). The effect of massage on pain in cancer patients. *Applied Nursing Research, 3*, 140–145.

Wilkinson, S. (1995). Aromatherapy and massage in palliative care. *International Journal of Palliative Nursing, 1*, 21–30.

Zerinsky, S. (1987). *Introduction to pathology for the massage practitioner*. New York: Swedish Institute.

5

Massage therapy for chemotherapy-induced emesis

Buford T. Lively, Monica Holiday-Goodman,
Curtis D. Black, Bhakti Arondekar

INTRODUCTION

This study was an economic evaluation of the cost savings of massage therapy in alleviating high-dose chemotherapy-induced nausea and vomiting. The study sample was comprised of women undergoing peripheral stem cell transplant for breast or ovarian cancer. Alleviating such nausea and vomiting has become a highly desired goal in the treatment of cancer patients.

The goal of this study was to answer the following question related to controlling nausea and vomiting in women undergoing stem cell transplant procedures for breast or ovarian cancer. From the perspective of an institution, is massage therapy as an adjunct to anti-emetic drug therapy a more cost-effective treatment therapy than anti-emetic drug therapy used alone?

Nausea and vomiting are two of the three components of the emetic process described by Borison & Wang (1953). The three components of the emetic process are:

1. Emesis, or vomiting: the forceful expulsion of gastrointestinal (GI) contents through the mouth, accomplished by the coordination of diaphragmatic contraction, sustained abdominal muscle action, and the opening of the gastric cardia.

2. Nausea: a 'subjective, unpleasant feeling that may signal imminent vomiting.' Signs and symptoms of automatic nervous system stimulation, e.g., flushing, pallor, tachycardia accompany it. Other symptoms are diminished gastric tone, reduced peristalsis, and retrograde duodenal peristalsis.

Because nausea is such a subjective phenomenon, only the patient is able to describe its existence.

3. Retching: the synchronized movements of the diaphragm, chest wall, and abdominal muscles that may precede or follow emesis. Retching and nausea may occur independently of emesis; their frequency, severity, and duration are separable phenomena.

High-dose chemotherapy presents many risks to patients, some life threatening, others mundane. Among the most feared side effects are nausea and vomiting, which can be so distressing that their prospect often dominates discussions of the risks and benefits of high-dose chemotherapy and stem cell rescue (Meisenberg, 1997). Thus, the control of nausea and vomiting is an important factor predicting patient compliance and acceptance of high-dose chemotherapy regimens.

Cancer is one of the leading causes of mortality in America. One of every four deaths in the United States is from cancer (Center for Disease Control, 1998). Given such a high estimation of cancer prevalence, it is not surprising to know that cancer treatments consume a major portion of US health care expenditures.

Stem cell transplant after dose intensive chemotherapy is an increasingly used treatment modality for selected patients with hematologic or solid tumors. When the stem cells used for the transplant are obtained from the patients' circulating peripheral blood, it is called an autologous peripheral stem cell transplant (PSCT). Autologous PSCT enables patients to receive potentially lethal doses of chemotherapy and rescues them with a viable source of new blood cells. The transplanted stem cells migrate to the patients' bone marrow, where they repopulate the marrow, and reinitiate normal hematopoiesis. This in turn decreases the expected morbidity and mortality from the high doses of chemotherapy (Jassak & Riley, 1994).

Beyond the therapeutic benefit, the effective control of nausea and vomiting also leads to more cost-effective therapy. These costs include indirect consequences of nausea and vomiting, such as the need to provide total parenteral nutrition (TPN), since nutrients cannot be tolerated orally. Reduced costs could be translated into significant savings for managing the cost of cancer chemotherapy.

The increasingly accepted field of alternative medicine has had an impact on every facet of the health care system, including oncology (American Cancer Society, 1996). Massage therapy, a type of alternative therapy, offers one potential solution for reducing costs associated with high-dose chemotherapy-induced nausea and vomiting.

Cancer patients, particularly inpatients and those undergoing bone marrow transplantation, experience a significant amount of anxiety and emotional distress due to the intensity of treatment, the uncertainty of response, and severe side effects of chemotherapy agents and immuno-suppression. These side effects, especially when uncontrolled, exacerbate the unpleasantness of an inherently stressful situation and significantly affect patients' quality of life. Moreover, the psychological sequelae of rigorous cancer treatment can interfere with patients' performance of self-care behaviors, such as mild exercise and appropriate food intake, which are assumed to assist in recovery from stressful cancer treatment. Massage can be used in an effort to maintain or improve the patients' quality of life, especially during rigorous treatment (Massie & Shakin, 1993). In clinical studies, massage has been shown to help reduce anxiety and depression. Therefore, massage may also be a useful component in oncology settings.

METHODS

The data analyzed in this study were collected at a large primary care and teaching medical center in Toledo, Ohio, during an 18-month period from September 1996 to February 1998. The research site has an active Oncology Department, including a peripheral stem cell transplant service. The small number of patients with breast or ovarian cancer who were undergoing PSCT procedures was 31, so the whole group was included in this study. Out of the total study population, a control group of 14 patients was treated only with anti-emetics for nausea and vomiting. An experimental group of 17 patients received massage therapy as an adjunct to anti-emetic drug therapy for nausea and vomiting.

An instrument was designed for collection of data for each of the two groups. The instrument is shown in Appendix A. The costs of hospital room and board, anti-emetic therapy, TPN, and massage therapy, shown in Appendices B-1 and B-2, were calculated separately for each group.

The data collection instrument contained four major sections that included data such as: the demographic characteristics of the sample; direct costs such as the cost of anti-emetic drugs; indirect costs associated with the therapies such as the cost of hospitalization; and information related to the effectiveness of drug therapy alone and massage therapy as an adjunct to drug therapy, which included the amount of total parenteral nutrition needed, reduced episodes of nausea and vomiting, and increased caloric intake.

Section I of the data collection instrument contained relevant patient information including demographic data. Demographic data assisted in documenting the relationship of factors such as age, race, marital status, and transplant physician to the emetogenic experience of patients.

The history of the patient before PSCT was collected in Section II. Information about the patients' admitting diagnosis (breast cancer stage I, II, III, or metastatic breast cancer; stage I ovarian cancer, or advanced ovarian cancer) was obtained. Other relevant variables such as the previous chemotherapy and number of cycles of previous kind of chemotherapy were also noted. Previous chemotherapy sometimes causes anticipatory emesis that was considered an important variable.

Section III included information about the patients while they were undergoing PSCT procedures. Information about the patients' length of stay in the hospital was assessed. This section also consisted of variables used to identify the first day of nausea or vomiting, the total days of nausea and vomiting, and the extent of nausea and vomiting.

Section IV, massage therapy, contained relevant data for the experimental group only. Data obtained in this section included the first day of massage therapy, number of days of massage therapy, number of massage sessions, and the type of massage therapy applied.

An Excel chart was attached to the data collection instrument. This chart was used in listing the different anti-emetics given, the number of units per day, the cost per dose of each anti-emetic medication, the total cost of anti-emetic medication per day, amount of total parenteral nutrition (TPN) administered, and the cost for TPN.

The cost perspective adopted for the purpose of this study was that of the hospital. As a result, all the costs were obtained from the department of pharmaceutical care at the institution.

DATA PROCESSING

The demographic data were analyzed using the PC version of the Statistical Package for Social Sciences (SPSS-PC). The cost data collected for this study were entered into the Microsoft Excel version 97. Microsoft Excel was used for the calculation of the total cost of treatment therapies, and to evaluate treatment effectiveness. Since the PSCT program was relatively new at the institution, the sample size was small. As a result, it was not possible to determine the content and criterion-related validity of the instrument.

A descriptive analysis, including frequency distributions, was done to characterize the demographic variables. An independent samples *t*-test was used to compare the days of nausea/vomiting, length of stay, and days of TPN. The independent samples *t*-test helped in determining significant relationships between the two groups' other variables such as the effect of massage on the days of nausea and vomiting.

Sensitivity analyses were performed to examine the sensitivity of the study results to potential changes in the cost parameters used. The cost for massage therapy, the cost for hospital room and board, and the cost for the anti-emetic regimen were the variables that were increased and decreased, while all the other costs were held constant. A range of values for these manipulated economic variables was obtained from the literature and from the research data using minimum, maximum, and average values.

Those simulated increases and decreases helped in assessing the study's impact to determine if future price fluctuations would still yield the same relative, significant costs savings.

DATA ANALYSIS AND RESULTS

The ages of the patient population ranged from 32 years to 60 years. The mean age of the control population was 46 years, with a range of 34–60 years. The mean age of the treatment group was 45 years, with a range of 32–58 years. Both groups were primarily comprised of white women (92.9% in the control group, and 64.7% in the treatment group). The remaining subjects were African American. Most subjects were married (85.7% of the control group and 70.6% of the treatment group).

Most respondents had health insurance. Private insurance agencies covered the cost of care for 85.7% of the treatment group and 82.4% of the control group. The remaining respondents were covered primarily by government agencies. Only one patient paid for treatment with personal funds. One physician transplanted approximately 40% of all patients, and four additional physicians transplanted the remaining patients in almost equal numbers. Although different physicians performed the PSCT procedures, the same protocol was used for all the patients.

Pre-peripheral stem cell transplant patient history

Patients with breast cancer in stages I, II, or III, accounted for 64.3% of the control group and 47.1% of the treatment group. Patients with metastatic breast cancer accounted for 21.4% of the control group and 35.3% of the treatment group. The remaining patients, 14.3% of the control group and 17.6% of the treatment group, were advanced ovarian cancer cases.

One of the criteria for a patient being selected to undergo PSCT is their response to chemotherapy. The underlying principle of PSCT is that if a patient is responsive to chemotherapy in small doses, subsequent treatment with high-dose chemotherapy can help in complete or a partial remission. However, since the patient was exposed to chemotherapy previously, it was important to measure the extent to which the previous chemotherapy might influence the incidence of nausea and vomiting.

The chemotherapeutic regimen followed by the patients before they underwent PSCT was classified into four groups:

1. cyclophosphamide, doxorubicin (Adriamycin) and 5-fluorouracil (CAF)
2. paclitaxel (Taxol), and doxorubicin (Adriamycin) (TA)
3. paclitaxel
4. CAF and paclitaxel.

A majority of the patients in both the groups (76.9% in the control group and 53.3% in the treatment group) had CAF as their chemotherapeutic drug regimen. TA was used for 7.7% of the control group and 13.3% of the treatment group. Approximately 15% of the patients in the control group were administered cycles of paclitaxel only, and 33.3% of the patients in the treatment group were administered cycles of CAF and paclitaxel.

The number of cycles of the different chemotherapeutic regimen was also recorded. Patients in the control group were administered an average of 3.92 cycles per patient. Patients in the treatment group were administered an average of 4.64 cycles per patient.

Patient peripheral stem cell transplant record

The data collection instrument contained information about the patients' progress while they were undergoing PSCT procedures. Data concerning the total number of days in the PSCT program, days of nausea and vomiting, days of total parenteral nutrition, and number of sessions of massage were collected.

Independent samples t-tests were performed to determine any statistically significant differences between the two groups of patients in terms of: length of stay in the hospital, first day of nausea/vomiting, days with no vomiting, number of days where vomiting was controlled by anti-emetics, number of days with nausea and no vomiting, total number of days with nausea/vomiting, and days of TPN.

The total number of days in the PSCT program was calculated using the date of admission and the date of discharge, as shown in the medical records. The mean number of days in the PSCT program for patients in the control group was 20.29 days. The mean number of days in the PSCT program for patients in the treatment group was 17.82 days. The independent samples t-test for the total number of days in the PSCT program revealed a statistically significant difference between the two groups [$t(14.74) = 2.872, (p < 0.05)$].

Nausea and vomiting in the patients was assessed using a scale in which '0' indicated no nausea or vomiting during that day, '1a' indicated vomiting controlled by anti-emetics, '1b' indicated nausea without vomiting, '2' indicated intractable vomiting for less than two weeks, '3a' indicated intractable vomiting (unable to retain water in spite of maximal anti-emetic therapy) lasting for more than two weeks, and '3b' indicated Mallory-Weiss tear with life-threatening hemorrhage or esophageal perforation. There were no patients in either group with a score of '3'. There was only one patient in the treatment group with a score of '2' for 3 days.

Results of the independent samples t-test indicated that there was no statistically significant difference in the first day of nausea or vomiting for the control group (3.29) and the treatment group (4.12) [$t(29) = -0.945$,

$(p > 0.05)$]. The total number of days with no nausea and vomiting for both groups of patients was also recorded. Patients in the control group had a mean of 8.86 days with no nausea or vomiting, as compared with 12.12 days for patients in the treatment group [$t(29) = -0.204$ ($p = 0.05$)].

Patients in the control group had a mean of 8.21 days of vomiting controlled by anti-emetics. Patients in the treatment group had a mean of 3.65 days of vomiting controlled by anti-emetics. An independent samples t-test revealed that patients in the control group had significantly more days of vomiting requiring control by anti-emetics than patients in the treatment group [$t(29) = 4.55$, $p < 0.05$)].

When the number of days of nausea without vomiting was compared, the control group had a mean of 3 days as compared with 2 days for patients in the treatment group. However, based on the t-test, there was no significant difference between the two groups [NS, $t(19.94) = 1.06$, ($p > 0.05$)].

The total number of days of nausea and vomiting was considered as the sum of the number of days with nausea or vomiting or both (days with scores of 1a + days with 1b + days with 2). The treatment group had approximately 50% fewer days of nausea and vomiting than the control group. The mean number of days of nausea and vomiting was calculated as 11.21 for the control group and 5.82 for the treatment group. This difference was significant based on the independent samples t-test [$t(28.37) = 4.41$, ($p < 0.05$)].

Some patients in the PSCT program were administered TPN because of the severe nausea and vomiting that limited their oral nutritional intake. As a result, the need for TPN served as an indirect outcome measure with respect to the severity of patients' nausea and vomiting. Therefore, data concerning the number of times that TPN was administered were collected. Only 29.4% of patients in the treatment group received TPN as compared with 92.9% of patients in the control group. Patients in the treatment group required TPN for a mean of 1.0 day, while those in the control group required TPN for a mean of 10.6 days. The t-test revealed a statistically significant difference in the number of days of TPN required for the two groups [$t(29) = 9.23$, ($p < 0.05$)]. A summary of all independent samples t-test with the means, statistical significance, and confidence intervals is given in Table 5.1.

Patient massage history

Section IV of the data collection instrument noted the number of times that massage was administered to patients in the treatment group. All treatment group patients received massage along the vagal nerve pathway, and to the hands and legs. There were times when the masseuse went to administer the massage, but because of severe nausea and vomiting, some patients refused the massage. Refused sessions were not considered in the total

Table 5.1 Independent samples *t*-test

Parameter	Mean (patients without massage)	Mean (patients with massage)	Statistical significance	95% confidence interval of the mean	
				Lower	Upper
1. Total number of days in the PSCT program	20.29	17.82	$t(14.74) = 2.672, p < 0.05$	0.50	4.43
2. First day of nausea/vomiting	3.29	4.12	$t(29) = -0.945, p > 0.05$	−2.63	0.97
3. Days with no nausea/vomiting	8.86	12.12	$t(29) = -2.04, p = 0.05$	−6.53	4.7
4. Number of days of vomiting controlled by anti-emetics	8.21	3.65	$t(29) = 4.55, p < 0.05$	2.51	6.62
5. Number of days of nausea without vomiting	3	2	$t(19.94) = 1.06, p > 0.05$	−0.96	2.96
6. Total days of nausea/vomiting	11.21	5.82	$t(28.37) = 4.41, p < 0.05$	2.89	7.9
7. Days of total parenteral nutrition	10.64	1	$t(29) = 9.23, p < 0.05$	7.51	11.91

number of massage sessions. When the massage was started on a trial basis, it was not noted in the medical records for the first four patients. A number of sessions equal to the mean number of sessions for the remaining 13 patients were allocated to those four patients. Slightly over 50% of patients in the treatment group were administered five massage sessions.

Cost calculation and analysis

The cost data collected were analyzed using Microsoft Excel 97. Outcome costs were calculated based on the cost for anti-emetic medications, the cost for TPN, the cost for hospitalization, and the cost for massage therapy.

The average costs to the hospital for anti-emetic medications were obtained from the purchasing agent in the Pharmacy Department at the institution. The average cost of anti-emetic medications for patients in the control group was $2106.84, and the average cost of anti-emetic medications for patients in the treatment group was $1361.61.

The cost for TPN was calculated using the cost of the ingredients to the pharmacy and the hourly rate of the pharmacy technician and the pharmacist to the pharmacy. The average cost to the hospital for TPN was $865.59 for control group patients, and $66.00 for treatment group patients.

The cost for massage therapy was calculated as the cost to the hospital in reimbursement to the masseuse. The hospital paid $18 per massage session to the masseuse. The average cost to the hospital per patient for massage therapy was $90.

The total cost for nausea and vomiting treatment was the sum of the cost for anti-emetic medication, the cost of TPN, and the cost for massage therapy. The average cost for treating nausea and vomiting due to high-dose chemotherapy was $2972.43 for patients in the control group, and $1517.61 for patients in the treatment group. Table 5.2 shows the total cost to the institution and average cost per patient of nausea and vomiting treatment for both groups.

The length of stay in the hospital was another outcome measure compared between the two groups of patients. The average cost of a hospital room was obtained for the year 1990, and was calculated for 1998 using the inflation rates for hospital services provided by the Consumer Price

Table 5.2 Calculated costs of nausea and vomiting treatment

Patient group	Total cost of anti-emetic therapy, TPN & massage[a]	Average cost of anti-emetic therapy, TPN & massage per patient
Control group	$41,613.96	$2972.43
Treatment group	$25,799.39	$1517.61

[a]Massage was only administered to the treatment group.

Index (CPI, 1998). The average cost of a hospital room was $567.90 per day for the North Central region in the United States. The average cost of the hospital stay per patient was calculated as follows:

$$\begin{array}{ccccc} \text{Total cost of} & = & \text{Number of days} & \times & \text{Cost to hospital} \\ \text{hospital room} & & \text{in the hospital} & & \text{per day} \end{array}$$

The average cost of the hospital room was $11,520.26 per patient in the control group as compared with $10,121.98 per patient in the treatment group.

The average cost of nausea and vomiting treatment was then added to the average cost of the hospital room. When added together, these costs were $14,492.69 per patient for the control group, and $11,639.59 for the treatment group. The net incremental cost of not using massage therapy in patients, over using massage therapy as an adjunct to anti-emetic medications was found to be $2853.10 per patient.

Cost savings

There were 31 women who were treated with PSCT for breast or ovarian cancer between September 1996 and February 1998. The total cost of nausea and vomiting treatment and hospital room and board for both groups was $400,770.65, as shown in Table 5.3.

For the 17 patients in the treatment group, the use of massage therapy for nausea and vomiting resulted in significant cost savings of $2853.10 per patient in cost avoidance to the hospital. Projections would indicate that had the 14 patients in the control group received massage therapy the potential cost savings to the hospital would have been an additional $39,943.40 ($2853.10 × 14).

Sensitivity analyses

As mentioned earlier, sensitivity analyses were performed to examine the sensitivity of the study results to potential changes in the cost parameters

Table 5.3 Total costs to the hospital

Patient group	Total cost for nausea and vomiting (A)	Total cost of hospital room (B)	(A) + (B)	Total costs to the hospital
Patients without massage	$41,613.96	$161,283.60	$202,897.56	$400,770.65
Patients with massage	$25,799.39	$172,073.70	$197,873.09	

used. These analyses help in assessing the impact of different assumptions on the study's results.

Massage therapy

Sensitivity analyses help in assessing the impact of different assumptions on the study results. The cost of massage therapy was varied, while other economic parameters were held constant. This calculation was done to reflect a more realistic dollar amount for the massage sessions. Since massage was started on an experimental basis at the hospital, the masseuse was reimbursed at $18 per session, a rate lower than the average rate for such therapy. The typical rate for massage therapy was calculated at $45 per session. Therefore, $45 was considered as the extreme negative value for the worst-case estimate. The best case estimate considered the values obtained from the study. As revealed by the sensitivity analysis, the lower price scenario showed a net benefit of $2853.10, as mentioned previously. The higher price scenario showed a net benefit of $2718.09.

Hospital room and board

A sensitivity analysis was also performed by varying the cost of the hospital room. Hospital room costs were varied, while other economic parameters, such as the cost of massage therapy, cost of TPN, and direct drug costs to the hospital, were held constant. Hospital room costs were allowed to shift simultaneously to their most positive value, and alternatively to their most negative value. The extreme positive and negative values of cost of hospital room for the United States were obtained from the Medstat (Hass, 1995) data. The 'best case estimate' and 'worst case estimate' were then calculated taking into account the cost to the hospitals at $386.35 and $755.24 per day, per patient, respectively. The higher price scenario projected a net benefit of $3309.15 for patients with massage therapy. Similarly, the lower price scenario projected a net benefit of $1660.98 for patients with massage therapy. Thus, the benefit in regard to savings in hospital room and board were found to be stable between the extreme ranges.

Anti-emetic therapy

Only four patients out of the total 31 patients were given an ondansetron (Zofran) anti-emetic regimen, while the remaining patients were given granisetron (Kytril) anti-emetic regimen. Since ondansetron had a higher acquisition cost than granisetron, a sensitivity analysis was done to determine if there would still be an incremental cost benefit if the patients on ondansetron regimen were excluded. Sensitivity analyses showed that when the patients on ondansetron were excluded, the net cost savings was $3016.11, as compared with the best-case estimate of $2847.89.

Regression analysis

A regression analysis was done to determine the extent to which the independent variables accounted for the observed variability in the total number of days of nausea and vomiting. A multiple step-wise regression was done with a number of independent variables and total days of nausea and vomiting as the dependent variable. The independent variables used were patient group (massage vs no massage), age, race, marital status, insurance information, transplant physician, admitting diagnosis, previous chemotherapy, and number of cycles of previous chemotherapy. Table 5.4 summarizes the results of the stepwise multiple regression.

The results of the regression analysis indicate that 40.5% of the observed variability in the total days of nausea and vomiting was explained by the patient group. Thus, the presence or absence of massage therapy accounted for 40.5% of the observed variability in the total days of nausea and vomiting.

The regression model used was a stepwise multiple regression. This model helps in removing variables whose importance diminishes as additional predictors are added or removed. The first model used the group of patients as the predictor variable, as mentioned above. The second model used the transplant physician along with the group of patients as the predictor variable. The analysis indicates that 51.7% ($r^2 = 0.517$) of the observed variability in the total days of nausea and vomiting can be explained by patient group (massage vs no massage) and transplant physician.

The remaining independent variables (race, age, insurance information, previous chemotherapy, number of cycles of previous chemotherapy, marital status, and admitting diagnosis) were excluded by the stepwise multiple

Table 5.4 Summary of regression analysis

Model	Variable	r	r square	Adjusted r square	Standard error of estimate	Significance
1	Group of patients (massage vs no massage)	0.636[a]	0.405	0.381	3.40	$p < 0.05$
2	Transplant physician	0.719[b]	0.517	0.477	3.13	$p < 0.05$

[a]Predictors: (constant), group of patients (massage vs no massage).
[b]Predictors: (constant), group of patients (massage vs no massage), transplant physician.
[c]Dependent variable: total days of nausea and vomiting.

regression model. This indicates that there was no significant accountability towards the observed variability in the total days of nausea and vomiting because of the remaining independent variables.

DISCUSSION

The results of this study indicate that the cost to the institution for anti-emetic drug therapy and parenteral nutritional support (TPN) for the patient undergoing stem cell transplantation for the treatment of breast cancer averaged $2972.43. When thrice weekly massage therapy was added to the patient care plan as an adjunct to anti-emetic medication, the cost of anti-emetic therapy and nutritional support was $1517.61. The cost to the hospital for the massage therapy was an average of $90 per patient (five massage sessions @ $18 per session); thus, using massage therapy for nausea and vomiting in PSCT patients generated cost savings of $1454.82 per patient. This finding indicates that massage therapy is a valuable adjunct to anti-emetic medications in treating high-dose chemotherapy-induced nausea and vomiting in women undergoing PSCT procedures for breast or ovarian cancer.

Length of stay in the hospital was another index measured to determine the impact of massage therapy on the outcome of patients receiving high-dose chemotherapy for PSCT. There was a significant ($p < 0.05$) decrease in the total length of stay for patients with massage therapy as compared with patients without massage therapy. The average length of stay for the control group was 20.29 days as compared with 17.82 days for patients with massage therapy. Given that all other treatment variables were held constant, this infers that massage therapy was instrumental in reducing the length of stay in the hospital. When adding the cost of room and board for the patient to the cost of the anti-emetic medication, the cost of massage therapy and the mean cost for TPN therapy, there was a net incremental benefit to the hospital of $2853.10 per patient, or a cost avoidance of 19.69% associated with massage therapy.

Sensitivity analyses revealed that significant trends in cost avoidance associated with massage therapy held across a number of assumptions with each of the measured variables.

Additional study observations

The total number of patient charts reviewed for this study was 31, out of which 14 patients received only anti-emetic medication, and 17 patients received massage therapy as an adjunct to anti-emetic medications. A majority of the patients in both the groups were breast cancer patients (85.7% in the control group and 82.4% in the treatment group). All other patients were diagnosed with advanced ovarian cancer. A subsequent study by

Anantharaman et al. (2000) extended the massage therapy population to include 34 patients receiving high-dose chemotherapy for PSCT. In the Anantharaman study 91% of patients received PSCT for the treatment of breast cancer while the remaining patients were treated for advanced ovarian cancer.

A majority of the patients in the present study were married women, and had private insurance agencies covering the expenses for the PSCT procedures. A majority of the patients from both groups were administered CAF (cyclophosphamide, doxorubicin, and 5-fluorouracil) as pretransplant chemotherapy.

Five physicians were responsible for contributing patients to the study. However, once enrolled in the PSCT program, patients were subject to the same procedures and conditions as agreed to by the entire group of physicians. Also, all the patients received the same chemotherapy (STAMP V) and the same dosage of the chemotherapeutic agents.

Multiple stepwise regression analyses were performed to determine the extent to which the demographic variables accounted for the variability in the total days of nausea and vomiting. The results indicated that the variable 'massage therapy' accounted for 40.5% of the observed variability in the days of nausea and vomiting while the second 'step' of the model indicated that the 'transplant physician' accounted for 11.2% of the remaining observed variability in the total days of nausea and vomiting. The stepwise regression model excluded the remaining variables.

The study by Anantharaman et al. revealed that the variable 'transplant physician' was related to pretransplant exposure to chemotherapy and the anti-emetic regimens used in that setting. Specifically, the use of a single agent therapy to control nausea and vomiting associated with the chemotherapy in the pretransplant phase of the program (which is individualized by the 'transplant physician' and performed in a private office setting) was directly proportional ($r^2 = 0.299$, $p < 0.05$) to the post-transplant days of nausea and vomiting. When pretransplant chemotherapy-associated anti-emetic therapy was further evaluated, singularly and in combination, the use of high-dose ondansetron (32 mg IV) was the only variable in addition to massage therapy that was significantly predictive of post transplant days of nausea and vomiting. Although not evaluated specifically in this study, these observations are consistent with literature that describes the increased likelihood of nausea and vomiting in patients with prior emetic experiences and may infer the presence of anticipatory nausea and vomiting.

The study by Anantharaman et al. also spoke to the durability of the findings in this study, in that the mean length of stay for patients receiving massage therapy was 18.25 days, and that nausea and vomiting were experienced in the massage therapy group for a mean duration of 4.92 days. Correlative studies of factors significantly associated with the presence of massage therapy included fewer days of nausea and vomiting ($r^2 = 0.401$, $p < 0.01$), shorter length of stay ($r^2 = 0.433$, $p < 0.01$) and the likelihood to experience nausea, but no vomiting ($r^2 = 0.613$, $p < 0.01$). Slightly less than five massage sessions were provided to each patient in the intervention group. Cost analysis revealed that the net incremental cost avoidance in the massage intervention group compared with the control was $3727 in the study by Anantharaman et al. (2000).

CONCLUSIONS

Massage therapy as an adjunct to anti-emetic medication was found to be more cost saving and effective in controlling high-dose chemotherapy-induced nausea and vomiting in women undergoing PSCT procedures for breast or ovarian cancer, under a number of assumptions. The extent of savings was dependent on the length of stay in the hospital, days of TPN, amount of anti-emetic medication administered, and number of massage sessions.

The realization by the health care administrators of the potential cost savings and effectiveness of massage therapy, as shown by this study, would prove to be beneficial for the institution. These savings could then be directed to other necessary treatment therapies in the health care system. This type of analysis helps institutional policy makers prioritize funding to maximize the net health benefit from a fixed amount of resources.

Besides the economic benefit of massage therapy, it has several other benefits. Nausea and vomiting are some of the most dreaded side effects of chemotherapy. Massage therapy, along with anti-emetic medication, alleviated these chemotherapy-related side effects to a certain extent, and thus helped the patient in better tolerating high doses of chemotherapy. Also, most patients are apprehensive about undergoing PSCT procedures because of the nausea and the vomiting associated with it. Massage therapy would prove to be beneficial in improving patient participation and compliance in such high-dose chemotherapy alternatives, which offer a hope for a potential cure or at least a partial remission from cancer.

Assumptions

The assumptions made in the study are:

1. This retrospective study was done by an examination of medical records. Different physicians and interns noted these records. The study assumes that the different interns reporting the patient status and physician orders were consistent in recording the information about nausea and vomiting.

2. The study assumes that each physician was consistent in prescribing anti-emetic medications for all the patients. A protocol was established, but variances were allowed.

3. The same masseuse administered the massage to all the patients in the study, and the type of massage administered was also the same for all the patients. So it was assumed that the quantitative therapy rendered through the massage was the same in all the patients.

Limitations

The limitations of the study are:

1. The sample size for this study was small. The study results could have been different in the presence of a larger patient population.

2. Only one masseuse administered the massage. Had the massage been administered by a different masseuse, there could have been a difference in the results.

3. The study did not take into account the cost of nursing for the episodes of nausea and vomiting. The extent of care required for the nausea and vomiting does not determine the nursing cost. This made it difficult to identify the exact time invested by the nurse for nausea and vomiting in these patients. It was assumed that since nursing cost is paid immaterial of the extent of care required, it must be proportional to the length of stay in the hospital, and hence the study was not biased in this respect. But the identification of nursing cost to the hospital may have changed the results of the study.

4. The reliability and validity of the study instrument could not be determined since the sample was too small ($n = 31$) to do a pre-test.

5. The study did not quantify the intangible aspects of massage therapy, such as the anxiety and stress relieved by massage.

6. Only one type of chemotherapy regimen (STAMP V) was considered. The results of the study could have been different if different types of high-dose chemotherapy regimen were used, because of the different emetogenic potential of the different therapies. Also, only breast and ovarian cancer patients were considered. The effect of massage could have been different for the different types of cancer.

7. The study did not investigate whether other factors, such as infection, could have affected hospital length of stay.

REFERENCES

Anantharaman, R., Siganga, W., Black, C., & Lively, B. (2000). Relationship and economic evaluation of emesis and its control associated with pre- and post-PSCT high-dose chemotherapy for breast and ovarian cancer. *Journal of the American Pharmaceutical Association, 40*, 294–295.

American Cancer Society (1996). Cancer — alternative and complementary therapies. *Cancer, 77.*

Borrison, H. L., & Wang, S. C. (1953). Physiology and pharmacology of vomiting. *Pharmacology Review, 5,* 193–230.

Center for Disease Control. (1998). *Cancer Prevention.* [On-line]. Available: http://www.cdc.gov/nccdphp/dcpc/index.html

Consumer Price Index (1998). *CPI.* [On-line]. Available: http//www.stats.bls.gov/cpifaq.html

Haas, S. (1995). *Analysis.* Trius, Inc.: Pharmacia and Upjohn, Inc. [A private insurer database].

Jassak, P. F., & Riley, M. B. (1994). Autologous stem cell transplant — an overview. *Cancer Practice, 2,* 141–145.

Massie, M. J., & Shakin, E. J. (1993). Management of depression and anxiety in cancer patients. In W. Breitbert, & J. C. Holland (Eds.), *Psychiatric aspects of symptom management in cancer patients.* Washington, DC: American Psychiatric Press.

Meisenberg, B. G. (1997). Prevention of nausea and vomiting following high-dose chemotherapy and stem rescue. *Health Care Innovations,* 11–14.

FURTHER READING

American Cancer Society. *Cancer facts and figures — 1998: Basic cancer facts.* [On-line]. Available: http://www.cancer.org/statistics/cff98/basicfacts.html

Balmer, C., & Valley, A. W. (1993). Basic principles of cancer treatment and cancer chemotherapy. In J. T. DiPiro, R. L. Talbert, P. E. Hayes, G. C. Yee, G. R. Matzke, & M. Posey, (Eds.), *Pharmacotherapy: a pathophysiologic approach* 2nd ed. (pp. 1894–1903). Connecticut: Simon & Schuster.

Bongflio, T. A., & Terry, R. (1983). The pathology of cancer. In Rubin, P. (Ed.), *Clinical oncology — a multidisciplinary approach* 6th ed. (pp. 20–29). New York: American Cancer Society.

Bonneterre, J., Chevallier, B., Metz, R. et al. (1990). A randomized double-blind comparison of Ondansetron and Metaclopramide in the prophylaxis of emesis induced by Cyclophosphamide, Fluorouracil, and Doxorubicin therapy. *Journal of Clinical Oncology, 8,* 1063–1069.

Bootman, J., Townsend, R., & McGhan, W. (1996). *Principles of pharmacoeconomics.* Cincinnati, Ohio: Harvey Whitney Books Company.

Burtness, B. (1997). High-dose chemotherapy for breast cancer. *Principles and Practice of Oncology, 11,* 1–11.

Calabresi, P., & Parks, R. E. (1930). Antiproliferative agents and drugs used for immunosuppression. In A. G. Gilman, & L. S. Goodman (Eds.). *The pharmacologic basis of therapeutics* 6th ed. (pp. 1256–1313). New York: Macmillan.

Chabner, B. A. (1990). Clinical strategies for cancer treatment: The role of drugs. In B. A. Chabner, & J. M. Collins (Eds.), *Cancer chemotherapy: principles and practice* (pp. 1–15). Philadelphia, PA: J. B. Lippincott.

Cheson, B. D., Lacerna, L., Leyland-Jones, B., et al. (1989). Autologous bone marrow transplantation, current status and future directions. *Annals of Internal Medicine, 110,* 51–56.

Coates, A., Abraham, S., Kaye, S. B., et al. (1983). On the receiving end — patient perception of the side effects of cancer chemotherapy. *European Journal of Cancer Clinical Oncology, 19,* 203–208.

Coia, L. R., & Moylan, D. J. (Eds.). (1984). *Therapeutic radiology for the house officer.* Baltimore, MD: Williams and Wilkins.

Dalton, W. S. (1991). Management of systemic metastases and sequential therapy for advanced disease. In K. I. Bland, & E. M. Copeland (Eds.). *The breast* (pp. 877–899). Philadelphia, PA: W. B. Saunders.

Daly, J. M., & DeCosse, J. J. (1985). Principles of surgical oncology. In P. Calabresi, P. S. Schein, & S. A. Rosenberg (Eds.), *Medical oncology: basic principles and clinical management of cancer* (pp. 261–279). New York: Macmillan.

Domenico, G. D., & Wood, E. C. (1997). *Beards massage* (4th ed.). Philadelphia, PA: W. B. Saunders.

Eye, G. C. (1996). Bone marrow transplantation. In J. T. DiPiro, R. L. Talbert, P. E. Hayes, G. C. Yee, G. R. Matzke, & M. L. Posey (Eds.). *Pharmacotherapy — a pathophysiologic approach* 3rd ed. (pp. 2651–2670). Connecticut: Simon & Schuster.

Gralla, R. J., Tyson, L. B., Kris, M. G., et al. (1987). The management of chemotherapy-induced nausea and vomiting. *Medical Clinics of North America, 71,* 289–301.

Griffin, A. M., Butow, P. N., Coodes, A. S., et al. (1993). On the receiving end. V: Patient perception of the side effects of cancer chemotherapy. *Annals of Oncology, 7,* 189–195.

Henderson, C. I., Harris, J. R., Kinne, D. W., et al. (1989). Cancer of the breast. In V. R. Devita (Ed.), *Cancer principles and practice of oncology* (pp. 1197–1258). Philadelphia, PA: J. B. Lippincott.

Hesketh, P. M., Harvey, W. H., Harker, T. M., et al. (1994). A randomized, double-blind comparison of intravenous ondansetron alone and in combination with intravenous Dexamethasone in the prevention of high-dose cisplatin-induced emesis. *Journal of Clinical Oncology, 2,* 596–600.

Jassak, P. F., & Riley, M. B. (1994). Autologous stem cell transplant — an overview. *Cancer Practice, 2,* 141–145.

Kaasa, S., Kvaloy, S., Dicato, M. A., et al. (1990). A comparison of Ondansetron with Metoclopramide in the prophylaxis of chemotherapy-induced nausea and vomiting: A randomized, double-blind study. International Emesis Study Group. *European Journal of Cancer, 26,* 311–314.

Kirchner, V. (1993). Clinical studies to assess the economic impact of new therapies: pragmatic approaches to measuring costs. *Anti-Cancer Drugs, 4*(3), 13–20.

Marschner, N. W., Adler, M., Nagell, G. A., et al. (1991). Double-blind, randomized trial of the anti-emetic efficacy and safety of Ondansetron and Metoclopramide in advanced breast cancer patients treated with Epirubicin and Cyclophosphamide. *European Journal of Cancer, 27,* 1137–1140.

McGuire, T. R. (1993). Breast cancer. In J. T. DiPiro, R. L. Talbert, P. E. Hayes, G. C. Yee, G. R. Matzke, & M. L. Posey (Eds.). *Pharmacotherapy: A pathophysiologic approach* 2nd ed. (pp. 1930–1945). Connecticut: Simon & Schuster.

Meek, S. S. (1993). Effects of slow stroke back massage on relaxation in hospice clients. *IMAGE: Journal of Nursing Scholarship, 25,* 17–21.

Morrow, G. R., Hickok, J. T., & Rosenthal, S. N. (1995). Progress in reducing nausea and emesis: comparisons of ondansetron (Zofran), granisetron (Kytril), and tropisetron (novoban). *Cancer, 76,* 343–357.

Navari, H. G., Kaplan, R. J., & Gralla, R. J. (1994). Efficacy and safety of granisetron, a selective 5-hydroxytryptamine-3 receptor antagonist, in the prevention of nausea and vomiting induced by high-dose cisplatin. *Journal of Clinical Oncology, 12,* 2204–2210.

Parker, S. L., Tong, T., Zbolden, S., et al. (1997). Cancer statistics. *CA Cancer Journal Clinics, 47,* 5–27.

Perez, R., et al. (1993). Mechanism and modulation of resistance to chemotherapy in ovarian cancer. *Cancer, 71,* 1571–1580.

Peters, W. P., Shpall, E. J., Jones, R. B., et al. (1988). High-dose combination alkylating agents with bone marrow support as initial treatment of metastatic breast cancer. *Journal of Clinical Oncology, 6,* 1368–1376.

Rosenberg, S. A. (1989). Principles of surgical oncology. In V. T. Devita, Jr., S. Hellman, & S. A. Rosenberg (Eds.), *Cancer: Principles and practice of oncology* 3rd ed. (pp. 236–246). Philadelphia, PA: J. B. Lippincott.

Sims, S. (1986). Slow stroke back massage for cancer patients. *Nursing Times, 82,* 140–145.

Tannock, I. (1989). Principles of cell proliferation: Cell kinetics. In V. T. Devita, Jr., S. Hellman, & S. A. Rosenberg (Eds.), *Cancer: Principles and practice of oncology* 3rd ed. (pp. 3–13). Philadelphia, PA: J. B. Lippincott.

Tonato, M., Roila, F., Del Favero, A., et al. (1996). Methodology of trials with anti-emetics. *Support Care Cancer, 4,* 281–286.

US Congress, Congressional Budget Office. (1992). *Economic implications of rising health care costs.* Washington, DC: Government Printing Office.

APPENDICES

Appendix A: Instrument for data collection

Patient Information

---

1) Age   Patient Code
2) Date of Birth
3) Race
     1. White   2. Black   3. Hispanic   4. Asian
     5. Native American   6. Mixed   7. Other
4) Marital Status
     1. Married   2. Single   3. Widowed
     4. Divorced   5. Separated
5) Insurance Information
     1. Payer 1 (Government)
     2. Payer 2 (Private)
6) Transplant Physician
     1. Dr A.   2. Dr B.   3. Dr C.
     4. Dr D.   5. Dr E.   6. Dr F.

Patient Pre-PSCT History

7) Admitting Diagnosis
     1. Breast Cancer (Stage I, II, III)
     2. Metastatic Breast Cancer
     3. Stage I Ovarian Cancer
     4. Advanced Ovarian Cancer
8) Previous Chemotherapy
     1. CAF [cyclophosphamide, Adriamycin, Fluorouracil]
     2. TA [Taxol (paclitaxel), Adriamycin]
     3. Taxol (paclitaxel)
     4. CAF & Taxol
9) Number of Cycles of Previous Chemotherapy:
     1.   2.   3.   4.

PSCT Information

10) Date of Admission into PSCT Program
11) Last Date in PSCT Program
12) Number of Days in PSCT Program
13) First Day of Nausea/Vomiting
14) Days of Nausea/Vomiting
15) Anti-emetic Medication Regimen
     1. IV   2. Oral   3. Sublingual
     1. Ativan   2. Kytril   3. Compazine   4. Reglan
     5. Zofran   6. Haxadrol   7. Metacloprin   8. Torecan

Massage Therapy

16) First Day of Massage Therapy
17) Number of Days of Massage Therapy
18) Number of Massage Sessions
19) Kind of Massage Therapy
20) Additional Comments

Appendix B-1: Cost calculations for patients with anti-emetic drug therapy without massage therapy

PSCT No.	Length of stay	Hospital room & board (A)	Anti-emetic cost (B)	Cost of TPN (C)	Cost of massage (D)	Total Cost (A + B + C + D)
1	19	$10,790.10	$1782.59	$982.80	$0.00	$13,555.49
2	30	$17,037.00	$4219.71	$1036.15	$0.00	$22,292.86
6	25	$14,197.50	$2351.10	$1246.28	$0.00	$17,794.88
7	19	$10,790.10	$2400.39	$1020.00	$0.00	$14,210.49
9	18	$10,222.20	$4207.14	$688.50	$0.00	$15,117.84
10	19	$10,790.10	$2586.85	$998.75	$0.00	$14,375.70
11	21	$11,925.90	$1154.67	$851.95	$0.00	$13,932.52
12	19	$10,790.10	$2541.66	$918.00	$0.00	$14,249.76
13	19	$10,790.10	$883.52	$1035.30	$0.00	$12,708.92
14	19	$10,790.10	$1080.48	$0.00	$0.00	$11,870.58
15	19	$10,790.10	$1322.47	$683.40	$0.00	$12,795.97
16	20	$11,358.00	$2594.75	$856.80	$0.00	$14,809.55
19	20	$11,358.00	$1233.22	$882.30	$0.00	$13,473.52
21	17	$9654.30	$1137.18	$918.00	$0.00	$11,709.48
Sum		$161,283.60	$29,495.73	$12,118.23	$0.00	$202,897.56
Average	20.28	$11,520.26	$2106.84	$865.59	$0.00	$14,492.68

Appendix B-2: Cost calculations for patients with massage therapy as an adjunct to anti-emetic drug therapy

PSCT No.	Length of stay	Hospital room & board (A)	Anti-emetic cost (B)	Cost of TPN (C)	Cost of massage (D)	Total Cost (A + B + C + D)
20	18	$10,222.20	$2725.39	$0.00	$90.00	$13,037.59
22	18	$10,222.20	$590.89	$102.00	$90.00	$11,005.09
23	20	$11,358.00	$1318.21	$0.00	$90.00	$12,766.21
26	17	$9654.30	$1328.56	$0.00	$90.00	$11,072.86
31	17	$9654.30	$1313.58	$102.00	$90.00	$11,159.88
33	17	$9654.30	$1377.98	$0.00	$90.00	$11,122.28
34	18	$10,222.20	$1460.45	$0.00	$90.00	$11,772.65
36	17	$9654.30	$1314.33	$0.00	$90.00	$11,058.63
38	17	$9654.30	$1325.95	$0.00	$90.00	$11,070.25
39	18	$10,222.20	$1744.73	$688.50	$72.00	$12,727.43
44	17	$9654.30	$812.94	$229.50	$90.00	$10,786.74
46	20	$11,358.00	$1360.75	$0.00	$108.00	$12,826.75
47	18	$10,222.20	$1337.09	$0.00	$90.00	$11,649.29
48	18	$10,222.20	$1432.20	$0.00	$108.00	$11,762.40
52	18	$10,222.20	$1332.76	$0.00	$72.00	$11,626.96
54	18	$10,222.20	$964.67	$0.00	$90.00	$11,276.87
56	17	$9654.30	$1406.91	$0.00	$90.00	$11,239.72
Sum		$172,073.70	$23,147.39	$1122.00	$1530.00	$197,873.09
Average	17.82	$10,121.98	$1361.61	$66.00	$90.00	$11,639.59

6

Massage therapy following spinal cord injury

Sandra L. Rogers

INTRODUCTION

Increased vulnerability of individuals who have sustained a traumatic spinal cord injury (SCI) to a host of potentially preventable illnesses including pressure ulcers, urinary tract infections, and respiratory tract infections is commonly recognized (Eastwood et al., 1999; Whiteneck et al., 1992). Considerable investigation has been undertaken by medical professionals to understand the causative factors underlying these conditions and to educate affected individuals and their caregivers on reasonable and cost-effective strategies to prevent these maladies. Typically, immediate causative factors are explored (i.e., incomplete bladder emptying, prolonged sitting, absence of cough) and countered with pragmatic solutions (i.e., intermittent catheterization, pressure relief, assisted cough). One thread common to all these illnesses is a failure of the immune system to adequately protect the individual following SCI. Unfortunately, there is sparse data on immunological changes which persist in chronic SCI, and even less on how the immune function might be augmented in following SCI.

Long-term health consequences of spinal cord injury

Clinically, dysregulation of the autonomic nervous system is manifested by the occurrence of apneic bradycardia, autonomic dysreflexia, thermoregulation, orthostatic hypotension, and endocrine dysregulation (Daverat et al., 1995). In cervical SCI, an additional disruption of the sympathetic nervous system signaling outflow to lymphoid tissues and their blood vessels is present (Cruse et al., 1996a). Other common occurrences of illness, which reflect immunosuppression, are respiratory tract infections, pneumonia, urinary tract infections and pressure ulcers. Depression, a psychosocial stressor, following SCI is also common, nearly 80% of individuals with SCI have mild to severe levels of depression (Heinemann et al., 1997; Kliesch et al., 1996; Lu & Yarkony, 1996; Saboe et al., 1997). Depression following neurological damage has been linked to further immunosuppression, placing the SCI population at greater risk for infection (Irwin et al., 1987; MacHale et al., 1998). All of these illnesses indicate that a dysregulation of sympathetic nervous system activity, impaired signaling from the periphery to the CNS, and multiple stressors may be present (Daverat et al., 1995). Taken together, the evidence for altered immune regulation following SCI is convincing. This places survivors of SCI at a greater risk for disease and thus encourages rehabilitation professions to design interventions which can improve health and wellness.

Immunological consequences of spinal cord injury

Dysregulation of immune function is often caused by disruptions among the critical pathways between the nervous, endocrine and immune systems. Evidence suggests that individuals with acute SCIs have compromised natural and adaptive immune functioning as a result of their injuries (Cruse & Lewis, 1989, 1997; Cruse et al., 1992, 1993, 1996a,b; Kliesch et al., 1996; Smith et al., 1987). Neuroendocrine and cellular immune functions are altered following acute SCI (Cruse et al., 1996a). Alterations in the cellular immune functions following SCI indicate that there is a reduction in natural killer (NK) cell-mediated lysis and diminished lymphocyte transformation/IL-2R levels, with the tetraplegic subjects significantly more impaired than paraplegics (Cruse et al., 1993, 1996a; Kliesch et al., 1996). These changes persisted for up to 1 year following injury (Cruse et al., 1992). Furthermore, participation in a generalized rehabilitation program appeared to improve immune status in all subjects, however it is not clear what aspect of the rehabilitation program contributed to these changes (Kliesch et al., 1996).

Other reports indicate that adrenal reserve in men ($n = 20$) with chronic tetra- or paraplegia SCI was significantly impaired on a low dose ($1 \mu g$) adrenocorticotrophic hormone (ACTH) test when compared with controls, but reported no data for differences on level of injury (Wang, 1999). Cortisol and dehydroepiandrosterone sulfate (DS) were reported to be elevated in another group of chronic SCI participants when compared with controls, but no differences were seen between the tetraplegic participants and paraplegic subjects (Campagnolo et al., 1999). Campagnolo and colleagues found no difference on measures of dehydroepiandrosterone (DHEA), ACTH or prolactin between SCI and healthy controls. Patterns of differences emerged however, when tetra and paraplegic response levels where compared, with individuals in the tetraplegic group showing higher levels of DS and DHEA, but no significant differences in cortisol, ACTH or prolactin levels. In another study, levels of adrenaline (epinephrine), noradrenaline (norepinephrine), and dopamine were measured at rest and during exercise in chronic SCI with the SCI population divided into four groups [C3–C7 ($n = 30$); T1–T4 ($n = 15$); T5–T10 ($n = 15$); T10 & below ($n = 15$)] and controls (Schmid et al., 1998). Only the C3–C7 group (tetraplegic) showed significantly lower E and NE at rest when compared with controls with only slight elevations with exercise. Individuals with T1–T4 levels of injury showed lower levels of E and NE at rest and exercise when compared with those with paraplegia distal to T5. Questions about the consistency of findings and clinical implications remain.

Influence of perceived health, disability and immunological status

The above patterns of neuroendocrine and cellular immune dysfunction following chronic SCI are likely to be influenced by alterations in the neuroendocrine axis and by varying degrees of interruption of the tonic firing of the efferent and afferent fibers of the sympathetic nervous system as a direct result of SCI. However, emotional states/mood and levels of stress can also modify neuroendocrine and cellular immune. The occurrence of extraordinary stress and depression following SCI are unfortunately common (Daverat et al., 1995). And, as stated earlier, the immune system alterations seen following SCI are strikingly similar to those found in individuals who have chronic stress conditions (Cacioppo et al., 1998a; Coe, 1993; Dhabhar & McEwen, 1997; Esterling et al., 1994; Fleming et al., 1987; Irwin et al., 1987; Pike et al., 1997). Perhaps SCI, by its very nature, induces a state of chronic stress which then has a negative impact on overall health. For example, negative psychosocial states are known to influence immune competence, which may alter and delay wound healing, a critical issue following occurrence of pressure ulcers in SCI (Cruse et al., 1996b; Glaser et al., 1999a; Kiecolt-Glaser et al., 1995). There is striking evidence supporting the role emotional states play in ultimately affecting the immune system (Esterling et al., 1996; Glaser et al., 1990, 1998, 1999a; Kiecolt-Glaser et al., 1996, 1998). For example, depressive thoughts and moods depress neuroendocrine and autonomic functioning, which in turn has a significant negative effect on immunity (Irwin et al., 1987). Since there are consistent immunosuppressive effects across different populations and kinds of stressors, it is reasonable to assume that persons with

SCI who bear negative emotions would display immunosuppressive effects as well (Watkins & Maier, 1999). This is of paramount importance to therapists, since a great portion of SCI patients experience mild to severe depression after their injury. Taken together, individuals with SCI have multidimensional stressors, which make them ideal candidates for application of stress reduction modalities in therapy.

In addition, the immune system alterations seen in acute SCI are strikingly similar to those found in individuals who have chronic stress conditions (Dhabhar & McEwen, 1997). Furthermore, while there is extensive evidence that chronic levels of stress reduces the effectiveness of the immune system (Burleson et al., 1998; Cacioppo et al., 1998b; Dura et al., 1990; Esterling et al., 1994; Glaser & Kiecolt-Glaser, 1997, 1998; Glaser et al., 1998, 1999b; Kiecolt-Glaser et al., 1991, 1996; Uchino et al., 1992; Wu et al., 1999), there is little rigorous scientific evidence of what types of interventions could enhance the immune system responses once they have been altered (Rabin, 1999).

Massage as a modality to positively enhance immune function

Spinal cord injured patients are an important part of the rehabilitation population. There are approximately 200,000 people alive in the United States today with spinal cord injuries, and approximately 11,000 new cases arise each year. Theoretically, a method of intervention to effectively and predictably decrease stress could also lead to improved immune responses in individuals with SCI (Cruse et al., 1996a,b). One therapeutic technique touted by popular literature to enhance immune system function is massage.

Despite the broad use of complementary and alternative medicine (CAM) treatments there is a relative paucity of data that convincingly demonstrates safety, efficacy, effectiveness, and mechanism of CAM practices (Eisenberg et al., 1998). Many of these remedies lack scientific evidence of their curative effects, discouraging health professionals from utilizing any medicine labeled 'alternative' (Rabin, 1999; Watkins, 1997). While massage may be an alternative, and therefore an unproven, treatment in rehabilitation medicine it is an often recommended and used intervention. Fortunately, there is some convincing evidence that suggests massage may enhance certain immune parameters (Field, 1995; Field et al., 1996a,b,c, 1997a,b, 1998a,b; Ironson et al., 1996; Prodromidis et al., 1995; Scafidi & Field, 1996; Scafidi et al., 1996). As health care approaches change rapidly, rehabilitation professionals need to document the impact we have on our clients. Little has been done to convince skeptics about how therapeutic techniques work, for whom they work best, and for how long these techniques must be used in order to foster change (Fletcher & Fletcher, 1997; Ottenbacher & Maas, 1999).

Studies that used massage intervention report primarily psychological benefits to numerous patient groups. These benefits include enhanced positive emotionality, decreased anxiety, increased attention (to math computation), and induction of a state of relaxation which persists after the massage intervention ceases (Field et al., 1996a,b, 1997a,b, 1998a; Ironson et al., 1996; Lang et al., 1996; Scafidi & Field, 1996, 1997; Scafidi et al., 1996, 1997; Wheeden et al., 1993). The range of populations positively affected by massage includes healthy adults, infants in a neonatal intensive care unit, children with autism, depressed adolescents, adolescent mothers, healthy adolescents and mothers of sick infants (Field et al., 1996a,b, 1997a,b, 1998a,b; Ironson et al., 1996; Lang et al., 1996; Scafidi & Field, 1996, 1997; Scafidi et al., 1996, 1997; Wheeden et al., 1993). Since the reported psychological benefits are attributed to relaxation it is reasonable to infer that a state of lowered sympathetic activation is being induced. This inference is supported by the few studies that have utilized physiological outcome measures, which show reductions in the levels of norepinephrine and cortisol in depressed adolescents, HIV+ and HIV− gay men, child psychiatric patients, and healthy adults when treated with massage (Ironson et al., 1996). Other physiological evidence for the benefits of massage include enhanced effects on the circulatory system (Goats, 1994). Goats has demonstrated increases in the rate of blood flow and cardiac stroke volume, implying enhanced venous return. Critically, the immunological benefits to a group of HIV+ gay men following an intensive massage protocol significantly enhanced natural killer cell numbers and cytotoxicity, and the activity of the cytotoxic CD8 T cells (Ironson et al., 1996).

In order to investigate the relationship between immunological status following chronic spinal cord injury and to examine the effectiveness of massage on this population we have undertaken two studies. The specific aims of the first of these studies was to investigate whether altered immunological and neuroendocrine regulation deficits persists in chronic SCI, to determine whether an intensive massage treatment enhances cellular immunity, and if so, how long after treatment the effects persist. The second pilot study was developed to assess whether there are greater benefits for individuals who have a cervical verses a thoracic level spinal cord injury. Study 2 methodology was identical to the first study. However, in this pilot study we compared the long-term consequences of living with paraplegia and tetraplegic spinal cord injury (SCI) and examined the responses of two differing populations to massage. The data presented here represent a compilation of these two studies findings.

RESEARCH METHODS AND MASSAGE PROCEDURE
General research methods

Subjects

Subjects were recruited through a database of active, wheelchair-reliant individuals with spinal cord injury. All participants signed an institutional review board (IRB)-approved informed consent prior to their participation in this study. Individuals who were age 18 years or older and initially injured at least 6 months prior to the study were invited to participate. To answer the question as to whether those with chronic SCI have different immunologic profiles than normals, a group of age (±3 years) matched, gender and life-style (smoking and marital status) matched controls were recruited. Controls were recruited from general advertisement. To ensure the selection of healthy controls and generally healthy SCI participants, potential subjects were screened using a slightly modified version of a self-report health questionnaire, the Survey of Immunological and General Health (SIGH) (Kang et al., 1997; Strauman et al., 1993). Any potential subject with a history of multiple spinal cord injuries, malignant, autoimmune, or chronic infectious disease, as well as those who were using immuno-suppressive or anti-psychotic medications, was excluded. Seventeen SCI subjects with paraplegia and 12 SCI subjects with tetraplegia met these criteria and were recruited for the studies. Of this sample, 25 were male and four were female, representing the United States spinal cord injured population (82% male) (National Spinal Cord Injury Statistical Center, 2000). The mean age was 32.5 with a range of between 25 and 55. Thirteen of the participants had paraplegia, four had tetraplegia. Fifteen age and gender matched, healthy, non-spinal cord-injured individuals comprised the control group, and two individuals served as the control for two of the SCI participants, given the demographic similarities of the subjects (Table 6.1).

Design overview

To determine whether immunologic profiles were different between subjects and controls, blood was drawn at the same time in the morning and compared. Both groups also completed health questionnaires at the same time of the day. The normal control subjects were not used again in any other part of this study. To test the effect of massage on immunologic profile amongst SCI individuals, a before and after intervention design was used. All SCI participants received the massage and were asked to provide a one month post-massage follow-up. The study was conducted in either a massage therapy clinic or in an outpatient rehabilitation clinic. Data was collected at three time points: prior to initiation of the study (baseline), at

Table 6.1 Demographic information on participants

	SCI participants	Controls
Age mean (SD)	32.41 (4.53)	31.65 (8.8)
Level of injury		
Tetraplegia (C3–C5)	12	
Paraplegia (T1–T5)	12	
Paraplegia (T5–T10)	5	
Gender		
Males	25	13
Females	4	2
SIGH Mean (SD)		
UTI	0.71 (0.59)	0.00 (0.00)
RTI	0.47 (0.51)	0.00 (0.00)
Pressure Ulcers	0.59 (0.62)	0.00 (0.00)
FIM	101.47 (25.41)	125.60 (1.55)

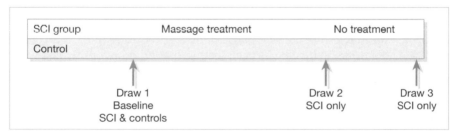

Figure 6.1 Study design with blood collection time points.

the end of the month of massage (prior to the massage being given that final day to eliminate immediate treatment effects), and at the end of the no-treatment month (Fig. 6.1).

Survey of immunological and general health (SIGH)

A modified version of a self-report health questionnaire, the SIGH, was used to screen participants. The SIGH is used to document demographic as well as a detailed health history and information about current health. The modifications included gathering information on the use of alternative therapies, herbs, and food/dietary supplements. Individuals report demographic data, the frequency of common respiratory and immune-related illnesses (e.g. dermatological, allergic) during the preceding two-month period at baseline with subsequent administrations using only the intervening one-month periods, as well as any family history of more severe immunological disorders (including asthma, autoimmune and neoplastic conditions (Kang et al., 1991; Strauman et al., 1993).

Functional independence measure (FIM)

A FIM score was determined for each subject. The FIM is a widely-used standardized assessment tool designed to measure the functional abilities of individuals in six areas of self-care, including, grooming, bathing, dressing, toileting, bowel and bladder management, mobility, locomotion, communication, and social cognition. Levels of functional independence measurement include (1) total assistance, (2) maximum assistance, (3) moderate assistance, (4) minimum assistance, (5) supervision; (6) modified independence and (7) complete independence. Levels 1–5 require the assistance of a helper whereas level 6 and 7 do not require the assistance of a helper (Deutsch et al., 1996; Ota et al., 1996; Watson et al., 1995).

Profile of mood states (POMS)

The POMS is a reliable and valid self-administered survey that is designed to measure individuals' transient, fluctuating affective states. It uses an inventory of 65 adjectives; each rated on a five-point scale, which measures six identifiable moods. The participant is asked to read each adjective and rate how often he or she has been feeling that mood over the past week with $0 =$ not at all, and $4 =$ always. The moods or affective states include anger-hostility, vigor-activity, fatigue-inertia, confusion-bewilderment, tension-anxiety, and depression-dejection (McNair et al., 1992).

Blood collection and cell preparation

Ten ml of blood were drawn by venipuncture into a heparinized vacutainer tube for functional immune assays and 5 ml into vacutainer tubes containing EDTA for complete blood count (CBC) analysis and phenotypic analysis of lymphocyte subsets. A medical center clinical laboratory (Columbus, OH) performed the CBC analysis. All cellular assays were conducted on the day of sampling. Plasma extracts were frozen at $-70°C$ until the day of assay for cortisol and cAMP assays. Peripheral blood mononuclear cells (PBMC) were isolated by centrifugation over Histopaque-1077. PBMC were washed twice in calcium- and magnesium-free Dulbecco's phosphate buffered saline (DPBS) and resuspended in Iscoves's modified Dulbecco's medium (IMDM) supplemented with 5% heat-inactivated fetal bovine serum, 1% GMS-S, and, 1% antibiotic/antimycotic solution (IMDM-C).

Lymphocyte proliferation

Mitogen-stimulated peripheral blood lymphocyte (PBL) activity was assessed via a colormetric assay that determines the number of viable proliferating cells and results in data comparable with those obtained through radioactive isotope incorporation procedures. Proliferative responses to phytohemagglutinin (PHA) were analyzed. PBMC (1×10^5/ml) were cultured in quadruplicate in 96-well flat-bottom microtiter plates (200 μl total volume/well), in the presence of PHA at (2 doses of 25 μg/ml and 50 μg/ml) at 37°C/5% CO_2 for a total of 96 hours. At 24 h, 20 μl of a colormetric oxidation-reduction (RedoxA) indicator, AlmarBlue dye was added to each well. At 96 h, the cells absorbance was measured at 570 nm and 600 nm on a microplate. The mean specific absorbance OD of triplicates of respective groups was calculated. This assay indicates the amount of t-cell proliferation after stimulation that a population of t-cells is able to induce. The higher the proliferation the more effective the t-cells are against a pathogen.

Phenotypic analysis of lymphocyte subsets

EDTA-treated whole blood (100 μl) was stained with 20 μl of the following fluorescein isothiocyanate (FITC) or phycoerythrin (PE) labeled antibodies in pairs: CD3-FITC/CD19-PE, CD4-FITC/CD8-PE, CD16-FITC/CD56-PE, and Pan gamma/delta-FITC/CD25-PE, along with the appropriate isotype controls. Samples were incubated for 15 minutes at room temperature in the dark. Lyse and Fix IO Test reagents were used to prepare the whole blood samples for flow cytometry. Percentages of cell subsets were enumerated within 1–3 days on a Coulter EPICS XL Flow Cytometry System (OSU Medical Center, Columbus, OH). Phenotypic analysis provides information regarding the number of different cell populations of lymphocytes that are present in the peripheral blood.

Plasma adenosine 3′,5′ -monophosphate (cAMP)

Plasma cyclic AMP was quantified using a standardized radioimmunoassay (RIA). Cyclic AMP levels were determined by extrapolation from a standard curve of count bound cAMP in counts per minute/total counts per minute vs cAMP concentration (log scale in nmol/min). Radioactivity was measured using an Isoflex automated gamma counter. Cyclic AMP is believed to indicate the level of sympathetic nervous system activation occurring. Higher levels are indicative of greater sympathetic nervous system activation.

Cortisol

Plasma levels of cortisol were measured by a standardized human cortisol enzyme-linked immunoassay (ELIZA). Absorbance was read at 450 nm, using a microplate reader. Cortisol levels were determined by extrapolation from a standard curve of absorbance vs cortisol concentration reported in μg/dl. Cortisol is an indication of how much sympathetic nervous system reactivity is occurring.

sIL-2R Levels

Plasma levels of sIL-2R were measured by the quantitative sandwich enzyme immunoassay technique. Optical density was read at 450 nm and 540 nm using a microplate reader and is reported in pg/ml concentrations. Higher levels of sIL-2R indicate that the immune system has recently been activated, one would expect low levels of sIL-2R in healthy adults.

Natural killer cell (NK) assay

A whole blood chromium-release assay against K562 target cells (established from a patient with chronic myelogenous leukemia) is used. Briefly, 2×10^6 K562 cells are incubated with 100 μCi sodium chromate (^{51}Cr) at 37°C for 2 hours, washed twice with RPMI, and resuspended at a final concentration of 2×10^6 cells/ml in RPMI. Fifty microliters of target cells and 150 μl of effector cells are added in quadruplicate to a 96-well round-bottom microtiter plate. The concentration of effector cells (PBMC) is varied to produce four effector:target ratios (12.5, 25, 50, and 100:1). Spontaneous and maximal release is determined by incubating 50 μl of target cells with 150 μl RPMI or 5% triton-x, respectively. Plates are then centrifuged to create a buffy coat layer of leukocytes and target cells on top of the red blood cells. The plate is incubated for 4 h at 37°C in a humidified 5% CO_2 incubator. Plates are then centrifuged again and 10-μl aliquots of the supernatants are collected. The released ^{51}Cr was quantified using a gamma counter (TiterTek, Austin, TX). Lysis of target cells at each of the four ratios is calculated using the following formula:

$$\frac{(\text{cpm} - b) \times \dfrac{V_t - (V_b \times \text{Hct})}{V_t} - (\text{SR} - b)}{(\text{MR} - b) - (\text{SR} - b)}$$

Natural killer cells (NK) are believed to be more sensitive to psychological pertubations and indicates that the cells are functional and that they should be able to contribute to the resistance to viral infections and react appropriately should cells become malignant.

Data analysis

A statistical analysis software program (SPSS) was used for data analysis. A one-way analysis of variance (ANOVA) was used to determine whether statistically significant differences existed between the control group and the experimental group on the functional, immunological, and psychological data. Results are reported with means, standard deviations, and the *f*-statistic. To compare the variables within the SCI experimental massage group between the three trials (baseline, post-massage, post no-treatment), a general linear model-repeated measures ANOVA was used for both the immune and psychological and clinical health data. To avoid problems with violations of sphericity the statistical significance of the resultant F ratios were evaluated based on degrees of freedom that were corrected according to the Huynh-Feldt epsilon.

Massage procedure and specialized techniques

Each massage therapist was instructed in and demonstrated competence in wheelchair transfer techniques, the signs and symptoms of autonomic dysreflexia, and the placement of urinary collection bags. Therapists who elected to participate in this study were provided with a two-hour mandatory training session to ensure that each therapist would follow a similar procedure. While we attempted to provide a uniform massage protocol there was no attempt to alter the typical therapeutic massage session. This frequently would include communication between the client and therapist, requests by the client to focus more intensively on painful tissues (i.e., neck, back), the use or disuse of lubricants, and the use of greater or less pressure. Unscented lubricants were typically offered to reduce the friction and a medium to deep pressure was applied and adjusted to each individual's comfort level.

The 60-minute, massage was eclectic in design. It included aspects of Swedish, Trager, Polarity, Accupressure, and Craniosacral Therapy (Fritz, 1999; Tappan & Benjamin, 1997). Several types of strokes were used, including effleurage, petrissage, stretching, holding, stroking, rocking, and squeezing. The subjects transferred to a mat table, and were situated in a supine position, alternating to a prone position during the massage. The subjects received a full-body massage, regardless of their injury level. The full body massage included, head, neck, upper and lower extremities, and trunk. Abdominal massage was excluded from this study because of its unpredictable effect on the gastrointestinal tract motility. The intent of the massage session was to provide a relaxing and soothing experience. Consequently, the massage was conducted with reduced lighting and soothing music.

Baseline session

The evening prior to the first session, subjects were contacted by phone and reminded to refrain from caffeine, nicotine, alcohol, or cold medications on the morning of the massage appointment. Subjects were scheduled between 9 am and 11 am to control for circadian rhythm variations. Upon arrival at the clinic for the first session, the SCI subjects and a healthy control were asked to provide a blood sample and complete the FIM, POMS, and SIGH evaluations. The SCI participants then received their standardized 45 minute massage. Control subjects were debriefed and dismissed from the study.

Massage therapy sessions

SCI subjects received massages three times per week for 60 minutes each session, for four consecutive weeks. Massage session time did not include dressing or transferring time. While the initial massage took place in the morning, each subsequent session occurred at a convenient time for the participant. The subjects were scheduled with either a licensed massage therapist or a student who was in the advanced stages of training (completing residence training). The principle investigator and the clinical massage instructor supervised the massage therapy sessions. To reduce the influence of a single individual's response to a specific massage practitioner, subjects were randomly assigned to a massage therapist. Massage therapists were rotated among the participants. The massage therapists were blind to the study's outcome measures.

RESEARCH FINDINGS

General immunological findings with individuals with spinal cord injuries

In comparing the individuals with SCI with the healthy controls, immunological data analysis provided us with a greater understanding of the differences which persist in individuals with SCI. Analysis of the SIGH identified that the SCI population experienced significantly more incidents of urinary tract infections, respiratory tract infections, and pressure ulcers, $F [1, 43] = 21.54$, $p = 0.001$, $F [1, 43] = 12.50$, $p = 0.001$, and $F [1, 43] = 13.52$, $p = 0.001$, respectively. Means and standard deviations are presented in Table 6.2. No other areas identified by the SIGH were significantly different between the SCI and control group. The spinal cord-injured participants had significantly lower FIM scores than the control group, $F [1, 43] = 13.43$, $p = 0.001$. The differences in FIM scores were due to difficulties with mobility in the community and decreased independence in activities of daily living.

Differences seen on the lymphocyte subsets included a significantly lower percentage of NK cells seen in the SCI groups compared with the controls, $F [1, 43] = 16.10$, $p \geq 0.001$; as well as a significantly lower percentage of

Table 6.2 Immune changes over the course of the month-long massage period

Measure	Baseline Mean (SD)	Post-massage Mean (SD)	N
% NK cells[a]			
Controls	16.47 (1.23)		15
Paraplegic	15.35 (1.32)[b]	19.62 (1.19)	17
Tetraplegic	10.60 (1.52)[c]	14.26 (1.07)[c]	12
% CD3+ T cells[a]			
Controls	74.15 (0.90)		15
Paraplegic	76.49 (1.20)[b]	82.49 (1.42)	17
Tetraplegic	65.80 (0.70)[c]	79.35 (0.85)[c]	12
% CD4+ T cells[a]			
Controls	50.59 (1.24)		15
Paraplegic	40.70 (1.28)[b]	45.31 (0.83)	17
Tetraplegic	29.60 (0.94)[c]	34.58 (0.75)[c]	12
% CD8+ T cells[a]			
Controls	24.16 (1.04)		15
Paraplegic	26.80 (1.14)	32.85 (0.82)	17
Tetraplegic	22.61 (1.22)	28.23 (1.01)[c]	12
Mean % WB NK cytotoxicity ± SEM (E:T ratio 10:1)[a]			
Controls	70.54 (11.68)		15
Paraplegic	60.24 (9.22)	70.53 (8.07)	17
Tetraplegic	44.90 (7.37)	58.45 (8.27)	12
Lymphocyte proliferation			
Controls	0.2245 (0.03)		15
Paraplegic	0.1656 (0.04)[b]	0.2190 (0.03)[a]	17
Tetraplegic	0.1437 (0.03)[b]	0.2258 (0.06)[a]	12
sIL-2R levels			
Controls	654.33 (251.16)		15
Paraplegic	1428.82 (633.09)[b]	1499.64 (875.57)[a]	17
Tetraplegic	2090.08 (690.03)[c]	1323.58 (509.61)[ac]	12
CAMP			
Controls	624.67 (475.92)		15
Paraplegic	3037.07 (282.13)[b]	1881.93 (697.48)[a]	17
Tetraplegic	4005.92 (500.97)[b]	1473.33 (626.49)[a]	12
Cortisol			
Controls	9.34 (4.74)		15
Paraplegic	12.36 (3.12)	8.91 (4.68)[a]	17
Tetraplegic	13.62 (4.38)[b]	11.17 (3.19)[a]	12

[a]Baseline to post-massage condition significant at 0.001.
[b]Significantly different from controls $p \geqslant 0.01$.
[c]Significantly different from controls and/or paraplegic group $p \geqslant 0.01$. WB NK = (E:T ration at 10:1) whole blood natural killer.

CD4+ T-helper cells compared with controls, $F [1, 43] = 261.37$, $p \geqslant 0.001$. A significantly higher percentage of CD3+ T-cells for the SCI groups compared with the control group $F [1, 43] = 5.37$, $p = 0.027$. On the cellular immune measures taken at baseline, the SCI group showed a significantly higher sIL-2R levels than the control group, F [1, 43] = 19.65, $p \geq 0.001$. The SCI groups also displayed significantly higher levels of cortisol than controls, F [1, 43] = 4.64, $p = 0.04$. Furthermore, the SCI groups had significantly higher levels of cAMP when compared with the controls F [1, 43] = 47.18, $p \geq 0.001$, and significantly lower lymphocyte proliferation verses the controls F [1, 43] = 24.48, $p \leq 0.001$. (Fig. 6.2).

The baseline NK assay showed that both paraplegic and tetraplegic subjects showed significantly lower cytotoxicity than the healthy controls, F [2, 42] = 5.52, $p \leq 0.001$, at all four effector to target ratios. Post hoc analysis revealed that the tetraplegic group had significantly lower levels of cytotoxicity when compared with the individuals with paraplegia (Fig. 6.3).

Comparison of tetraplegic subjects to paraplegic subjects following massage intervention

Here we analyzed the data for significant effects of the massage treatment condition between baseline, treatment and follow-up, as well as for differences between tetra- and paraplegia. The means and standard deviations

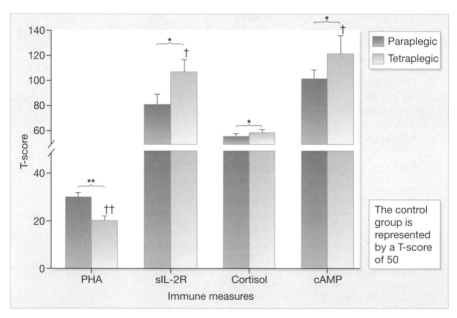

Figure 6.2 Baseline comparison of tetra- and paraplegic participants across immune measures. The control group is represented by a score of 50, indicated by the horizontal bar. Individuals with SCI had significantly higher (*) cAMP, sIL-2R, cortisol levels, and significantly lower (**) levels of lymphocyte proliferation, when compared with healthy controls. Individuals with tetraplegia had significantly lower (††) lymphocyte proliferation, and higher (†) cAMP and (†) sIL-2R but not cortisol levels when compared with paraplegic participants.

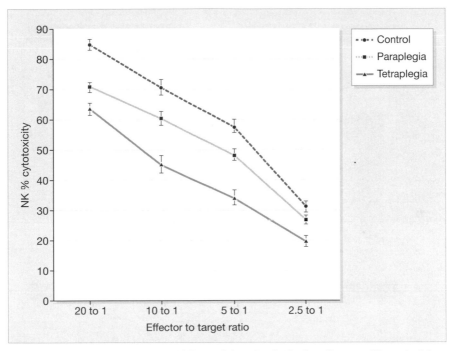

Figure 6.3 Comparison of natural killer cell function in the baseline condition, at all four effector to target ratios, individuals with SCI in either the paraplegia or tetraplegic group are significantly lower than healthy controls.

for the immune measures at baseline and in the post-massage condition are displayed in Table 6.2. Changes identified on lymphocyte subsets included a significant increase in the percentage of NK cells seen following massage in the SCI group when compared with baseline, F [1, 28] = 107.78, $p \geq 0.001$; as well as a significant increased percentage of CD4+ T-helper cells, F [1, 28] = 85.54, $p \geq 0.001$, and CD3+ T-cells, F [2, 30] = 25.76, p ≥ 0.001. Tetraplegic participants were also significantly different than controls and paraplegics on CD8+ subsets, F [1, 28] = 54.60, $p = 0.001$. Means for all the lymphocyte populations returned to baseline levels, yielding no significant differences by post hoc analysis between the post-treatment and baseline conditions.

The effects of the month-long intervention on cellular immune measures are presented in Figure 6.4. Cyclic AMP levels were significantly decreased after the month of massage and the no-treatment condition, F [1, 28] = 48.55, $p = 0.001$, for both groups. Additionally, the tetraplegic subjects showed significantly different levels of cAMP at baseline and post-massage when compared with the paraplegic subjects. The levels of cAMP between post-massage and non-treatment were not significantly different,

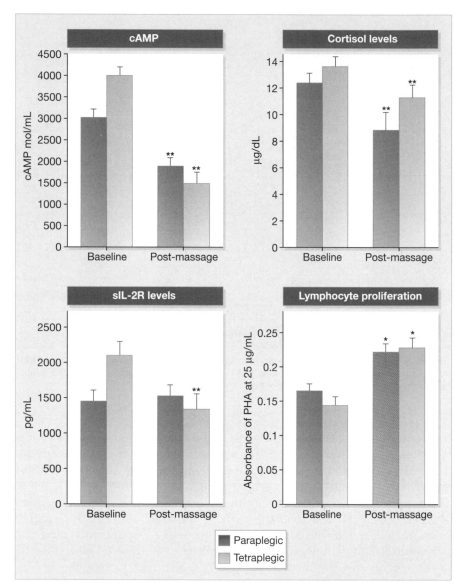

Figure 6.4 Comparison of the SCI groups, paraplegic and tetraplegic participants at the post-massage time point. Both groups of SCI participants showed significantly lower (**) levels of cAMP and cortisol at the post-massage time point. Individuals with tetraplegia also showed a significant reduction (**) of sIL-2R levels that the paraplegic subjects did not show. Both groups also showed a significant improvement (*) of lymphocyte proliferation to PHA at the 25 μg/ml dose.

although the levels measured at non-treatment appeared to be returning to baseline levels.

SIL-2R levels show a significant decrease during the massage intervention for the tetraplegic but not the paraplegic subjects, $F[1, 28] = 10.55$, $p = 0.003$.

Panel C of Figure 6.4 displays the changes in blood cortisol level over the three samples. Cortisol levels decreased significantly from the baseline measure to the post treatment measure, $F[1, 28] = 11.96$, $p = 0.002$, of both subject groups. No differences were seen between groups at either condition. After the month of no treatment, cortisol levels were higher than both post-massage and baseline but not significantly so.

In panel D of Figure 6.4, lymphocyte proliferation to PHA at the 25 µg/ml dose increased significantly after the month of massage, $F[1, 28] = 33.18$, $p \le 0.001$, when compared with baseline. Again there were no differences between subject groups by condition. Post-hoc revealed no significant differences between proliferation levels from baseline and post-no treatment condition.

In Figure 6.5, panel B, shows the change in NK cytotoxicity following the massage protocol for both the paraplegic and tetraplegic subjects.

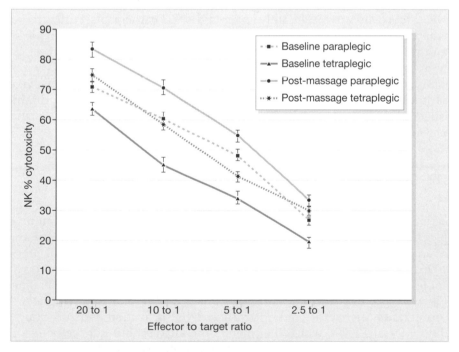

Figure 6.5 Comparison of paraplegic or tetraplegic groups following the massage protocol also show a significant increase of cytotoxicity at all four effector to target ratios following massage.

There is a significant increase in cytotoxicity in both SCI groups following the massage intervention at all four effector to target ratios. There were no differences between the paraplegic or tetraplegic groups on the post-massage condition.

Psychological profile and benefits of massage

The profile of mood states showed significant differences between the experimental and control groups on the axes of anger-hostility and vigor-activity. The SCI group had significantly lower anger-hostility scores with a mean 6.59 (s.d. = 2.62) compared with the control group with a mean of 11.73 (s.d. = 5.02), F [1, 43] = 13.67, $p = 0.001$. Additionally, the SCI group had a higher vigor-activity score with a mean of 22.88 (s.d. = 3.22) while the control group had a mean of 18.80 (s.d. = 6.12), $F = 5.77$, $p = 0.023$ (Fig. 6.6).

In summary, the cellular immune responses and neuroendocrine functioning showed that the SCI participants displayed diminished proliferative responses to PHA, and higher soluble IL-2 receptor (sIL-2R) levels, plasma cortisol levels and plasma cAMP levels when compared with healthy controls (Fig. 6.3). Quantitative measures of T cells demonstrated differences in CD3+, CD4+, and NK cells (Table 6.2). Additionally NK cytotoxicity was significantly lower in the SCI participants. Furthermore, when SCI participants were divided into either paraplegic or tetraplegic groups, the individuals in the tetraplegic group were significantly lower on lymphocyte proliferation, NK cytotoxicity, sIL-2 and cAMP levels when compared with the paraplegic group (Figs 6.3 and 6.4). The massage protocol was associated with enhanced proliferative responses, diminished soluble IL-2 receptor (sIL-2R) levels, plasma cortisol levels and plasma cAMP levels.

DISCUSSION

These results demonstrate that even fit, psychologically healthy, sports-active individuals with SCI have persistent alterations in immune function, which is consistent with other reports of cellular immune dysregulation following SCI (Campagnolo et al., 1999; Cruse et al., 1993, 1996a; Schmid et al., 1998; Wang, 1999). The elevations in cAMP and cortisol levels in the SCI group suggest chronic activation of sympathetic tone. Likewise the high levels of sIL-2R, cortisol, cAMP and low lymphocyte proliferation are consistent with chronic t-cell activation and sub-clinical illness (Nash, 2000), which the phenotypic analysis but not the hematology panels support. The SCI subjects had been screened to be otherwise healthy and at least based on self-report there was no overt evidence for higher levels of infectious illnesses during the preceding two months.

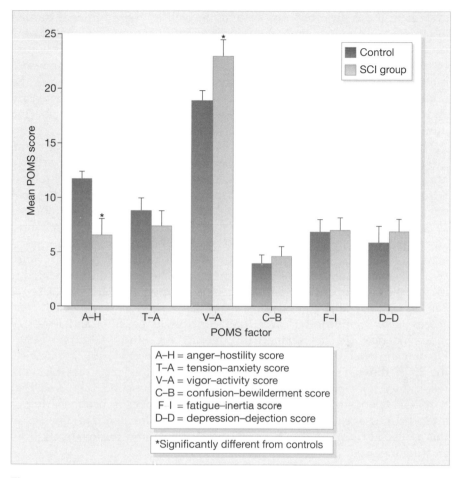

Figure 6.6 Mean scores on the profile of mood states (POMS) (+SE) for controls and SCI group. Individuals with SCI scored significantly different (*) from healthy controls.

It is notable that the majority of the participants in this study were several years post-injury, suggesting that alterations in the immune profile can persist for long periods following the injury.

It is known that lymphocytes and monocytes will respond more poorly in vitro to interleukin and interferon stimulation, which may be associated with the increased cytokine activity in vivo (Esterling et al., 1996). Higher cortisol levels and dysregulation of immune function is routinely demonstrated in chronic stress conditions, supporting the notion that SCI can be equated to a chronic stress condition (Cruse et al., 1996a; Kliesch et al., 1996; Pariante et al., 1997). Disruption of the autonomic pathways and the subsequent loss of afferent signals from the peripheral sympathetic nervous system to the central nervous system, as well as the additional burden of stress, could reduce the volume or intensity of immune signals to the central nervous system resulting in persistent immune alterations (Cruse et al., 2000). The immune alterations identified by this study represent multiple immune compartments; consequently this study supports the notion that SCI creates immune alterations by influencing the intensity and localization of immune responses versus influencing any specific immune component (Nash, 2000).

The psychological health of the SCI group is striking. Despite the group's spinal cord injuries, SCI subjects scored higher on vigor-activity and lower on anger-hostility than matched controls on the POMS (otherwise their scores were comparable). This contrasts with other studies that suggest that SCI increases vulnerability to depression which persists several years post-injury (Daverat et al., 1995). The key question remains: Are psychologically fit people with SCI more likely to participate in sports activity or does higher activity lead to psychological health in SCI? Since psychological health, fitness, and immune function are all inter-related it is difficult to tease out cause from effect (Cacioppo et al., 1998a; Glaser & Kiecolt-Glaser, 1997; Kiecolt-Glaser & Glaser, 1995). As expected, FIM scores were significantly lower than controls at baseline and levels of independence did not change throughout the study (Ditunno, 1997; Heinemann et al., 1995; Lu & Yarkony, 1996; Saboe et al., 1997). Likewise, the SIGH showed significantly higher incidences of urinary tract infection, respiratory tract infections and pressure ulcers at baseline. It is likely that the SIGH is not sufficiently sensitive to detect changes in health during or after the massage intervention because of the low incidence of illnesses in this unusually healthy group of SCI participants and the relatively brief treatment period.

Massage may be an effective tool to improve cellular immune responses in some individuals with chronic spinal cord injury, as is the case with HIV+ gay men (Ironson et al., 1996). Given that the massage protocol robustly improved the cellular immune responses in an unusually healthy sports active SCI population it would be important to study the effects on a more typical SCI population. Utilizing massage as a modality prior to purposeful activity or done by a massage therapist in conjunction with other therapies may decrease susceptibility to common illnesses associated with SCI. Massage may also lessen negative emotions, which can interfere with treatment. Massage may help to ready a patient for therapy, increasing his or her emotional and physical ability to participate fully.

Questions that must be answered before massage becomes standard therapy in SCI treatment include the required intensity and duration of treatment needed to produce a benefit and the cost-effectiveness of this treatment. Unfortunately, the immunological benefits of massage appear to be short-lived, with most gains reversed four weeks following the cessation of treatment.

Informal reports from the participants showed excitement over the individual benefits massage had for them during the course of this study. SCI participants began to spontaneously offer reports of improvement during the course of the protocol. These comments, which can only be considered anecdotal, are none the less intriguing. Twelve subjects reported decreased pain at the level of injury and one subject reported being pain-free for the first time since his injury three years ago. Five participants noted an increased feeling of circulation in their legs, which was confirmed by therapist reports of increased warmth and color in the lower extremities of these subjects. Three patients noted that their range of sensation had broadened, seven reported less spasticity, and eight reported sleeping better as a result of reduced spasticity and/or pain. A more rigorous trial would be needed to confirm these findings and attribute them to massage as opposed to suggestion or placebo effects.

Limitations

Because the SCI participants in these studies were all willing, highly motivated, sports-active individuals, it is difficult to generalize these results to the wider SCI population. However, the fact that these otherwise healthy and active individuals with SCI had immune dysfunction that resembled that of more typical SCI survivors, and that they responded to massage suggests that the general SCI population might show the same response. Because the design of this study did not include a group that received similar social and personal attention, one cannot exclude social support as the critical factor affecting immunologic change. Finally, this study did not explore the physiologic mechanisms that cause improved immunologic profiles nor was it demonstrated that massage actually led to improved function or decreased morbidity in SCI. These important questions await further large-scale investigations.

CONCLUSIONS

One could predict the implications for improved health and wellness of individuals with SCI would be substantial, including shorter lengths of stay in rehabilitation programs or hospital settings, improved wound healing, fewer respiratory illnesses, fewer urinary tract infections, and a more swift transition to productive work. Research is critical in order to provide the evidential data needed to verify complementary rehabilitation modalities as a rational alternative to traditional rehabilitation medicine. Many treatment techniques theoretically foster a reduction in sympathetic tone through their influence of the central nervous systems to allow for a greater impact of the specific treatment.

If one accepts this, then we should be able to see this change as a reduction in physiological reactivity and measure this change through physiological systems. Consequently, we should have a way to more directly evaluate central nervous system activity. Physiological measures have the potential to more directly measure underlying sympathetic tone, and are relatively noninvasive and easily measured. One of the ways to document the impact of rehabilitation is to have accurate ways for measuring the connection between nervous system activity and changes in physiological and psychological conditions. Development of immunological and physiological measures may guide therapeutic intervention and allow better prediction of which treatment modalities will be most effective in producing change. The findings of this project will provide us with information about how massage influences the health and wellness of a patient population frequently seen in rehabilitation.

REFERENCES

Burleson, M. H., Malarkey, W. B., Cacioppo, J. T., et al. (1998). Postmenopausal hormone replacement: effects on autonomic, neuroendocrine, and immune reactivity to brief psychological stressors. *Psychosomatic Medicine, 60*(1), 17–25.

Cacioppo, J. T., Berntson, G. G., Malarkey, W. B., et al. (1998a). Autonomic, neuroendocrine, and immune responses to psychological stress: the reactivity hypothesis. *Annals of the New York Academy of Sciences, 840*(May 1), 664–673.

Cacioppo, J. T., Poehlmann, K. M., Kiecolt-Glaser, J., et al. (1998b). Cellular immune responses to acute stress in female caregivers of dementia patients and matched controls. *Health Psychology, 17*(Mar), 182–189.

Campagnolo, D., Bartlett, J., Chatterton, R. J., & Keller, S. (1999). Adrenal and pituitary hormone patterns after spinal cord injury. *American Journal of Physical Medicine and Rehabilitation, 78*(Jul–Aug), 361–366.

Coe, C. L. (1993). Social stressors and immune function. *Psychosomatic Medicine, 55,* 298–308.

Cruse, J., & Lewis, R. (1997). Immunologic renaissance in the 21st century. *Immunologic Research, 16*(Feb), 1–2.

Cruse, J. M., Keith, J. C., Bryant, M. L., & Lewis, R. E. (1996a). Immune system-neuroendocrine dysregulation in spinal cord injury. *Immunologic Research, 15*(4), 306–314.

Cruse, J. M., Lewis, R., Bishop, G., et al. (1992). Neuroendocrine-immune interactions associated with loss and restoration of immune system function in spinal cord injury and stroke patients. *Immunologic Research, 11*(2), 104–116.

Cruse, J. M., & Lewis, R. E. (1989). Immunologic equinox — between two centuries. *Year in Immunology, 4,* 1–22.

Cruse, J. M., Lewis, R. E., Bishop, G. R., et al. (1993). Decreased immune reactivity and neuroendocrine alterations related to chronic stress in spinal cord injury and stroke patients. *Pathobiology, 61*(3–4), 183–192.

Cruse, J. M., Lewis, R. E., Bishop, G. R., et al. (1996b). Adhesion molecules and wound healing in spinal cord injury. *Pathobiology, 64,* 193–197.

Cruse, J. M., Lewis, R. E., Roe, D. L., et al. (2000). Facilitation of immune function, healing of pressure ulcers, and nutritional status in spinal cord injury patients. *Experimental and Molecular Pathology, 68,* 38–54.

Daverat, P., Petit, H., Kemoun, G., et al. (1995). The long term outcome in 149 patients with spinal cord injury. *Paraplegia, 33*(11), 665–668.

Deutsch, A., Braun, S., & Granger, C. (1996). The functional independence measure (FIM) and the functional independence measure for children (WeeFIM). *Critical Reviews in Physical and Rehabilitation Medicine, 8*(4), 267–281.

Dhabhar, F. S., & McEwen, B. S. (1997). Acute stress enhances while chronic stress suppresses cell-mediated immunity in vivo: A potential role for leukocyte trafficking. *Brain, Behavior, & Immunity, 11,* 286–306.

Ditunno, J. F., Jr. (1997). Functional outcomes in spinal cord injury (SCI): quality care versus cost containment. *Journal of Spinal Cord Medicine, 20*(1), 1–7.

Dura, J. R., Stukenberg, K. W., & Kiecolt-Glaser, J. K. (1990). Chronic stress and depressive disorders in older adults. *Journal of Abnormal Psychology, 99*(3), 284–290.

Eastwood, E. A., Hagglund, K. J., Ragnarsson, K. T., et al. (1999). Medical rehabilitation length of stay and outcomes for persons with traumatic spinal cord injury. *Archives of Physical Medicine and Rehabilitation, 80,* 1457–1463.

Eisenberg, D., Davis, R., Ettner, S., et al. (1998). Trends in alternative medicine use in the United States, 1990–1997: Results of a follow-up national survey. *JAMA, 280*(Nov 11), 1569–1575.

Esterling, B. A., Kiecolt-Glaser, J. K., Bodnar, J. C., & Glaser, R. (1994). Chronic stress, social support, and persistent alterations in the natural killer cell response to cytokines in older adults. *Health Psychology, 13*(4), 291–298.

Esterling, B. A., Kiecolt-Glaser, J. K., & Glaser, R. (1996). Psychosocial modulation of cytokine-induced natural killer cell activity in older adults. *Psychosomatic Medicine, 58*(3), 264–272.

Field, T. M. (1995). Massage therapy for infants and children. *Journal of Developmental & Behavioral Pediatrics, 16*(2), 105–111.

Field, T. M., Estroff, D. B., Yando, R., et al. (1996a). 'Depressed' mothers' perceptions of infant vulnerability are related to later development. *Child Psychiatry & Human Development, 27*(1), 43–53.

Field, T. M., Grizzle, N., Scafidi, F., & Schanberg, S. (1996b). Massage and relaxation therapies' effects on depressed adolescent mothers. *Adolescence, 31*(124), 903–911.

Field, T. M., Henteleff, T., Hernandez-Reif, M., et al. (1998a). Children with asthma have improved pulmonary functions after massage therapy. *Journal of Pediatrics, 132*(5), 854–858.

Field, T. M., Hernandez-Reif, M., Seligman, S., et al. (1997a). Juvenile rheumatoid arthritis: benefits from massage therapy. *Journal of Pediatric Psychology, 22*(5), 607–617.

Field, T. M., Ironson, G., Scafidi, F., et al. (1996c). Massage therapy reduces anxiety and enhances EEG pattern of alertness and math computations. *International Journal of Neuroscience, 86*(3–4), 197–205.

Field, T. M., Lasko, D., Mundy, P., et al. (1997b). Brief report: autistic children's attentiveness and responsivity improve after touch therapy. *Journal of Autism & Developmental Disorders, 27*(3), 333–338.

Field, T. M., Quintino, O., Hernandez-Reif, M., & Koslovsky, G. (1998b). Adolescents with attention deficit hyperactivity disorder benefit from massage therapy. *Adolescence, 33*(129), 103–108.

Fleming, I., Baum, A., Davidson, L. M., et al. (1987). Chronic stress as a factor in physiologic reactivity to challenge. *Health Psychology, 6,* 221–237.

Fletcher, R. H., & Fletcher, S. W. (1997). Evidence-based approach to medical literature. *Journal of General Internal Medicine, 12*(Suppl.), s5–s12.

Fritz, S. (1999). *Mosby's Fundamentals of Therapeutic Massage* 2nd ed. St. Louis, MO: Mosby-Year Book.

Glaser, R., Kennedy, S., Lafuse, W. P., et al. (1990). Psychological stress-induced modulation of interleukin 2 receptor gene expression and interleukin 2 production in peripheral blood leukocytes. *Archives of General Psychiatry, 47*(8), 707–712.

Glaser, R., & Kiecolt-Glaser, J. (1998). Stress-associated immune modulation: relevance to viral infections and chronic fatigue syndrome. *American Journal of Medicine, 105,* 35S–42S.

Glaser, R., & Kiecolt-Glaser, J. K. (1997). Chronic stress modulates the virus-specific immune response to latent herpes simplex virus type 1. *Annals of Behavioral Medicine, 19,* 78–82.

Glaser, R., Kiecolt-Glaser, J. K., Malarkey, W. B., & Sheridan, J. F. (1998). The influence of psychological stress on the immune response to vaccines. *Annals of the New York Academy of Sciences, 840,* 649–655.

Glaser, R., Kiecolt-Glaser, J. K., Marucha, P. T., et al. (1999a). Stress-related changes in proinflammatory cytokine production in wounds. *Archives of General Psychiatry, 56,* 450–456.

Glaser, R., Rabin, B., Chesney, M., et al. (1999b). Stress-induced immunomodulation: implications for infectious diseases? *Journal of the American Medical Association, 281,* 2268–2270.

Goats, G. (1994). Massage — the scientific basis of an ancient art: Part 1. The techniques. *British Journal of Sports Medicine, 28*(Sep), 149–152.

Heinemann, A. W., Hamilton, B., Linacre, J. M., et al. (1995). Functional status and therapeutic intensity during inpatient rehabilitation. *American Journal of Physical Medicine & Rehabilitation, 74*(4), 315–326.

Heinemann, A. W., Kirk, P., Hastie, B. A., et al. (1997). Relationships between disability measures and nursing effort during medical rehabilitation for patients with traumatic brain and spinal cord injury. *Archives of Physical Medicine & Rehabilitation, 78*(2), 143–149.

Ironson, G., Field, T., Scafidi, F., et al. (1996). Massage therapy is associated with enhancement of the immune system's cytotoxic capacity. *International Journal of Neuroscience, 84*(1–4), 205–217.

Irwin, M., Daniels, M., Bloom, E. T., et al. (1987). Life events, depressive symptoms, and immune function. *American Journal of Psychiatry, 144*(4), 437–441.

Kang, D. H., Coe, C. L., McCarthy, D. O., & Ershler, W. B. (1997). Immune responses to final exams in healthy and asthmatic adolescents. *Nursing Research, 46*(1), 12–19.

Kang, D. H., Davidson, R. J., Coe, C. L., et al. (1991). Frontal brain asymmetry and immune function. *Behavioral Neuroscience, 105*(6), 860–869.

Kiecolt-Glaser, J. K., Dura, J. R., Speicher, C. E., et al. (1991). Spousal caregivers of dementia victims: longitudinal changes in immunity and health. *Psychosomatic Medicine, 53*(4), 345–362.

Kiecolt-Glaser, J. K., & Glaser, R. (1995). Psychoneuroimmunology and health consequences: data and shared mechanisms. *Psychosomatic Medicine, 57*(3), 269–274.

Kiecolt-Glaser, J. K., Glaser, R., Cacioppo, J. T., & Malarkey, W. B. (1998). Marital stress: immunologic, neuroendocrine, and autonomic correlates. *Annals of the New York Academy of Sciences, 840*(May 1), 656–663.

Kiecolt-Glaser, J. K., Glaser, R., Gravenstein, S., et al. (1996). Chronic stress alters the immune response to influenza virus vaccine in older adults. *Proceedings of the National Academy of Sciences, 93*(7), 3043–3047.

Kiecolt-Glaser, J. K., Marucha, P. T., Malarkey, W. B., et al. (1995). Slowing of wound healing by psychological stress. *Lancet, 346*(8984), 1194–1196.

Kliesch, W. F., Cruse, J. M., Lewis, R. E., et al. (1996). Restoration of depressed immune function in spinal cord injury patients receiving rehabilitation therapy. *Paraplegia, 34*(2), 82–90.

Lang, C., Field, T., Pickens, J., Martinez, A., et al. (1996). Preschoolers of dysphoric mothers. *Journal of Child Psychology & Psychiatry & Allied Disciplines, 37*(2), 221–224.

Lu, A. C., & Yarkony, G. M. (1996). Benefits of rehabilitation for traumatic spinal cord injury: a case report. *Journal of Spinal Cord Medicine, 19*(1), 17–19.

MacHale, S. M., O'Rourke, S. J., Wardlaw, J. M., & Dennis, M. S. (1998). Depression and its relation to lesion location after stroke. *Journal of Neurology, Neurosurgery & Psychiatry, 64*(3), 371–374.

McNair, D. M., Lorr, M., & Droppleman, L. F. (1992). *Profile of Mood States, Revised (POMS)* Revised ed. San Diego, CA: EdITS.

Nash, M. S. (2000). Known and plausible modulators of depressed immune functions following spinal cord injuries. *The Journal of Spinal Cord Medicine, 23*(4), 111–119.

National Spinal Cord Injury Statistical Center (2000). *Spinal cord injury factsheet* (Report). Birmingham: University of Birmingham.

Ota, T., Akaboshi, K., Nagata, M., et al. (1996). Functional assessment of patients with spinal cord injury: measured by the motor score and the Functional Independence Measure. *Spinal Cord, 34*(9), 531–535.

Ottenbacher, K. J., & Maas, F. (1999). How to detect effects: Statistical power and evidence-based practice in occupational therapy research. *American Journal of Occupational Therapy, 53*(2), 181–188.

Pariante, C. M., Carpiniello, B., Orru, M. G., et al. (1997). Chronic caregiving stress alters peripheral blood immune parameters: The role of age and severity of stress. *Psychotherapy and Psychosomatics, 66*, 199–207.

Pike, J. L., Smith, T. L., Hauger, R. L., et al. (1997). Chronic life stress alters sympathetic, neuroendocrine, and immune responsivity to an acute psychological stressor in humans. *Psychosomatic Medicine, 59*, 447–457.

Prodromidis, M., Field, T., Arendt, R., et al. (1995). Mothers touching newborns: a comparison of rooming-in versus minimal contact. *Birth, 22*(4), 196–200; discussion 201–203.

Rabin, B. S. (1999). *Stress, immune function and health: The connection.* New York, NY: Wiley-Liss.

Saboe, L. A., Darrah, J. M., Pain, K. S., & Guthrie, J. (1997). Early predictors of functional independence 2 years after spinal cord injury. *Archives of Physical Medicine & Rehabilitation, 78*(6), 644–650.

Scafidi, F., & Field, T. (1996). Massage therapy improves behavior in neonates born to HIV-positive mothers. *Journal of Pediatric Psychology, 21*(6), 889–897.

Scafidi, F., & Field, T. (1997). Brief report: HIV-exposed newborns show inferior orienting and abnormal reflexes on the Brazelton Scale. *Journal of Pediatric Psychology, 22*(1), 105–112.

Scafidi, F. A., Field, T., Prodromidis, M., & Rahdert, E. (1997). Psychosocial stressors of drug-abusing disadvantaged adolescent mothers. *Adolescence, 32*(125), 93–100.

Scafidi, F. A., Field, T. M., Wheeden, A., et al. (1996). Cocaine-exposed preterm neonates show behavioral and hormonal differences. *Pediatrics, 97*(6 Pt 1), 851–855.

Schmid, A., Huonker, M., Stahl, F., et al. (1998). Free plasma catecholamines in spinal cord injured persons with different injury levels at rest and during exercise. *Journal of Autonomic Nervous System, 68*, 96–100.

Smith, R. R., Clower, B. R., Cruse, J. M., et al. (1987). Constrictive structural elements in human cerebral arteries following aneurysmal subarachnoid haemorrhage. *Neurological Research, 9*(3), 188–192.

Strauman, T. J., Lemieux, A. M., & Coe, C. L. (1993). Self-discrepancy and natural killer cell activity: immunological consequences of negative self-evaluation. *Journal of Personality & Social Psychology, 64*(6), 1042–1052.

Tappan, F. M., & Benjamin, P. J. (1997). *Tappan's Handbook of Healing Massage Techniques: Classic, Holistic and Emerging Methods* 3rd ed. Upper Saddle, NJ: Prentice Hall.

Uchino, B. N., Kiecolt-Glaser, J. K., & Cacioppo, J. T. (1992). Age-related changes in cardiovascular response as a function of a chronic stressor and social support. *Journal of Personality & Social Psychology, 63*(5), 839–846.

Wang, Y. H. (1999). Impaired adrenal reserve in men with spinal cord injury: Results of low- and high-dose adrenocorticotropin stimulation tests. *Archives of Physical Medicine and Rehabilitation, 80*, 863–866.

Watkins, A. (Ed.). (1997). *Mind-body medicine: a clinician's guide to psychoneuroimmunology.* New York: Churchill Livingstone.

Watkins, L. R., & Maier, S. F. (1999). Implications of immune-to-brain communication for sickness and pain. *Proceedings of the National Academy of Science, 96*(Jul 6), 7710–7713.

Watson, A. H., Kanny, E. M., White, D. M., & Anson, D. K. (1995). Use of standardized activities of daily living rating scales in spinal cord injury and disease services. *American Journal of Occupational Therapy, 49*(3), 229–234.

Wheeden, A., Scafidi, F. A., Field, T., et al. (1993). Massage effects on cocaine-exposed preterm neonates. *Journal of Developmental & Behavioral Pediatrics, 14*(5), 318–322.

Whiteneck, G. G., Charlifue, S. W., & Frankel, H. L. (1992). Mortality, morbidity, and psychosocial outcomes of persons spinal cord injuried more than 10 years ago. *Paraplegia, 30*, 617–630.

Wu, H., Wang, J., Cacioppo, J., et al. (1999). Chronic stress associated with spousal caregiving of patients with Alzheimer's dementia is associated with downregulation of B-lymphocyte GH mRNA. *Journals of Gerontology, Biological Sciences and Medical, 54*, M212–215.

Massage across the life-span

SECTION CONTENTS

INTRODUCTION TO SECTION 3

Developmental psychologists have established an extensive set of empirical studies demonstrating the physical, intellectual, personality, and social changes that occur as people develop from infancy through old age (Papalia & Olds, 1995). This 'cradle to grave' approach to development indicates that perhaps massage therapy will have different applications and different effects depending upon to which age group it is applied.

As usual, Tiffany Field at the Touch Research Institute has been a leader in the relevant research literature. Trained as a developmental psychologist, Field is keenly aware of developmental issues, and her studies have frequently focused on the use and impact of massage therapy for one age group or another (Field, 2000). For instance, Field has examined the effects of massage, or 'tactile-kinesthetic stimulation,' on preterm infants, on other high risk infants, such as cocaine-exposed and HIV-exposed infants, and on 'normal' infants. She has examined massage for labor in childbirth as well. In a fascinating study, she examined the impact of massage as an intervention for post-traumatic stress in children following Hurricane Andrew. In children and adolescents she has examined the utility of massage for other conditions, such as attention deficit hyperactivity disorder. In adolescents she has found beneficial effects of massage for clients with depression, and for teenagers with eating disorders such as anorexia and bulimia. In adults, she has examined massage therapy as a useful procedure for such populations as breast cancer patients and HIV positive adults. Finally, with the elderly, Field has found beneficial effects for elder volunteer lay massage therapists (mean age = 70) who gave massages to infants (Field, 2000). Clearly massage therapy is a procedure which has beneficial effects across the lifespan, though how and why it is used changes as a person ages.

The following two chapters examine two 'endpoints' in the lifespan. Dieter and Emory examine touch therapy for preterm infants, reviewing much of Field's seminal work in the area. Remington examines hand massage as an intervention for the agitated elderly in nursing home residents with dementia. Using an easy to administer 10-minute (five minutes for each hand) massage, Remington finds a decrease in agitation in comparison to a control group. The author notes that agitation is a common problem in nursing homes, impacting between 64% and 93% of residents. Her work suggests that her intervention may be useful for other types of people with agitation problems, such as AIDS dementia and brain injury patients, but further research will need to examine these hypotheses in detail. Her work also makes an interesting comparison to calming music interventions, which also appear to reduce agitation. Future studies, using other outcome variables such as anxiety, depression, and cognitive efficacy measures, may point to differences in efficacy in the two types of treatments that were not apparent in the present study.

Since studies indicate that people over age 85 are one of the fastest growing demographics in the United States (Papalia & Olds, 1995), there will be an increase in demand for quality research on this age group. Much research indicates that many elderly are likely to suffer from chronic ailments, such as hypertension and diabetes (Taylor, 1999). Depression is also common among the elderly, and elderly men over the age of 85 have one of the highest rates of suicide (Papalia & Olds, 1995). While massage therapy is not a cure-all, already studies exist which show some positive effects for massage on glucose levels in children with diabetes (Field, 2000), and for mood in the elderly (Field, 2000). Some research indicates massage therapy may be useful for cardiac and hypertensive patients (Yates, 1999). Of course, future research should examine massage therapy for elderly populations in a systematic manner. Much anecdotal evidence from practicing clinicians suggests that effective techniques vary as clients and their bodies age. Theoretically techniques that are useful and appropriate with an adult population may be ineffective or dangerous with a pediatric or elderly population. Recent research on 'successful aging,' such as the seminal MacArthur Foundation Study of Aging in America (Rowe & Kahn, 1998), suggests that positive outcomes in late life are less determined by genetics, as was once believed, and are more influenced by lifestyle decisions regarding diet, exercise, intellectual stimulation, and social interaction. Perhaps massage therapy can become a standard component of the health intervention arsenal for the elderly. Certainly, studies with adults indicate massage therapy increases positive mood and boosts cognitive ability at least temporarily. And massage therapy is by nature a social interaction, an interaction many lonely widows and widowers lack. Future researchers and funders would be wise to consider the importance of quality research with this growing and understudied population.

REFERENCES

Field, T. (2000). *Touch therapy*. Edinburgh: Churchill Livingstone.
Papalia, D., & Olds, S. (1995). *Human development*. New York: McGraw Hill.
Rowe, J., & Kahn, R. (1998). *Successful aging*. New York: Pantheon Books.
Taylor, S. (1999). *Health psychology*. Boston: McGraw Hill.
Yates, J. (1999). *A physician's guide to therapeutic massage*. Vancouver, BC: Massage Therapists' Association of British Columbia.

7

Supplemental tactile and kinesthetic stimulation for preterm infants

John N. I. Dieter,   Eugene K. Emory

THE PROBLEM OF PREMATURITY

Prevalence and etiology

A normal course of pregnancy lasts approximately 40 weeks. Between 5% and 15% of all live births in the United States are premature (Wittenberg, 1990). Preterm deliveries are disproportionately represented among African American women. Almost 20% of all live births delivered by Black women are premature, whereas less than 9% of live White births are preterm (CDC, 1992). Furthermore, African American neonates account for 31% of all preterm infant deaths.

The etiology of prematurity is not well understood. The contributors to preterm birth are multifarious and include: fetal abnormalities, maternal illness, the mother being very young, a short interval between pregnancies, multiple births, low socioeconomic status, parental education level, maternal cigarette smoking, alcohol and illicit drug use, and number of previous pregnancies (Goldberg & Divitto, 1983; Siegel et al., 1982). In addition, Levin & DeFrank (1988) suggested that poor prenatal care and stressful life events contribute to the over representation of preterm deliveries among African American and minority women. Despite such factors, there is no readily apparent cause for 50% of premature births (Wittenberg, 1990).

The impact of prematurity on development

Modern neonatology, particularly the development of the neonatal intensive care unit (NICU), has substantially increased the survival rate of preterm infants. For infants whose gestational age is 25 weeks or more, the survival rate is between 15% and 66% (Hack & Fanaroff, 1989). The prognosis remains very poor if the infant's length of gestation is less than 24 weeks or the birthweight is less than 600 grams. Furthermore, these infants exhibit the most severe medical complications and developmental deficits (Pettett, 1986).

Over the last half century, numerous studies report that prematurity can be associated with substantial developmental impairment. Early postnatal difficulties include problems with autonomic nervous system control, behavioral state organization, and attentional regulation (Als, 1986; Doussard-Rossevelt et al., 1996). At 40 weeks post-conception, approximately 15% of preterm infants, across various gestational ages and birthweights, exhibit abnormal neurologic, motor, and cognitive functioning (Aylward et al., 1987). A wide range of long-term problems have been documented and include: delays in cross-modal transformations and auditory and visual deficits (Friedman et al., 1981; Herrgard et al., 1995; Luoma et al., 1998; Parmelee, 1985; Rose et al., 1978); motoric problems such as abnormal reflexes (Howard et al., 1976; Modanlou, 1988), hypotonia, and inferior grasping and hand use (Gorga et al., 1985, 1991; Prechtl et al., 1979; Touwen et al., 1988); cognitive deficits such as lower IQs, language and reading difficulties, and academic underachievement (Caputo & Mandell, 1970; Cohen et al., 1986; Francis-Williams & Davis, 1974; Kok et al., 1998; Lane et al., 1994; Wright, 1971), as well as emotional and behavioral problems such as hyperactivity and internalizing disorders (Chapieski & Evankovich, 1997; Rose et al., 1992; Schothorst & van Engeland, 1996). Understanding the etiology of these developmental problems has proved difficult. In many investigations, preterm infants with varying gestational ages, birthweights, and medical complications have been treated as a homogeneous group. Even when these variables are considered, it is difficult to determine to what degree factors such as the early extrauterine environment (e.g., the NICU), and subsequent family and socioeconomic factors, contribute to later developmental deficits.

Preterm infant supplemental stimulation

In an effort to compensate for environmental deprivation, or to accelerate development, researchers have provided preterm infants with various forms of supplemental stimulation. Intervention is usually directed towards only one or two of the infant's sensory systems. The major types of stimulation have included tactile (e.g., extra holding, passive touch, gentle stroking, rubbing), vestibular (e.g., spinning hammocks, rockerbeds, oscillating water-beds), kinesthetic (i.e., passive limb movements), oral (i.e., pacifiers), and auditory (e.g., recorded heartbeat, intrauterine sounds, music, maternal speech). Supplemental stimulation is generally provided several times per day, for a period or days or weeks, while the preterm infant resides in the hospital.

Although the impact that supplemental stimulation has upon long-term development has been questioned (Ferry, 1981; Russman, 1986), the inter-ventions do produce immediate and short-term benefits that include: decreased apnea, more stable behavioral state organization, increased weight gain, a decrease in abnormal reflexes, and enhanced sensory and motor performance on neurobehavioral assessments (Dieter & Emory, 1997; Field, 1980; Field, 1988; Harrison, 1985; Schaefer et al., 1980). Furthermore, supplemental stimulation has recently been shown to affect the biochem-istry of preterm infants through increases in urinary excretion of nora-drenaline (norepinephrine) and adrenaline (epinephrine), reductions in plasma cortisol levels, and increases in bone width, mineral density, and content (Acolet et al., 1993; Kuhn et al., 1991; Moyer-Mileur et al., 1995). A practical benefit reported by Field and her colleagues is that tactile/kinesthetic stimulation leads to earlier hospital discharge and a substan-tial reduction in hospital cost (Scafidi et al., 1986). Finally, supplemental stimulation of preterm infants is a salient research avenue for furthering our knowledge of the relationship between human brain plasticity and the impact of the environment on early development (Dieter & Emory, 1997).

PRETERM INFANT TACTILE AND KINESTHETIC STIMULATION

Historical perspective and the concept of maternal deprivation

It was only with the invention of the incubator, in the early part of the last century, that it became possible to save preterm infants from death by hypothermia. Prior to the 1960s, it was generally believed that preterm infants were too fragile to sustain any but minimal forms of handling (Korner, 1990). Findings from both animal studies and examinations of institutionalized children suggested that a more serious threat to preterm infants might be that their early environment is sensory deprived. Furthermore, it was this belief that precipitated the early supplemental stimulation studies (e.g., Hasselmeyer, 1964; Neal, 1968).

The argument that tactile supplemental stimulation is essential to develop-ment lies in the concept of 'maternal deprivation'. Both Ribble (1944) and Spitz (1945) found that children who were reared in orphanages, or were separated from their mothers during infancy, demonstrated profound developmental and emotional retardation that Spitz labeled 'hospitalism'. This notion of maternal deprivation contributing to developmental problems and psychopathology was widely adopted and took on near mystical nuances, especially by psychoanalytic and object relational thinkers.

The idea of providing preterm infants with supplemental tactile stimulation was borrowed from research on institutionalized full-term neonates conducted by White et al. (1964). From the sixth to the 30th day of life, nurses administered up to 20 minutes of extra holding per day. Although the treatment had little effect upon growth or health parameters, extra holding appeared to soothe the infants and facilitate visual exploration. The benefits reported were interpreted as arising from supplemented 'maternal contact'.

From research with animals, the work of Levine (1958), Harlow (1958), and to a lesser extent, Mason (1968) has been offered as support that the preterm infant's early environment is maternally deprived and might be enhanced by extra handling or rocking. More recently, a group of rodent studies undertaken by Schanberg and his colleagues attempted to reconfirm that sensory deprivation is harmful to the human preterm neonate (Pauk et al., 1986; Schanberg et al., 1984; Schanberg & Field, 1987). Furthermore, these authors concluded that the specific absence of maternal contact is the pernicious agent as demonstrated in rats by reductions in ornithine decarboxylase (ODC — a primary growth hormone and sensitive index of tissue growth and differentiation). ODC reductions, which are normally corrected by the dame rat licking her pup, were elevated through supplemental tactile stimulation (i.e., stroking the pup with a brush whose texture was similar to that of the mother's tongue). Field (1988) accepted this finding as supporting the use of massage for stimulating human preterm infants.

Research findings

'Touch Therapy' for preterm infants

Varieties of techniques have been developed to provide supplemental tactile and kinesthetic stimulation to hospitalized preterms. Most protocols reflect minor derivations of the method introduced by White & Labarba (1976). Tactile (rubbing and/or stroking) and kinesthetic (flexing and extending the limbs) stimulation are administered sequentially during a session and the procedural sequence is often quite precise. Other researchers have relied upon less intense forms of tactile stimulation such as gentle strokes (Adamson-Macedo et al., 1994) or passive touch. Passive or 'gentle human touch' (GHT) consists of laying hands upon the infant's head, lower back, and buttocks for 10 or 15 minutes at a time (Harrison et al., 1996).

The most standardized approach for massaging preterms has been developed and investigated over a number of studies by Field and her colleagues (Field et al., 1986). Sessions of tactile/kinesthetic stimulation (T/K) are provided for three 15-minute periods per day, five days per week. The first treatment occurs about one hour after the morning feeding, the second about one-half hour after the mid-day feeding, and the third approximately 45 minutes after the completion of the second period. Each treatment session consists of five minutes of tactile stimulation [i.e., six 10-second strokes to the head, shoulders, back (no contact with the spine), arms, and legs], followed by five minutes of kinesthetic stimulation (i.e., six 10-second passive extensions/flexions of each arm and leg, followed by six extensions/flexions for both legs simultaneously), and concluding with another five-minute period of tactile stimulation.

The effect of T/K stimulation on the behavior and state regulation of preterm infants

There has been some debate between researchers who study tactile stimulation over how disruptive it is to the preterm neonate. This debate is complicated since the forms of tactile stimulation provided to preterm infants have differed across studies.

Early tactile stimulation studies focused on stroking and rubbing. Although they failed to include formal state analysis, there was evidence that intervention led to heightened alertness and increased activity. Using a procedure that consisted of nonrhythmic massage of the neck, back, and arms for five minutes each hour of the day for ten days, Solkoff et al. (1969) found that stimulated low birth weight (LBW) infants were more often awake and moving than controls. Solkoff & Matuszak (1975) reported that participants who received ten days of stroking were more alert and changed state more often during the Brazelton neonatal examination (Brazelton, 1973). Adamson-Mecedo (1986) found that providing cephala-caudal massage to sleeping very low birth weight preterms produced a state change that ranged from drowsy to alert and led to some behavioral disorganization. Subsequently, she became a vocal advocate against rubbing preterms and now limits her intervention to a procedure of gentle strokes she calls TAC-TIC (Adamson-Macedo & Alves-Attree, 1994).

Recent studies suggest that tactile stimulation is quite safe for preterm infants. Acolet et al. (1993) found that massage was well tolerated by extremely low birth weight preterms (e.g., 630 g) once they were medically stable. Adamson-Mecedo and her associates (1994) found that gentle strokes failed to disturb oxygen tension in high-risk preterm infants. Harrison et al. (1996) found that during GHT, newly born preterm infants exhibited significantly less active sleep, motor activity, and behavioral distress.

Regardless of recent findings, tactile and kinesthetic stimulation have not been widely adopted on NICUs. This reflects a 'minimal touch' policy that still is maintained by many neonatologists and NICU staff (Morrow et al., 1991). This view arose from a frequently cited study conducted by Long et al. (1980) whereby procedures such as feedings, diaper changes, and examinations were sometimes associated with significant decreases in transcutaneous oxygen saturation. The widespread acceptance of these findings has hindered the introduction of procedures that are beyond standard nursery care.

To date, only Scafidi et al. (1986, 1990) and Dieter (1999) have undertaken comprehensive behavioral analyses of the effects of tactile and kinesthetic stimulation on preterms across the ten-day treatment period. Behavioral analyses used Thoman's (1975) criteria to define seven state categories: Quiet Sleep, Active Sleep, REM Sleep, Drowsy, Quiet Alert, Active Alert, and Fussy/Crying. A number of motor behaviors were also recorded including: single and multiple limb movements, head-turns, gross body movement, startles, smiles, mouthing, facile grimaces, and clenched fists.

The Scafidi et al. (1986, 1990) studies found that during T/K, preterms became more active as evidenced by significant increases in multiple limb movements and facial expressions. Furthermore, kinesthetic stimulation produced significantly greater alertness and motor behavior than did tactile stimulation (Scafidi et al., 1986). At the conclusion of 10 treatment days, Scafidi et al. (1986) conducted a single 45-minute observation and found that infants who received T/K exhibited active alertness 14% of the time, while non-stimulated control infants failed to show the state. Although more active, T/K infants did not demonstrate a significant increase in crying. Furthermore, T/K infants did not exhibit significantly more stress behaviors (e.g., startles, facial grimaces, or clenched fists) than did control infants.

Utilizing a repeated-measures design, Dieter (1999) observed the influence of 10 days of T/K on behavioral state on 15 preterm infants (mean gestational age 30.1 weeks; mean birthweight 1359 g; mean assignment weight 1655.1 g) residing in an intermediate care NICU nursery and compared findings against those obtained from 15 controls (mean gestational age 31.1 weeks; mean birthweight 1421 g; mean assignment weight 1621.2 g). Infants were medically stable at time of assignment and were no longer receiving gavage feeds. Table 7.1 provides the demographic variables and medical history for the two groups.

The effects of T/K during actual stimulation were similar to those reported by Scafidi et al. (1986, 1990). In comparison to baseline, T/K increased the amount of time that infants spent in Active Sleep (i.e., sleep with movement) and decreased the amount of time spent in Quiet Sleep (i.e., sleep without movement) (Table 7.2). In addition, during T/K infants

Table 7.1 Means (and standard deviations) for the pre-assignment variables (Dieter, 1999)

Measures	T/K	Control	p value
Maternal age	26.9 (4.8)	28.1 (5.6)	0.52
Parity	2.0 (0.9)	2.7 (1.6)	0.23
Gestational age (weeks)	30.1 (2.5)	31.1 (2.8)	0.30
Birthweight (grams)	1359.3 (140.1)	1421.5 (91.9)	0.20
Ponderal index[a]	2.1 (0.3)	2.2 (0.3)	0.30
Apgar 1 minute	6.7 (1.7)	7.4 (1.3)	0.20
Apgar 5 minutes	8.1 (0.8)	8.4 (0.6)	0.36
Obstetric complications[b]	68.7 (14.7)	70.7 (9.9)	0.67
Postnatal complications[b]	75.1 (6.6)	74.9 (5.3)	0.93
NICU days	20.4 (12.3)	18.9 (12.2)	0.74
Days O_2 therapy	2.8 (1.6)	3.5 (1.7)	0.23
Days-to-gavage feeds	1.9 (1.5)	2.3 (0.8)	0.39
Days antibiotics	4.2 (1.0)	4.5 (1.8)	0.52
Days phototherapy	3.7 (1.4)	4.4 (1.1)	0.13
Days since birth	25.6 (11.7)	22.0 (5.8)	0.29
Assignment weight	1655.1 (89.9)	1621.2 (54.4)	0.21
Assignment head circumference (mm)	30.0 (1.2)	29.7 (1.1)	0.52
Pre-assignment weight gain (1 day, grams)	29.9 (14.0)	25.3 (11.9)	0.21
Pre-assignment formula intake (1 day, ml)	225.7 (51.9)	211.3 (34.0)	0.36
Pre-assignment ml/kg/d	149.5 (30.6)	135.2 (27.1)	0.36
Pre-assignment bowel movements (1 day, number)	1.9 (0.9)	2.0 (0.5)	0.63

[a]Ponderal Index = birthweight/length^3 × 100.
[b]Higher score is optimal.

showed an increase in the amount of multiple limb and gross body movements (Table 7.2). Contrary to the findings of Scafidi et al. (1986, 1990), kinesthetic stimulation was no more arousing than tactile stimulation. Of particular interest is that the immediate effects of T/K on behavior did not change significantly over the ten treatment days, suggesting that infants did not habituate to this form of supplemental stimulation. The theoretical implications of this finding are discussed below.

Dieter (1999) further examined the effects that ten days of T/K has on behavior during non-treatment periods in comparison to the control group. As shown in Table 7.3, there were no significant differences between the distribution of behavioral states across the two groups at assignment. Findings shed some light on the dose/response ratio with respect to the effects of T/K on the distribution of sleep/wake states. Following five days of treatment, T/K infants spent more time in the drowsy state (mean % time 16.8, SD 19.3) than did infants in the control group (mean % time 2.5, SD 3.8), t (1, 30) = 2.91, $p < 0.01$. At the conclusion of ten treatment days, T/K infants were fully awake more often and spent significantly less time

Table 7.2 Immediate impact of T/K on behavioral state and motor behavior (Dieter, 1999)

Variable	Mean % Time		
	Pre-T/K baseline	During T/K	p value
Quiet category[a]	63.6 (15.1)	48.5 (9.7)	<0.01
Active category[b]	26.7 (13.1)	50.8 (9.9)	<0.01
Quiet sleep[c]	46.5 (20.7)	32.0 (9.8)	<0.05
Active sleep[d]	13.3 (9.0)	27.2 (10.2)	<0.01
Multiple limb	8.4 (5.3)	12.7 (5.7)	<0.05
Gross body	7.9 (6.1)	21.9 (9.9)	<0.01

[a]Consisting of the total % time spent in quiet sleep, drowsiness, and quiet alert.
[b]Consisting of the total % time spent in active sleep, active awake, and crying.
[c]Sleep without movement.
[d]Sleep with movement.

Table 7.3 Between-group effects of T/K on behavioral state organization (Dieter, 1999)

Measures	Mean % time		
	T/K	Control	p value
Pre-assignment day			
Sleep[a]	89.2 (17.0)	90.4 (14.6)	0.89
Awake[a]	4.7 (7.9)	5.7 (10.6)	0.79
Day 10			
Sleep	53.0 (37.7	81.1 (34.5)	0.04
Awake	15.2 (21.9)	5.7 (9.2)	0.25
REM sleep	9.8 (5.8)	14.8 (7.9)	0.05

[a]Summation of the sleep and awake categories will not equal 100% since state 4 (i.e., drowsy) is not included in either category.

in REM sleep (Table 7.3). That T/K appeared to reduce REM sleep is important since many studies have found greater amounts of REM in younger and sicker pre- and full-term infants (Dinges et al., 1980; Dittrichova et al., 1985; Emory & Mapp, 1988), therefore suggesting that T/K may foster better health and possibly neurobehavioral development.

In an effort to evaluate the degree to which T/K may affect behavior, Dieter (1999) examined T/K and control infants during mid-day bottle-feedings. Findings obtained on the fifth and tenth days of participation revealed that T/K infants spent less time in the Drowsy/Sleep state (T/K mean 33.1%, SD 22.29; Control mean 59.6%, SD 26.0; $p<0.05$) and more time in the Quiet Alert state (T/K mean 63.1%, SD 23.1; Control mean 39.1%,

SD 25.1; $p < 0.05$) than did control infants. However, there was no significant difference in the % time the two groups spent feeding. Because infants commonly scan and engage the environment during Quiet Alertness, the effects of T/K on bottle feeding may promote the infant-caregiver relationship and increase the opportunity for incidental learning. Future studies need to confirm this.

The effect of T/K stimulation on the physiological reactivity of preterm infants

A few researchers studying tactile and kinesthetic stimulation have focused on physiological reactivity to assess the preterm infant. The immediate effects of stimulation have been examined through heart and respiration rate, and percentage of arterial oxygen saturation.

Tribotti (1990) found that during the first session, Gentle Human Touch (GHT) decreased arterial oxygen saturation and increased respiratory regularity in preterms whose gestational age ranged from 32 to 35 weeks. A second treatment session failed to disturb oxygen levels and continued to promote respiratory regularity. Using a systematized GHT protocol, Harrison found that passive touch had little influence on mean heart rate or oxygen saturation across the nine-day treatment period (Personal communication, L. Harrison, 1996). These findings suggest that GHT does not promote immediate physiological instability in very young preterm infants.

Several studies have examined the immediate physiological consequence of active tactile stimulation on preterm infants over the course of treatment. Kattwinkel et al. (1975) evaluated the effects of rubbing the extremities of six preterm infants for a total of 45 minutes per day from the second to the 35th post-natal day. Tactile stimulation reduced the occurrence of idiopathic apnea (i.e., the cessation of respiration longer than 15 seconds) by 35%. Oehler (1985) found no significant difference in heart rate response among 15 preterm infants following stroking; however, stroking did decrease transcutaneous oxygen saturation. Oehler concluded that active tactile stimulation might be too disruptive to preterm infants and might contribute to episodes of hypoxia. To the contrary, Morrow et al. (1991) found that T/K did not result in clinically significant decreases in transcutaneous oxygen tension when compared with a heel-stick procedure used for drawing blood from infants. Such contradictory findings may reflect more the clinical status of the preterms studied than any endemic dangers to tactile and kinesthetic stimulation. Dieter & Emory (1997) suggested that the effects a form of supplemental stimulation has upon the individual preterm should guide that infant's course of intervention. Adverse reactions to one form of simulation would herald the introduction of a less intense protocol. For instance, for preterms not tolerating T/K, GHT might be the appropriate first course of treatment.

Recent studies have shown that T/K does influence heart rate, but that the effects are safe for preterms residing in the grower nursery. Wheeden et al. (1993) found that preterms who received T/K exhibited significantly higher heart rates (i.e., T/K mean 158.8, Control mean 154.7), during non-stimulation periods, throughout the study. This finding suggests that the effects of T/K on physiological activity transcend the actual period of stimulation and further indicates that the benefits of stimulation may involve heightened arousal. A limitation of this study is that physiological data were obtained from daily nursing notes.

Dieter (1999) undertook a comprehensive examination of the effects of T/K on heart and respiration rate during both treatment and non-treatment periods. In comparison to baseline (mean 156.92 bpm, SD 7.05), T/K produced a significant increase in heart rate (mean 174.08 bpm, SD 9.57; F [1, 2] = 81.98, $p < 0.01$). However, the effect was short-lived since there was no significant difference between the baseline and immediate post-stimulation periods (mean 163.06 bpm, SD 5.57). As was the case with behavior, the immediate effects of T/K on heart rate did not significantly diminish over the ten days of treatment and there was no difference between the tactile and kinesthetic phases. T/K was not found to have a significant effect on respiration rate.

While Dieter (1999) observed that the immediate effects of T/K were associated with a significant rise in heart rate, on average it represented only about a 10% increase and the mean heart rate during stimulation was far below the clinically significant level. Also found was that the mean heart and respiration rates exhibited during T/K were not significantly different that those observed during physical examinations and diaper changes. Thus, it is safe to conclude that T/K is no more stressful than standard nursery care, which is well tolerated by most preterms long before they reach the grower nursery. Contrary to the findings of Wheeden et al. (1993) no significant difference was found between the basal heart and respiration rates observed in T/K infants during non-stimulation periods when compared with the control group.

The effect of T/K stimulation on the biochemistry of preterm infants

A few studies have examined biochemical variables assayed from preterm infant blood, urine, and saliva following stimulation. The aim of these investigations was directed towards determining if tactile and/or kinesthetic stimulation evokes or reduces stress responses and whether biochemical factors contribute to the observed weight gain and enhanced neurobehavioral performance.

In pilot work, Harrison (Personal communication, L. Harrison, 1996) found that nine days of GHT, provided for 15 minutes, three times per day, reduced salivary cortisol levels in three preterm infants. Since cortisol is a hormone released by the hypothalamic-pituitary-adrenal (H-P-A) axis, often in response to stress (Hole, 1981), the conclusion drawn was that GHT comforts the preterm and enhances adaptation.

Cortisol assay studies of infants receiving Field's T/K protocol have yielded mixed results. Kuhn et al. (1991) found that preterms who received ten days of treatment exhibited no significant change in blood cortisol levels when compared with controls. In pilot work, Acolet et al. (1993) did observe that T/K caused a significant reduction in serum cortisol levels. Therefore, the question as to how T/K may affect cortisol remains unanswered. Future research should focus on repeated pre- and post-T/K measures across the treatment period. Determining the influence of T/K on cortisol has important theoretical implications. If cortisol levels consistently drop across treatment, this suggests that T/K's biochemical effect is predominately stress reducing, despite findings of heightened behavioral arousal and physiological reactivity. An immediate cortisol increase which then decreases over the treatment period would support the hypothesis that some of the benefits of T/K arise from adaptation to the challenges of stimulation.

Two of the above studies looked at additional biochemical variables. Acolet et al. (1993) found that T/K was associated with a significant reduction in levels of serum beta-endorphin. Lower endorphin levels were interpreted as further reflecting the infant's ability to better cope with stressful or painful events. While Kuhn et al. (1991) reported that T/K was associated with significant increases in urine noradrenaline (norepinephrine) and adrenaline (epinephrine), no change was found in the serum human growth hormone levels of treatment and control infants.

The Kuhn et al. (1991) interpretation that increases in the urine catecholamines noradrenaline (norepinephrine) and adrenaline (epinephrine) reflect maturation of the sympathetic nervous system requires further elaboration. These catecholamines are released by the adrenal medulla (Hole, 1981). In adults, concentrations of these catecholamines often increase in reaction to physical or psychological stress in order to initiate sympathetic nervous system responses such as elevated blood pressure and blood glucose levels. If T/K is contributing to nervous system maturation, it may be limited to the H-P-A axis since Kuhn et al. (1991) failed to show that T/K affected urine dopamine levels. Furthermore, the behavioral arousal observed in infants receiving T/K may be mediated by the mobilizing effects of catecholamines. If subsequent research finds that T/K does not affect cortisol, but leads to increases in these catecholamines, maturational effects may be primarily related to the adrenal branch of the H-P-A axis. In order to establish a comprehensive model explaining the benefits of T/K, it is imperative that future studies obtain multiple biochemical samples. The paramount question is to what degree, and in which directions, behavioral, physiological, and biochemical variables co-vary.

The effect of T/K stimulation on preterm infant weight gain

As indicated, the most consistent benefit of T/K is the promotion of weight gain. At least seven investigations have demonstrated that treated preterms gained more weight than control infants over the ten-day stimulation period (Dieter, 1999; Field et al., 1986; Goldstein-Feber, 1997; Jinon, 1996; Scafidi et al., 1986, 1990; Wheeden et al., 1993). The average greater daily weight gains shown by T/K infants in these studies have ranged from 28% to 47%. That T/K promotes weight gain has great clinical significance, since once a preterm is medically stable, this variable determines when the infant is discharged. The faster a baby gains weight, the sooner it is released from the hospital. Indeed, both Field et al. (1986) and Scafidi et al. (1986, 1990) found that preterms receiving T/K left the hospital between five and six days earlier than control infants.

The question of how T/K promotes weight gain remains unanswered (Scafidi et al., 1990). Research has failed to support the most common-sensical explanations. For instance, studies have shown that infants receiving T/K do not consume more formula than control preterms (Field et al., 1986; Scafidi et al., 1986, 1990). Thus, the greater weight gain does not appear to be a function of increased caloric intake. Another discrepant finding discussed above is that preterms receiving T/K exhibit increased activity when compared with control infants. Intuitively, heightened activity might be expected to increase energy expenditure and lead to lesser weight gain (Scafidi et al., 1990).

The failure to find obvious reasons for explaining how T/K promotes weight gain has led researchers to propose hypotheses that entail a complex cascade of physiological and biochemical events. Field believes that T/K 'stimulates the vagus nerves which then triggers processes that aid digestion...' (Drummond, 1998). Others have suggested that vagal stimulation leads to an increase in growth hormones that then stimulate gastrointestinal growth, motor and secretory activity, and promote insulin release (Kuhn et al., 1991; Uvnas-Moberg et al., 1987).

Dieter (1999) also found that infants who received T/K showed a weight gain advantage. Across the 10 days of treatment, T/K infants gained an average of 334.6 grams (SD 48.2) and control infants 281.8 grams (SD 48.5), F $(1.28) = 7.12$, $p < 0.05$ (Fig. 7.1). Once again, no significant differences were observed between the amount of formula or kilocalories consumed across the two groups (Table 7.4). A previously unreported finding was that T/K infants showed a greater number of bowel movements per day than controls (Table 7.4). While possibly spurious, that T/K infants showed a greater number of bowel movements refutes the notion that the weight gain merely reflected fluid retention.

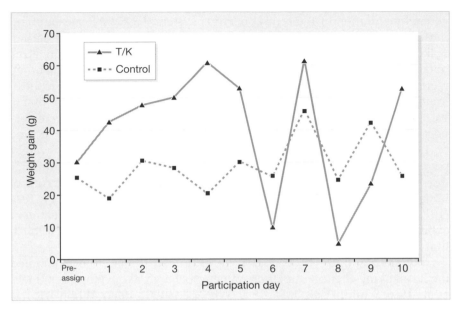

Figure 7.1 Effect of 10 days of T/K on weight gain (Dieter, 1999).

Table 7.4 Effects of T/K on daily weight gain and input/output variables (Dieter, 1999)

Measure	T/K	Control	p value
Weight gain (grams)	33.5 (4.8)	28.2 (4.9)	0.04
Volumetric intake (ml)	264.1 (54.2)	238.7 (42.3)	0.37
Kilocalories consumed	119.6 (10.8)	111.6 (12.3)	0.07
Bowel movements	3.2 (0.8)	2.2 (0.8)	0.01

The effect of tactile stimulation on preterm infant neurobehavioral maturation

The majority of investigations support that tactile stimulation promotes global development as measured by neurobehavioral examinations. Active forms of touch, such as T/K, may be superior to passive forms (e.g., GHT).

Little formal research has evaluated the influence of GHT on development. From preliminary pilot work, Harrison et al. (1996) found no difference in performance on the Brazelton Neonatal Behavioral Assessment Scale (BNBAS) between infants who did or did not received GHT from the 7th to the 16th post-natal day.

Post-treatment findings, from the early active tactile stimulation studies, all showed that infants receiving massage exhibited behaviors indicative of general maturation of the central nervous system (CNS). After examining participants who were discharged between six to nine months earlier, Solkoff et al. (1969) reported that each of the five stimulated preterms obtained scores on the Bayley Scales (Bayley, 1969) that indicated that they were 'active and physically healthy'. Contrarily, only one of the control infants was considered normal. The scores of the other four control infants were below the mean for their age on motor development; two were suspected of having cerebral palsy. Kramer et al. (1975) reported that at time of transfer from the incubator to the crib, healthy low birth weight preterms who received full body nonrhythmic stroking for 48 minutes per day for two weeks obtained significantly higher Bayley scores than control infants. Enhancement of motor development was also reported by Rice (1977). At four months, preterm infants who received 30 days of treatment exhibited fewer phylogenetic reflexes (i.e., those reflexes inherent at birth that indicate CNS immaturity) than controls.

Only Field and her colleagues have examined the effect of combined tactile and kinesthetic stimulation on neurobehavioral development (Field et al., 1986; Scafidi et al., 1986, 1990; Wheeden et al., 1993). While T/K has been shown to have a positive effect on development, statistically significant findings have varied somewhat across investigations.

At two days after the end of the ten-day treatment period, Scafidi et al. (1986) found that stimulated infants performed significantly better on the Lester Cluster Scales (Lester et al., 1982) of the BNBAS that measure habituation, orientation, motor behavior, and range of behavioral state. In their replicative effort, Scafidi et al. (1990) observed that treated preterms exhibited a superior performance only on the Habituation Scale. In their examination of cocaine-exposed preterms, Wheeden and her collaborators (1993) once again found that T/K infants exhibited superior motor maturity; additionally, these infants showed fewer stress behaviors than controls. In their one-year follow-up of the sample from the first study (i.e., Scafidi et al., 1986), Field et al. (1987) reported that T/K infants achieved a mean Bayley Mental Scale score of 101, while the mean score of the control group was 90. Treated preterm infants continued to exhibit superior motor performance (T/K motor scale mean 105, Control motor scale mean 90).

There may be several reasons for the inconsistent BNBAS findings across investigations. That there are seven separate BNBAS cluster scores, and that the sample sizes of T/K studies are relatively small (i.e., 15 to 20 participants per group), probably reduces the likelihood of obtaining statistically significant multivariate findings. In addition, it may be that the behaviors measured by the BNBAS are too complex, and therefore unlikely to consistently change with only 10 days of intervention, especially if there are no significant pre-treatment deficits. Perhaps the best test to what degree T/K improves BNBAS performance would be to examine a larger sample of preterms who clearly demonstrate improvised performance on the pre-treatment exam and then compare subsequent post-treatment findings against a matched control group. Furthermore, more than ten days of stimulation may be required to consistently improve BNBAS performance.

POSSIBLE MECHANISMS OF ACTION
Increased physical activity for promoting weight gain

As detailed previously, the most consistent findings across studies of active tactile stimulation are increased movement and alertness, and greater weight gain. Scafidi et al. (1990) were the first to suggest a causal relationship between weight gain and the increased alertness and movement observed in T/K infants during stimulation and nonstimulation periods. Although such a relationship appears intuitively paradoxical, there are a small number of animal and human studies supporting a link between increased physical activity and weight gain.

In two animal studies from the 1970s, Borer observed that free access to horizontal disc exercisers induced weight gain in adult hamsters (Borer, 1974; Borer & Kooi, 1975). In comparison to sedentary hamsters, the exercising animals showed an upward displacement of weight, length, and percentage of body fat. The onset of weight gain was rapid, and initially was not accompanied by an increase in food intake. Furthermore, the weight gain advantage persisted for three months after the cessation of exercise. These findings are remarkably similar to those observed in human preterms who received T/K.

Borer & Kooi (1975) argued that exercise reset the hamsters' weight regulatory mechanisms. Because the exercising hamsters demonstrated both increased weight gain and body length, Borer (1974) suggested that the underlying mechanism might include a rise in the secretion of growth hormone by the pituitary. If there is a casual relationship between physical activity and the enhanced weight gain observed in human preterms receiving tactile or kinesthetic stimulation, it is unlikely that the mediator is human growth hormone (HGH) since Kuhn et al. (1991) failed to find changes in HGH levels in those infants who received T/K.

Increased activity has been shown to promote weight gain in humans. A recent study by Kardel & Kase (1998) demonstrated greater weight gain in pregnant women carrying girls who exercised during the late second and third trimesters. Exercise consisted of muscle strength training, interval training, and endurance training. Results indicated that the more intense the exercise regimen the greater was the maternal weight gain. Furthermore, the weight gain advantage was not accounted for by the weight of the infant at birth.

In a well-controlled study, Moyer-Mileur et al. (1995) examined the effects of physical activity on bone mineralization and weight gain in preterm infants. The 'physical activity program' consisted of range of motion exercises and passive resistance to all extremities for 5 or 10 minutes a day for four weeks. This procedure appears comparable to the kinesthetic portion of T/K. Despite similar nutritional intake, treated preterms gained more weight than control infants (mean 17.8 vs 13.4 grams per day), and exhibited greater radial bone mass and density.

Moyer-Mileur et al. (1995) found that exercised preterms demonstrated lower serum levels of alkaline phosphatase (PTH). PTH plays an important role in calcium homeostasis by regulating the concentration of ionized calcium. Moyer-Mileur et al. reported that previous rodent studies found that exercising rats showed a positive calcium and phosphorous balance and an increase in skeletal mass. Furthermore, exercised rats did not eat more and did not differ from control rats in their urinary excretions of calcium and phosphorous. Similarly, the exercised human preterms did not differ from control infants in food intake, calcium intake, and urinary calcium output. The authors concluded that the increase in bone mineralization demonstrated by the exercise group might have resulted from enhanced metabolism, mediated by PTH, which promoted greater calcium absorption.

Dieter (1990) found mixed support that the weight gain advantage demonstrated by T/K infants is causally linked to the heightened physical activity observed during stimulation and non-stimulation periods. As predicted, infants did demonstrate a significant increase in active sleep, gross motor behavior, and heart rate during stimulation. However, no support was gained for the prediction that T/K infants would also show greater activity during non-stimulation observations. T/K infants were more often awake during non-treatment periods, but they were no more active than control infants and they did not demonstrate higher tonic heart and respiration rates. Finally, trend analyses failed to demonstrate any significant relationship between greater levels of physical activity and higher heart rates during stimulation and the weight gain advantage demonstrated by T/K infants. To the contrary, a significant linear relationship was found between the amount of time infants spent in the quiet alert state during T/K and the amount of weight they gained, $F (1, 13) = 5.07$, $p < 0.05$ (Fig. 7.2).

The above findings are preliminary and from a relatively small sample. Replication from a larger group is necessary and subjecting results to regression modeling vital. Because heightened physical arousal during T/K has been observed so consistently, it may be premature to dismiss it as a possible contributor to the weight gain advantage. Greater efforts should be dedicated to formulating the specific causal pathway between heightened physical activity and weight gain. The most obvious contender is the calcium absorption model proposed by Moyer-Mileur et al. (1995).

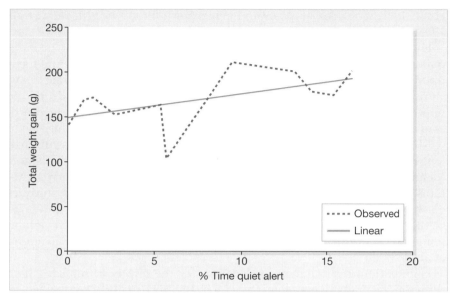

Figure 7.2 Relationship between the % time infants were in the quiet alert state during T/K and weight gain (Dieter, 1999).

Extra handling as a 'stress inoculator'

Since the early findings of Levine (1959, 1960) numerous animal studies show that supplemental stimulation or environmental enrichment accelerates development. The 'handling' paradigm has been widely applied in these investigations. Handling is a general term used to describe a variety of neonatal environmental alterations that are later found to modify adult animal behavior (Costela et al., 1993). Such studies usually consist of the experimenter separating the animal from its mother and literally holding it for a period of time. Subsequently, when handled young reach adulthood they are subjected to an environmental challenge, and their behavioral responses are compared with non-handled animals. Both animal groups are usually sacrificed and biochemical assays obtained. While most handling experiments study rats, other animals including mice and chickens have been examined (Cross & Labarba, 1978; Salvatierra et al., 1997).

The effects of handling on animal behavior appear far-reaching. Handled rats have been shown to demonstrate less fear in novel situations, greater exploratory behavior, shorter escape latencies from aversive stimuli, better performance during stressful challenges, lower emotional reactivity, greater weight gain, and even superior cognitive, learning, and memory performance in old age (Ader et al., 1968; Costela et al., 1993; Fernandez-Teruel et al., 1991; Gonzalez et al., 1990; Levine & Mullins, 1966; Meaney et al., 1988; Rocha & Vendite, 1990).

Handling is usually conceptualized as a form of stress that includes maternal separation and confinement. Biochemical assays frequently focus upon stress hormones produced by the H-P-A axis. Many studies have shown that handled rats secrete less corticosterone in adulthood than do non-handled rats, exhibit permanent increases in hippocampal glucocorticoid receptors, and show lower levels of corticotropin-releasing factor (CRF) and plasma adrenocorticotropin (ACTH) following stressful challenges (Denenberg et al., 1967; Meaney et al., 1987, 1988, 1989; Plotsky & Meaney, 1993). The effects of handling on the nervous and endocrine systems do not appear to be limited to the H-P-A axis. A recent study of chicks found that handling was associated with increases in forebrain GABA receptor density that ranged from 17% to 47% and was accompanied by superior performance on a food discrimination task (Salvatierra et al., 1997).

Habituation is a common explanation for the effects of repeated handling on the endocrine system. Initial handling is usually accompanied by a heightened H-P-A response that then diminishes over repeated exposures. For instance, Dobrakovova and colleagues observed that initial exposure of rats to brief handling led to rapid rises in ACTH, epine-phrine (EPI) and norepinephrine (NE) (Dobrakovoa et al., 1993). While EPI and NE elevations quickly returned to baseline, ACTH remained elevated throughout the 15-minute observation period. However, repeated handling during the three-hour experiment virtually eliminated the endocrine response.

Essentially, handling is viewed as a 'stress inoculator' whereby both the behavioral and endocrine reactions of the animal are shaped and this attenuated response generalizes to other stressful situations. While it might be expected that any form of repeated stress would inoculate the animal, handling appears to possess a unique quality. When compared with other forms of stress, only handling seems to promote superior behavioral and endocrine adaptation. In an early study, Ader et al. (1968) compared handling with electric shock. Rats who were repeatedly handled demonstrated an attenuated corticosterone response while rats who were repeatedly shocked failed to show habituation. More recently, Plotsky & Meaney (1993) compared handling with maternal separation (MS) on a restraint test. As adults, handled rats demonstrated significantly lower CRF levels than either MS or non-handled rats. Furthermore, restraint stress produced significantly lower plasma corticosterone in handled rats than in either MS or non-handled rats. These findings suggest that the tactile component inherent to handling may be key to its benefits. As will be discussed later, recent animal studies have found that sensorial qualities of touch, such as warmth and pressure, lower stress hormones and promote adaptation (Uvnas-Moberg, 1997).

That many of the immediate and subsequent effects of handling on animals are similar to those observed in human preterm infants receiving T/K are obvious. As reported above, studies have shown that infants demonstrate heightened behavioral and physiological arousal during T/K, but later exhibit greater weight gain, fewer stress signs, and superior performance on challenging neurobehavioral examinations. Therefore, procedures such as T/K may inoculate the infant against stress and promote general adaptation, presumably through their impact on the H-P-A axis. Crucial support for this model depends on how the preterm accommodates to tactile and kinesthetic stimulation over time.

Handling studies show that while animals initially exhibit both heightened behavioral and biochemical responses, repeated stimulation produces habituation and generalized adaptation. Scafidi et al. (1990) and Dieter (1999) found that preterms' behavioral reaction to T/K changed little over the 10 days. The few studies of the effects of T/K stimulation on the biochemistry of human preterms provide mixed support for the stress inoculation model. While Acolet et al. (1993) did observe that T/K caused a significant reduction in serum cortisol levels, Kuhn et al. (1991) reported that preterms who received 10 days of treatment exhibited no significant change in blood cortisol levels when compared with controls. Furthermore, Kuhn et al. found that post-treatment, T/K infants exhibited significantly higher epinephrine and norepinephrine levels than controls, a finding in direct contradiction to that observed in the animal model.

Dieter (1999) found little support for the stress inoculation model. As predicted, during T/K infants did show a significant rise in arousal as evidenced by increased heart rate and motor behavior. Contrary to the findings of animal studies, these behaviors did not diminish with repeated stimulation suggesting that the infants did not habituate to the arousing aspects of T/K. Furthermore, trend analysis failed to find any significant relationship between the arousal and few signs of stress demonstrated by infants during T/K and their weight gain advantage.

While Dieter (1999) failed to find behavioral support for the stress inoculation model, additional biochemical studies are needed to render a more definitive conclusion. In particular, the relationship between T/K and cortisol must be established. The two existing T/K studies have failed to demonstrate consistent results (Acolet et al., 1993; Kuhn et al., 1991). Biochemical support for the stress inoculation model would rest on two findings: T/K infants would initially show increased cortisol following stimulation which would diminish over time; when compared with controls, T/K infants would exhibit lower cortisol levels following stressful challenges.

The vagus nerves as the bridge between the nervous and endocrine systems

In recent years, much has been said about the role of the vagus nerves in behavior. The vagus or 10th pair of cranial nerves is mixed, containing both sensory and motor efferents (Tortora & Anagnostakos, 1990). The vagus has the greatest proliferation of branches throughout the body than any of the other cranial nerves. The motor portion originates in the medulla and terminates in muscles of the respiratory passages, lungs, esophagus, heart, stomach, intestines, and gall balder. Parasympathetic fibers innervate the involuntary muscles and glands of the gastrointestinal (GI) tract.

Porges (1983, 1995) maintained that since the vagus nerves are involved in the bidirectional communication between the heart and the sympathetic and parasympathetic nervous systems, heart rate variability has value as 'a potential diagnostic window to the brain'. Porges (1985) has developed a time-series method to measure cardiac vagal tone (CVT) through the quantification of respiratory sinus arrhythmia (RSA) amplitude. RSA arises from naturally occurring increases and decreases in heart rate that are associated with inhalation and exhalation. CVT values reflect proportional increases and decreases in RSA amplitude.

CVT has been widely applied to infant research as a physiological index of development, stress, emotional reactivity, and attachment (Fox, 1989; Izard et al., 1991; Porter et al., 1988). These studies have shown that vagal tone is highly correlated with autonomic reactivity and that infants with high CVT are better at regulating emotional and attentional processes; furthermore, these babies perform better on intellectual assessments such as the Bayley scales (Fracasso et al., 1994).

Cardiac vagal tone has been assessed in preterm infants. Findings indicate that preterm infants commonly exhibit lower CVT in comparison to full-term cohorts (e.g., 4.72 in healthy preterms vs 5.75 in healthy full-terms at 40 weeks); furthermore, preterm infants with lower CVT have been shown to be at greater risk for subsequent developmental deficits (Fox & Porges, 1985), and exhibit less adaptive behaviors (e.g., exploratory play) (DiPietro et al., 1992).

Field & Schanberg (1995) were the first to observe increases in vagal tone during T/K. Studying a sub-sample of preterms, Dieter (1999) found that during T/K vagal tone rose significantly from baseline levels and remained elevated during the 15-minute post-treatment period (Pre-T/K mean 2.2, SD 0.4; T/K mean 2.9, SD 0.7; Post-T/K mean 2.4, SD 0.5; F [2, 24] = 3.51, $p = 0.05$). Furthermore, trend analysis yielded a significant quadratic relationship between vagal tone activity during T/K and weight gain during the first treatment week, F (1, 6) = 20.69, $p < 0.05$ (Fig. 7.3). As already presented, a significant linear relationship was also found between weight gain and time spent in quiet alertness (a state positively correlated with higher CVT) during T/K. These findings preliminarily suggest that the promotion of weight gain may be best facilitated if some optimal range of vagal activity is achieved and maintained through the T/K session and the infant receives stimulation while in the quiet alert state. Gaining support for this hypothesis is possible by closely examining the relationship between behavioral state and CVT during T/K and the subsequent weight gain observed.

Uvnas-Moberg and colleagues proposed a vagal model of how tactile stimulation promotes weight gain (Uvnas-Moberg et al., 1987). They suggested that massage stimulates the activity of the vagus via peripheral afferent pathways. This heightened activity facilitates communication between the vagus and gastrointestinal (GI) tract through the efferent branch that terminates on, and is distributed across, the anterior and posterior surfaces of the stomach. Uvnas-Moberg et al. argued that vagal nerve parasympathetic activation stimulates the release of several peptide hormones including gastrin that then precipitates acid secretion and glucose-induced insulin release, the growth of the gastric mucosa, heightened GI functioning, and subsequent greater weight gain.

This vagal model can be elaborated upon by considering additional biochemical factors. Besides gastrin, insulin-like growth factor-I (IGF-I) is another peptide hormone that may be stimulated through heightened vagal activity. IGF-I has been implicated as mediating GI metabolism and

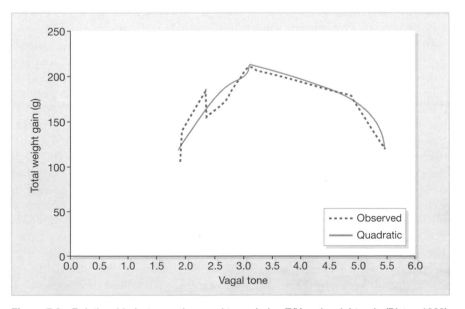

Figure 7.3 Relationship between the vagal tone during T/K and weight gain (Dieter, 1999).

growth. In both full-term and preterm infants, IGF-I is strongly correlated with placental weight, birthweight, body length, Ponderal index, and nutritional factors (Bennett et al., 1983; Colonna et al., 1996; Osorio et al., 1996; Yamasaki et al., 1989). Of relevance to the Kuhn et al. (1991) T/K study (see earlier) is that a strong inverse relationship has been demonstrated between IGF-I and human growth hormone (HGH) (Colonna et al., 1996). This may be why Kuhn et al. failed to find HGH increases in massaged preterms.

Xu (1996) proposed that IGF-I plays a role in the growth, morphological changes, and functional maturation of the GI tract during the immediate postnatal period. Furthermore, a positive relationship has been observed between levels of IGF-I, nutrient intake, and subsequent weight gain, suggesting enhanced metabolism (Díaz Gómez et al., 1996; Giniès et al., 1992; Smith et al., 1997). Collectively, these findings suggest that IGF-I might be another factor mediating the greater weight gain observed in massaged preterms.

Another peptide hormone that may mediate the benefits of preterm infant massage is oxytocin. Findings indicate that oxytocin is present in the human fetal pituitary glands as early as 14 weeks, and increases 50-fold over gestation (Khan-Dawood & Dawood, 1984). There is a significant positive correlation between birthweight and maternal oxytocin levels (Uvnas-Moberg et al., 1990). Oxytocin is produced by newborns and is released in a pulsatile fashion, reflecting fluctuations in hypothalamic cell activity (Marchini & Stock, 1996). Oxytocin has been implicated as playing a role in the maternal, attachment, feeding, bonding, and sexual behavior of both animals and humans (Insel, 1997; Nelson & Panksepp, 1998).

The rodent literature suggests that the stress encountered by human preterms on the NICU may lower levels of oxytocin that could then be elevated through massage therapy. Noonan and colleagues found that hippocampal oxytocin receptors decreased in rat pups following periods of maternal separation (Noonan et al., 1994). Uvnas-Moberg (1997) reported that repeated administration of oxytocin inoculated rats against stressful stimuli. This study also found that touch, light pressure, and warmth increased levels of both blood and cerebral spinal fluid oxytocin. Such increases in oxytocin were also linked to greater weight gain that persisted for several weeks. That increases in serum oxytocin are inversely related to cortisol secretion is also relevant since this adrenocorticotropic hormone inhibits IGF-I and subsequent growth (Chiodera et al., 1991). Uvnas-Moberg further suggested that oxytocin might mediate the effects of specific vagally controlled GI hormones such as gastrin and insulin that promote growth. In pilot work, Field & Schanberg (1995) found higher serum insulin levels in T/K infants following ten treatment days.

The potential effect that oxytocin has on attachment behavior may explain the finding that massaged preterms demonstrated superior performance on the Orientation Cluster of the Brazelton Neonatal Behavioral Assessment Scale: Massaged preterms were more engaged and exhibited a greater response to human and non-human stimuli (Scafidi et al., 1986). One year later, Field et al. (1987) found the massaged preterms performed better on the Mental and Motor Scales of the Bayley, suggesting that their post-discharge behavior enhanced the mother-infant relationship that facilitated development. That oxytocin is related to lower serum cortisol may also contribute to the enhanced neurobehavioral performance observed in massaged preterms. Considering the findings of animal studies that document the neurotoxic effects of adrenocorticotropin on the brain and particularly the hippocampus (Weinstock, 1997), a reduction of free cortisol within human preterms might not only reflect improved H-P-A axis function but also foster a hormonal environment that enhances neurobehavioral development.

Although inconclusive, one study has shown that preterms who received T/K demonstrated lower cortisol levels than controls (Acolet et al., 1993). The findings of Kuhn et al. (1991) of increased catecholamines levels may be additional evidence that massage enhances maturation of the neuroendocrine system, especially the H-P-A axis. Furthermore, Uvnas-Moberg and associates proposed that enhanced secretion of catecholamines might further increase the release of gastrin since it can be liberated by beta-adrenoreceptor stimulation (Uvnas-Moberg et al., 1984). In addition, it is known that increases in epinephrine and norepinephrine promote the release of fatty acid and enhance the rate of glycogen breakdown, thus increasing blood glucose levels (Holc, 1981). That massaged preterms have been observed to be more active than controls may be explained by the mobilizing effects of catecholamines.

The above research can be consolidated into a more comprehensive vagal model of how massage therapy promotes greater weight gain and neurobehavioral maturation in preterm infants:

1. Tactile stimulation transmitted via afferent peripheral nerves promotes parasympathetic vagal activity.

2. Direct communication between the vagus and GI tract is enhanced via the gastric branch thus evoking an increased release of hormones (e.g., gastrin and cholecystokinin) that stimulates insulin production, motor and secretory activity, inhibits somatostatin release, and promotes GI growth.

3. GI maturation and metabolic efficiency is further promoted through increases in both IGF-I and oxytocin.

4. The stress reducing benefits of oxytocin contribute to a reduction in serum cortisol levels and promote functioning of the H-P-A axis and neurobehavioral maturation (e.g., improved BNBAS performance and enhanced infant-caregiver relations).

5. Enhanced H-P-A axis functioning yields a greater release of cate-cholamines that in turn support the increase in GI peptides such as gastrin and may underlie changes in behavioral state organization (e.g., increased alertness).

The vagal model outlined above is complex and proposes a relationship between the activity of the vagus nerves, the H-P-A axis, the GI tract, and several peptide hormones. Conclusive support of the vagal model depends on future research. Along with vagal tone monitoring, these studies must include sophisticated biochemical assays in order to determine the rela-tionships between CVT, cortisol, catecholamines, and peptides such as IGF-I and oxytocin. Regression or structural equation modeling is needed to explore the interrelations between these variables and T/K benefits such as weight gain.

CONCLUSIONS AND CLINICAL GUIDELINES

Collectively, numerous studies strongly suggest that tactile and kinesthetic stimulation are safe for preterm infants and improve their hospital course. Passive forms of touch therapy have been shown to soothe young and sick infants residing in the NICU. For grower nursery infants, T/K facilitates weight gain and appears to enhance neurobehavioral maturation.

The value of passive tactile stimulation such as the Harrison et al. (1996) 'gentle human touch' (GHT) protocol should be investigated further. No research has examined the effects of supplemental stimulation that begins in the NICU and continues until the preterm infant is discharged from the hospital. A conjoint GHT and T/K regimen might be the first step in this direction since both procedures are easily administered. Infants would receive GHT as they resided in the NICU. T/K would begin upon transfer to the progressive care unit (PCU) or grower nursery and continue until discharge. Singular and additive treatment effects could be evaluated through three treatment conditions: singular NICU GHT, singular PCU/grower nursery T/K, and conjoint NICU GHT and PCU/grower nursery T/K. Treatment findings such as weight gain, neurobehavioral performance, and days to discharge could be compared with a control group.

Unfortunately, recent years have seen the number of supplemental stim-ulation studies diminish. Renewed efforts should be taken to revitalize this field of research. Preterm infant supplemental stimulation is of scien-tific interest for the contribution that it can make to our understanding of the relationship between the environment and early neurobehavioral development. It is also clinically relevant for its potential to shorten the hospital course of preterm infants and aid in the amelioration of some of the adversities of premature birth.

ACKNOWLEDGEMENTS

Dr. Dieter expresses his appreciation to Tiffany Field PhD and Maria Hernandez-Reif PhD for their invaluable assistance in completing the dissertation presented in this chapter.

REFERENCES

Acolet, D., Modi, N., Giannakoulopoulos, X., et al. (1993). Changes in plasma cortisol and catecholamine concentrations in response to massage in preterm infants. *Archives in Disease in Childhood, 68,* 29–31.

Adamson-Macedo, E. N. (1986). Effects of tactile stimulation on low and very low birthweight infants during the first week of life. *Current Psychological Research and Reviews, Winter,* 305–308.

Adamson-Macedo, E. N., & Alves-Attree, J. L. (1994). TAC-TIC therapy: The importance of systematic stroking. *British Journal of Midwifery, 2,* 264–269.

Adamson-Macedo, E. N., de Roiste, A., Wilson, A., et al. (1994). TAC-TIC therapy with high-risk, distressed, ventilated preterms. *Journal of Reproductive and Infant Psychology, 12,* 249–252.

Ader, R., Friedman, S. B., Grota, L. J., & Schaefer, A. (1968). Attenuation of the plasma corticosterone response to handling and electric shock stimulation in the infant rat. *Physiology and Behavior, 3,* 327–331.

Als, H. (1986). A synactive model of neonatal organization: Framework for the assessment of neurobehavioral and development in the preterm infant and for the support of infants and parents in the neonatal intensive care environment. *Physical and Occupational Therapy in Pediatrics, 6,* 3–53.

Aylward, G. P., Gustafson, N., Verhulst, J. A., & Colliver, S. J. (1987). Consistency in the diagnosis of cognitive, motor, and neurologic function over the first three years. *Journal of Pediatric Psychology, 12,* 77–98.

Bayley, N. (1969). *Bayley Scales of Infant Development: Birth to two years.* San Antonio: The Psychological Corporation.

Bennett, A., Wilson, D. M., Liu, F., et al. (1983). Levels of insulin-like growth factors I and II in human cord blood. *Journal of Clinical Endocrinology Metabolism, 57,* 609–612.

Borer, K. T. (1974). Absence of weight regulation in exercising hamsters. *Physiology and Behavior, 12,* 589–597.

Borer, K. T., & Kooi, A. A. (1975). Regulatory defense of exercise-induced weight elevation in hamsters. *Behavioral Biology, 13,* 301–310.

Brazelton, T. B. (1973). *Neonatal behavioral assessment scale.* Philadelphia: Lippincott.

Caputo, D. V., & Mandell, W. (1970). Consequences of low birth weight. *Developmental Psychology, 3,* 363–383.

Centers for Disease Control and Prevention. (1992). Reliability and validity assessment of the use of stressful life events in Black women of reproducing age. [200-92-0565 (P)] Section C, p. 3.

Chapieski, M. L., & Evankovich, K. D. (1997). Behavioral effects of prematurity. *Seminars in Perinatology, 21,* 221–239.

Chiodera, P., Salvarani, C., Bacchi-Modena, A., et al. (1991). Relationship between plasma profiles of oxytocin and adrenocorticotropic hormone during suckling or breast stimulation in women. *Cattedre di Endocrinologia, 35,* 119–123.

Ciafarani, S., Germani, D., Rossi, L., et al. (1998). *European Journal of Endocrinology, 138,* 524–529.

Cohen, S. E., Parmelee, A. H., Beckwith, L., & Sigman, M. (1986). Cognitive development in preterm infants: Birth to 8 years. *Developmental and Behavioral Pediatrics, 7,* 102–110.

Colonna, F., Pahor, T., de Vonderweid, U., et al. (1996). Serum insulin-like growth factor-I (IGF-I) and IGF binding protein-3 (IGFBP-3) in growing preterm infants on enteral nutrition. *Journal of Pediatric Endocrinology Metabolism, 9,* 483–489.

Costela, C., Tejedor-Real, P., Mico, J. A., & Gibert-Rahola, J. (1993). Effect of neonatal handling on learned helplessness model of depression. *Physiology and Behavior, 57,* 407–410.

Cross, M. S., & Labarba, R. C. (1978). Neonatal stimulation, maternal behavior, and accelerated maturation in BALB/c mice. *Developmental Psychobiology, 11,* 83–92.

Denenberg, V. H., Brumaghim, J. T., Haltmeyer, G. C., & Zarrow, M. X. (1967). Increased adrenocortical activity in the neonatal rat following handling. *Endocrinology, 81,* 1047–1052.

Díaz Gómez, N. M., Doménech Martínez, E., & Barroso Guerrero, F. (1996). Trace elements and growth factors in the perinatal period. *An Esp Pediatr, 44,* 351–356.

Dieter, J. N. I. (1999). The effects of tactile/kinesthetic stimulation on the physiology and behavior of preterm infants. *Dissertation Abstracts International,* B 60/05 (November), 2335.

Dieter, J. N. I., & Emory, E. K. (1997). Supplemental stimulation of premature infants: A treatment model. *Journal of Pediatric Psychology, 22,* 281–295.

Dinges, D. F., Davis, M. M., & Glass, P. (1980). Fetal exposure to narcotics: Neonatal sleep as a measure of nervous system disturbance. *Science, 209,* 619–621.

DiPietro, J. A., Porges, S. W., & Uhly, B. (1992). Reactivity and developmental competence in preterm and full-term infants. *Developmental Psychology, 28,* 831–841.

Dittrichova, J., Paul, K., & Vondracek, J. (1985). Rapid eye movements during sleep in premature infants. *Activitas Nervosa Superior, 27,* 137–138.

Dobrakovova, M., Kvetnansky, Oprsalova, Z., & Jezova, D. (1993). Specificity of the effect of repeated handling on sympathetic-adrenomedullary and pituitary-adrenocortical activity in rats. *Psychoneuroendocrinology, 18,* 163–174.

Doussard-Rossevelt, J., Porges, S. W., & McClenny, B. D. (1996). Behavioral sleep states in very low birth weight preterm neonates: Relation to neonatal health and vagal maturation. *Journal of Pediatric Psychology, 21,* 785–802.

Drummond, T. (1998). Touch early and often. *Time, 152* (July 27), 54.

Emory, E. K., & Mapp, J. R. (1988). Effects of respiratory distress and prematurity on spontaneous startle activity in neonates. *Infant Behavior and Development, 11,* 71–81.

Fernandez-Teruel, A., Escorihuela, R. M., Driscoll, P., et al. (1991). Infantile (handling) stimulation and behavior in young roman high- and low-avoidance rats. *Physiology and Behavior, 50,* 563–565.

Ferry, P. C. (1981). On growing new neurons: Are early intervention programs effective? *Pediatrics, 70,* 670–676.

Field, T. (1980). Supplemental stimulation of preterm infants. *Early Human Development, 4,* 301–314.

Field, T. (1988). Stimulation of preterm infants. *Pediatrics in Review, 10,* 149–153.

Field, T., Scafidi, F., & Schanberg, S. (1987). Massage of preterm newborns to improve growth and development. *Pediatric Nursing, 13,* 385–387.

Field, T., & Schanberg, S. M. (1995). Massage therapy effects on preterm infant vagal tone and serum insulin. Unpublished pilot data.

Field, T., Schanberg, S. M., Scafidi, F., et al. (1986). Tactile/kinesthetic stimulation effects on preterm neonates. *Pediatrics, 77,* 654–658.

Fox, N. (1989). Psychophysiological correlates of emotional reactivity during the first year of life. *Developmental Psychology, 25,* 364–372.

Fox, N. A., & Porges, S. W. (1985). The relation between neonatal heart period patterns and developmental outcome. *Child Development, 56,* 28–37.

Fracasso, M. P., Porges, S. W., Lamb, M. E., & Rosenberg, A. A. (1994). Cardiac activity in infancy: Reliability and stability of individual differences. *Infant Behavior and Development, 17,* 277–284.

Francis-Williams, J., & Davis, P. A. (1974). Very low birthweight and later intelligence. *Developmental Medicine and Child Neurology, 16,* 709–728.

Friedman, S. L., Jacobs, B. S., & Werthmann, M. W. (1981). Sensory processing in pre- and full-term infants in the neonatal period. In S. L. Friedman, & M. Sigman (Eds.), *Preterm birth and psychological development* (pp. 159–179). New York: Academic Press.

Giniès, J. L., Joseph, M. G., Chomiene, F., et al. (1992). Insulin-like growth factor I (somatomedin C) in premature infants on total parenteral nutrition. Relations with nutritional status and protein-energy intakes. *Arch Fr Pediatr, 49,* 429–432.

Goldberg, S., & Divitto, B. A. (1983). *Born too soon: Preterm birth and early development.* San Francisco: W.H. Freeman & Co.

Goldstein-Feber, S. (1997). *Massage in premature infants.* Paper presented at the Child Development Conference, Bar Ilan, Israel.

Gonzalez, A. S., Rodriguez Echandia, E. L., Cabrera, R., et al. (1990). Neonatal chronic stress induces subsensitivity to chronic stress in adult rats. I. Effects on forced swim behavior and endocrine responses. *Physiology and Behavior, 47*, 735–741.

Gorga, D., Stern, F. M., & Ross, G. (1985). Trends in neuromotor behavior of preterm and fullterm infants in the first year of life: A preliminary report. *Developmental Medicine and Child Neurology, 27*, 756–766.

Gorga, D., Stern, F. M., Ross, G., & Nagler, W. (1991). The neuromotor behavior of preterm and full-term children by three years of age: Quality of movement and variability. *Developmental and Behavioral Pediatrics, 12*, 102–107.

Hack, M., & Fanaroff, A. A. (1989). Outcomes of extremely-low-birth-weight infants between 1982 and 1988. *New England Journal of Medicine, 321*, 1642–1647.

Harlow, H. F. (1958). The nature of love. *American Psychologist, 13*, 673–685.

Harrison, L. (1985). Effects of early supplemental stimulation programs for premature infants. *Maternal Child Nursing Journal, 14*, 69–90.

Harrison, L., Olivet, L., Cunningham, K., et al. (1996). Effects of gentle human touch on preterm infants: Pilot study results. *Neonatal Network, 15*, 35–42.

Hasselmeyer, E. G. (1964). The premature neonate's response to handling. *American Nurses Association, 11*, 15–24.

Herrgard, E., Karjalainen, S., Martikainen, A., & Heinonen, K. (1995). Hearing loss at age 5 years of children born preterm — a matter of definition. *Acta Paediatrica, 10*, 1160–1164.

Hole, J. W. (1981). *Human anatomy and physiology.* Dubuque, IA: Wm. C. Brown.

Howard, J., Parmelee, A. H., Kopp, C. B., & Littman, B. (1976). A neurologic comparison of pre-term and full-term infants at term conceptual age. *Journal of Pediatrics, 88*, 995–1001.

Insel, T. R. (1997). A neurobiological basis of social attachment. *American Journal of Psychiatry, 154*, 726–735.

Izard, C. E., Porges, S. W., Simons, R. E., et al. (1991). Infant cardiac activity: Developmental changes and relations with attachment. *Developmental Psychology, 27*, 432–439.

Jinon, S. (1996). The effect of infant massage on growth of the preterm infant. In C. Yarbes-Almirante & M. De Luma (Eds.), *Increasing safe and successful pregnancy*, (pp. 265–269). Netherlands: Elsevier Science, B.Z.

Kardel, K. R., & Kase, T. (1998). Training in pregnant women: Effects on fetal development and birth. *American Journal of Obstetrics and Gynecology, 178*, 280–286.

Kattwinkel, J., Nearman, H. S., Fanaroff, A. A., et al. (1975). Apnea of prematurity-comparative therapeutic effects of cutaneous stimulation and nasal continuous positive airway pressure. *Journal of Pediatrics, 86*, 588–592.

Khan-Dawood, F. S., & Dawood, M. Y. (1984). Oxytocin content of human fetal pituitary glands. *American Journal of Obstetrics and Gynecology, 22*, 420–423.

Kok, J. H., den Ouden, A. L., Verloove-Vanhorick, S. P., & Brand, R. (1998). Outcome of very preterm small for gestational age infants: The first nine years of life. *British Journal of Obstetrics and Gynecology, 105*, 162–168.

Korner, A. F. (1990). Infant stimulation: Issues of theory and research. *Clinics in Perinatology, 17*, 173–185.

Kramer, L. T., Chamorro, I., Green, D., & Knudtson, F. (1975). Extra tactile stimulation of the premature infant. *Nursing Research, 24*, 324–334.

Kuhn, C. M., Schanberg, S. M., Field, T., et al. (1991). Tactile-kinesthetic stimulation effects on sympathetic and adrenocortical function in preterm infants. *Journal of Pediatrics, 119*, 434–440.

Lane, S. L., Attanasio, C. S., & Huselid, R. F. (1994). Prediction of preschool sensory and motor performance by 18-month neurologic scores among children born prematurely. *American Journal of Occupational Therapy, 48*, 391–396.

Lester, B. M., Als, H., & Brazelton, T. B. (1982). Regional obstetric anesthesia and new born behavior: A re-analysis towards synergistic effects. *Child Development, 53*, 687–692.

Levin, J. S., & Defrank, R. S. (1988). Maternal stress and pregnancy outcomes: A review of the psychosocial literature. *Journal of Psychosomatic Obstetrics and Gynecology, 9,* 3–16.

Levine, S. (1958). A further study of infant handling and adult avoidance learning. *Journal of Personality, 25,* 70–80.

Levine, S. (1959). The effects of differential infantile stimulation on emotionality at weaning. *Canadian Journal of Psychology, 13,* 243–247.

Levine, S. (1960). Stimulation in infancy. *Scientific American, 202,* 80–86.

Levine, S., & Mullins, R. F. (1966). Hormonal influences on brain organization in infant rats. *Science, 152,* 1585–1592.

Long, J. G., Alistair, G. S., Philip, M. B., & Lucey, J. F. (1980). Excessive handling as a cause of hypoxemia. *Pediatrics, 65,* 203–207.

Luoma, L., Herrgard, E., & Martikainen, A. (1998). Neuropsychological analysis of the visomotor problems in children born preterm at < or = 32 weeks of gestation: A 5-year prospective. *Developmental Medicine and Child Neurology, 40,* 21–30.

Marchini, G., & Stock, S. (1996). Pulsatile release of oxytocin in newborn infants. *Reproduction Fertility and Development, 89,* 163–165.

Mason, W. A. (1968). Early social deprivation in the non-human primates: Implications for human behavior in environmental influences. In D. C. Glass (Ed.), *Environmental influences.* New York: Rockefeller University Press and Russell Sage Foundation.

Meaney, M. J., Aitken, D. H., Bhatnagar, S., et al. (1988). Effect of neonatal handling on age-related impairments associated with the hippocampus. *Science, 239,* 766–768.

Meaney, M. J., Aitken, D. H., & Sapolsky, R. M. (1987). Thyroid hormones influence the development of hippocampal glucocorticoid receptors in the rat: A mechanism for the effects of postnatal handling on the development of the adrenocortical stress response. *Neuroendocrinology, 45,* 278–283.

Meaney, M. J., Aitken, D. H., Sharma, S., et al. (1989). Postnatal handling increases hippocampal glucocorticoid receptors and enhances adrenocortical negative-feedback efficacy in the rat. *Neuroendocrinology, 50,* 597–604.

Modanlou, H. D. (1988). Extension reflex of fingers in the newborn. *Pediatric Neurology, 4,* 66–67.

Morrow, C. J., Field, T. M., Scafidi, F. A., et al. (1991). Differential effects of massage and heelstick procedures on transcutaneous oxygen tension in preterm infants. *Infant Behavior and Development, 14,* 397–414.

Moyer-Mileur, L., Luetkemeler, M., Boomer, L. & Chan, G. M. (1995). Effect of physical activity on bone mineralization in premature infants. *Journal of Pediatrics, 127,* 620–625.

Neal, M. V. (1968). The relationship between a regimen of vestibular stimulation and the developmental behavior of the premature infant. *Nursing Research, 17,* 562.

Nelson, E. E., & Panksepp, J. (1998). Brain substrates of infant-mother attachment: contribution of opioids, oxytocin, and norepinephrine. *Neuroscience and Biobehavioral Review, 22,* 437–452.

Noonan, L. R., Caldwell, J. D., Li, L., et al. (1994). Neonatal stress transiently alters the development of hippocampal oxytocin receptors. *Developmental Brain Research, 80,* 115–120.

Oehler, J. M. (1985). Examining the issue of tactile stimulation for premature infants. *Neonatal Network, December,* 25–33.

Osorio, M., Torres, J., Moya, F., et al. (1996). Insulin-like growth factors (IGFs) and IGF binding proteins-1, -2, and -3 in newborn serum: relationships to fetoplacental growth at term. *Early Human Development, 46,* 15–26.

Parmelee, A. H. (1985). Sensory stimulation in the nursery: How much and when? *Developmental and Behavioral Pediatrics, 6,* 242–243.

Pauk, J., Kuhn, C. M., Field, T. M., & Schanberg, S. M. (1986). Positive effects of tactile verses kinesthetic or vestibular stimulation on neuroendrocrine and ODC activity in maternally-deprived rat pups. *Life Sciences, 39,* 2081–2087.

Pettett, G. (1986). Medical complications of the preterm infant. *Physical and Occupational Therapy in Pediatrics, 6,* 91–104.

Plotsky, P. M., & Meaney, M. J. (1993). Early, postnatal experience alters hypothalamic corticotropin-releasing factor (CRF) mRNA, median eminence CRF content and stress-induced release in adult rats. *Molecular Brain Research, 18,* 195–200.

Porges, S. W. (1983). Heart rate patterns in neonates: A potential diagnostic window to the brain. In T. M. Field, & A. M. Sostek (Eds.), *Infants born at risk: Physiological and perceptual responses.* (pp. 3–22). New York: Grune & Stratton.

Porges, S. W. (1985). *Method and apparatus for evaluating rhythmic oscillations in aperiodic physiological response systems.* US Patent. No: 4,510,944, April 16.

Porges, S. W. (1995). Cardiac vagal tone: A physiological index of stress. *Neuroscience and Biobehavioral Reviews,* 19, 225–233.

Porter, F. L., Porges, S. W., & Marshall, R. E. (1988). Newborn pain cries and vagal tone: Parallel changes in response to circumcision. *Child Development,* 59, 495–505.

Prechtl, H. F. R., Fargel, J. W., Weinmann, H. M., & Bakker, H. H. (1979). Postures, motility and respiration of low-risk pre-term infants. *Developmental Medicine and Neurology,* 21, 3–27.

Ribble, M. A. (1944). Infantile experience in relation to personality development. In J. M. Hunt (Ed.), *Personality and the behavior disorders (Vol. 2)* (pp. 621–651). New York: Ronald Press.

Rice, R. D. (1977). Neuropsychological development in premature infants following stimulation. *Developmental Psychology,* 1, 69–76.

Rocha, J. B. T., & Vendite, D. (1990). Effects of undernutrition and handling during suckling on shuttle avoidance and footshock escape behavior and on plasma glucose levels of young rats. *Developmental Psychobiology,* 23, 157–168.

Rose, S. A., Feldman, J. F., Rose, S. L., et al. (1992). Behavior problems at 3 and 6 years: Prevalence and continuity in full-terms and pre-terms. *Development and Psychopathology,* 4, 361–374.

Rose, S. A., Gottfried, A. W., & Bridger, W. H. (1978). Cross-model transfer in infants: Relationship to prematurity and socioeconomic background. *Developmental Psychology,* 14, 643–652.

Russman, B. S. (1986). Are stimulation programs useful? *Archives of Neurology,* 43, 282–283.

Salvatierra, N. A., Torre, R. B., & Arce, A. (1997). Learning and novelty induced increase of central benzodiazepine receptors from chick forebrain, in a food discrimination task. *Brain Research,* 757, 79–84.

Scafidi, F., Field, T. M., Schanberg, S. M., et al. (1986). Effects of tactile/kinesthetic stimulation on the clinical course and sleep/wake behavior of preterm neonates. *Infant Behavior and Development,* 9, 91–105.

Scafidi, F., Field, T. M., Schanberg, S. M., et al. (1990). Massage stimulates growth in preterm infants: A replication. *Infant Behavior and Development,* 13, 167–188.

Schaefer, M., Hatcher, R. P., & Barglow, P. D. (1980). Prematurity and infant stimulation: A review of the literature. *Child Psychiatry and Human Development,* 10, 199–212.

Schanberg, S. M., Evoniuk, G., & Kuhn, C. M. (1984). Tactile and nutritional aspects of maternal care: Specific regulators of neuroendocrine function and cellular development. *Proceedings of the Society for Experimental Biology and Medicine,* 175, 135–146.

Schanberg, S. M., & Field, T. M. (1987). Sensory deprivation stress and supplemental stimulation in the rat pup and preterm human neonate. *Child Development,* 58, 1431–1447.

Schothorst, P. F., & van Engeland, H. (1996). Long-term behavioral sequelae of prematurity. *Journal of the American Academy of Child and Adolescent Psychiatry,* 35, 175–183.

Siegel, L. S., Saigal, S., Rosenbaum, P., et al. (1982). Predictors of development in preterm and full-term infants: A model for detecting the at risk child. *Journal of Pediatric Psychology,* 7, 135–148.

Smith, W. J., Underwood, L. E., Keyes, L., & Clemmons, D. R. (1997). Use of insulin-like growth factor I (IGF-I) and IGF-binding protein measurements to monitor feeding of premature infants. *Journal of Clinical Endocrinology Metabolism,* 82, 3982–3988.

Solkoff, N., & Matuszak, D. (1975). Tactile stimulation and behavioral development among low-birthweight infants. *Child Psychiatry and Human Development,* 6, 33–43.

Solkoff, N., Yaffe, S., Weintraub, D., & Blase, B. (1969). Effects of handling on the subsequent development of premature infants. *Developmental Psychology,* 1, 765–768.

Spitz, R. A. (1945). An inquiry into the genesis of psychiatric conditions in early childhood. In: *The psychoanalytic study of the child (Vol. 1)* (pp. 53–74). New York: International University Press.

Thoman, E. (1975). Early development of sleeping behaviors in infants. In N. Ellis (Ed.), *Aberrant development in infancy* (pp. 132–138). Hillsdale, NJ: Erlbaum.

Tortora , G. J., & Anagnostakos, N. P. (1990). *Principles of anatomy and physiology, Sixth Edition.* New York: Harper Collins.

Touwen, B. C., Hadders-Algra, M., & Huisjes, H. J. (1988). Hypotonia at six years in prematurely-born or small-for-gestational-age children. *Early Human Development, 17,* 79–88.

Tribotti, S. J. (1990). Effects of gentle human touch on the premature infant. In Gunzenhauser (Ed.), *Advances in touch: New implications in human development* (pp. 80–89). Skillman, NJ: Johnson & Johnson.

Uvnas-Moberg, K. (1997). Oxytocin linked antistress effects — the relaxation and growth response. *Acta Physiologica Scandinavica Suppl, 640,* 38–42.

Uvnas-Moberg, K., Jarhult, J., & Alino, S. (1984). Neurogenic control of release of gastrointestinal peptides. *Scandinavian Journal of Gastroenterology, 19,* Suppl 89, 131–136.

Uvnas-Moberg, K., Widstrom, A. M., Marchini, G., et al. (1987). Release of GI hormones in mother and infant by sensory stimulation. *Acta Paediatrica Scandinavica, 76,* 851–860.

Uvnas-Moberg, K., Widstrom, A. M., Werner, S., et al. (1990). Oxytocin and prolactin levels in breast-feeding women. Correlation with milk yield and duration of breast-feeding. *Acta Obstetrica Gynecologica Scandinavica, 69,* 301–306.

Weinstock, M. (1997). Does prenatal stress impair coping and regulation of hypothalamic-pituitary-adrenal axis? *Neuroscience & Biobehavioral Reviews, 21,* 1–10.

Wheeden, A., Scafidi, F. A., Field, T., et al. (1993). Massage effects on cocaine-exposed preterm neonates. *Developmental and Behavioral Pediatrics, 14,* 318–322.

White, B. L., Castle, P., & Held, R. (1964). Observations of the development of visually-directed reaching. *Child Development, 35,* 349–364.

White, J. L., & Labarba, R. (1976). The effects of tactile and kinesthetic stimulation on neonatal development in the premature infant. *Developmental Psychobiology, 9,* 569–577.

Wittenberg, J. V. P. (1990). Psychiatric considerations in premature birth. *Canadian Journal of Psychiatry, 35,* 734–740.

Wright, L. (1971). The theoretical and research base for a program of early stimulation care and training of premature infants. *Exceptional Infant, 2,* 276–304.

Xu, R. J. (1996). Development of the newborn GI tract and its relation to colostrum/milk intake: a review. *Reproduction Fertility and Development, 8,* 35–48.

Yamasaki, A., Morikawa, H., Ueda, Y., & Mochizuki, M. (1989). Circulating forms of insulin-like growth factor-I (IGF-I)/Somatomedin C (SMC) in fetal life: relationship between changes in its binding proteins and growth delay during intrauterine and post-natal periods. *Nippon Naibunpi Gakkai Zasshi, 65,* 137–151.

8

Hand massage in the agitated elderly

Ruth Remington

BACKGROUND AND SIGNIFICANCE

Agitation is a widespread problem in the elderly that negatively affects their quality of life (Cohen-Mansfield & Billig, 1986; Teri et al., 1992). The effects of their agitation are also felt by their family caregivers for whom the presence of agitated behaviors predicts caregiver burden (Hamel et al., 1990) and increases the likelihood that the older person will enter a skilled nursing facility (Cohen-Mansfield, 1995; Cohen-Mansfield et al., 1989; Teri et al., 1992). There, agitation affects the cost of care by increasing the need for staff and for special environmental designs of nursing homes (Cohen-Mansfield et al., 1989).

Agitation is prevalent in the nursing home, affecting between 64% and 93% of residents (Cohen-Mansfield et al., 1989; Zimmer et al., 1984). The frequency of agitated behaviors is related positively to the level of cognitive impairment (Cariga et al., 1991; Cohen-Mansfield et al., 1990; Cooper et al., 1990; Swearer et al., 1988) and may serve as a dysfunctional coping mechanism to protect the cognitively impaired person from real or imaginary threats in the environment (Cohen-Mansfield et al., 1990).

Once in the nursing home, the quality of the agitated older person's life is imperiled still further. The presence of agitated behaviors increases the likelihood that the elderly resident will be physically restrained (Evans &

Strumpf, 1990; Werner et al., 1989), and/or chemically restrained by the use of psychotropic medications (Cariga et al., 1991). Research has shown that nursing home residents who experience falls are found to be more agitated (Cohen-Mansfield, 1986; Marx et al., 1989). Agitated residents are likely to be restrained to prevent falls. An estimated 66% of agitated nursing home residents are restrained at some time and the mean number of restraint days was 87 per year (Tinetti et al., 1991). In addition to loss of dignity and potential for injury (Lipowski, 1992), residents who are restrained exhibit the same or more agitated behaviors, disorientation, more incontinence and more falls than residents who are not restrained (Tinetti et al., 1991; Werner et al., 1989). These data indicate that agitation in nursing home residents leads to the use of restraints, which in turn leads to a further increase in agitation. Ironically, studies have shown that restraints do not prevent falls associated with serious injury in ambulatory nursing home residents (Evans & Strumpf, 1990) and restraint reduction can actually result in fewer falls and injuries (Meyer et al., 1994). Additionally, restraint use exposes residents to consequences of immobility such as urinary retention, constipation, osteoporosis, muscle atrophy, limb ischemia, protein-energy malnutrition and dehydration, as well as the potential for strangulation (Meyer et al., 1994; Werner et al., 1989).

The effectiveness of pharmacological interventions to control behavior is documented in the literature, however age-related changes in the older person may result in a longer duration of activity of the drug, a variable drug effect, and an increased incidence of adverse drug reactions (Chutka, 1997). Pharmacological interventions as a form of chemical restraint may paradoxically exacerbate the very behaviors they are intended to moderate, causing further cognitive or functional decline (Carlson et al., 1995). Additionally, these interventions introduce the potential for side effects such as gait impairment, falls, difficulty swallowing, anorexia, sedation, hypotension, diminished cognitive function and increased agitation (Carlson et al., 1995; Corrigan, 1989; Gardner & Garrett, 1997; Knopman & Sawyer-Demaris, 1990).

The Omnibus Budget Reconciliation Act (1987) requires that the nursing home resident's regimen be free from unnecessary physical and chemical restraint, but these standards did not address alternative measures to regulate agitated behavior. Thus, progress in the treatment of agitation has been slow (Williams-Burgess et al., 1996).

Several non-pharmacological management strategies for the reduction of agitated behaviors in nursing home residents that have been investigated include therapeutic touch and hand massage (Snyder et al., 1995a,b), the use of music (Gerdner & Swanson, 1993; Goddaer & Abraham, 1994; Ragneskog et al., 1996; Tabloski et al., 1995), restraint release (Moorse & McHutchion, 1991; Werner et al., 1989), and environmental modifications such as electronic security systems (Negley et al., 1990) and visual barriers (Chafetz, 1990; Dickinson et al., 1995; Hussian & Brown, 1987). While these studies consistently demonstrated a reduction in agitated behaviors in nursing home residents, most studies used differing definitions and measures of agitation, thereby limiting generalization about the effectiveness of these interventions in reducing agitation.

Nurses, in providing direct care to agitated nursing home residents, are in the position to identify agitated behaviors and intervene promptly, minimizing the escalation of agitation and the use of physical and chemical restraints. Reduction in agitated behaviors of nursing home residents would likely result in decreased costs associated with medications and associated adverse side effects, falls, special environmental designs, and increased staff-to-patient ratios. Because agitation is costly in terms of quality of life for the agitated nursing home resident, as well as in the direct and indirect costs of providing residential care for these persons, the purpose of this study was to compare hand massage and calming music as interventions to reduce agitated behavior in agitated nursing home residents with dementia. These interventions are feasible, cost-effective, easily administered, non-pharmacological treatments that can be administered by non-professional, as well as professional caregivers.

Agitation

The concept of agitation, its etiology and manifestations are not consistently defined in the literature (Cohen-Mansfield & Billig, 1986) and this is evidenced by the multiplicity of definitions and measures of agitation in the intervention research. Cohen-Mansfield & Billig (1986) proposed that agitation may be a construct of interrelated behavior problems, rather than a unified concept. They defined agitation as inappropriate verbal, vocal or motor activity that is not explained by needs or confusion. Although agitation may result from unmet needs or confusion, these may not be evident to the observer (Cohen-Mansfield & Billig, 1986). Agitation is manifested in three syndromes: physically aggressive behaviors, physically non-aggressive behaviors and verbally agitated behaviors (Cohen-Mansfield et al., 1989; Miller et al., 1995).

Agitated behaviors are a common occurrence in nursing home residents. In a sample of 408 nursing home residents in a single facility, irrespective of the presence of dementing illness, 93% exhibited agitated behaviors at least once a week and the mean number of agitated behaviors exhibited per resident, per week was 9.3 (SD = 8.6) (Cohen-Mansfield et al., 1989).

Touch

Healing through touch has been practiced in many cultures since ancient times. Philosophical and cultural differences have had a profound influence on the development of touch as a healing modality in different parts of the world. For example, the Oriental approach to healing touch involves the belief that healing energy is directed through the practitioner's hands to the patient. This is in stark contrast to the Western view of physiological effect of cellular changes that influences healing. The Puritan belief that equated touch with sex initiated the move away from the use of touch as a therapeutic intervention. This was furthered by the scientific advances in the nineteenth and twentieth centuries (Dossey et al., 1995). With the increasing complexity and demands of care involving life preserving machinery, nurses are faced with finding the right balance between 'high tech' and 'high touch' (Barnum, 1994).

In recent research, touch has been shown to produce a variety of therapeutic effects in diverse populations. Therapeutic touch was associated with a decrease in pain and increased relaxation in community residing adults (Heidt, 1991). When administered to psychiatric inpatients, therapeutic touch resulted in a significant reduction of anxiety, similar to that obtained with guided relaxation therapy. This supports the use of touch as a passive technique that can be used for the reduction of anxiety which can be utilized when the patient is unable to participate (Gagne & Toye, 1994).

In a descriptive study examining the relationship between agitation and touch in nursing home residents, results were differentially related to particular agitated behaviors. Verbally agitated and physically aggressive behaviors were manifested more often when the person was being touched, suggesting that this was in relation to a sense that their personal space was violated. Physically non-aggressive agitation was exhibited less frequently when the person was being touched, supporting the hypothesis that touch is a comforting form of communication (Marx et al., 1989). In this study the type of touch was not controlled for and included both comforting touch as well as touch involved in administering care and treatments, which may have influenced the differing response.

It has been suggested that the elderly are the most deprived of touch, particularly if they are dependent on others for physical care in nursing homes (Fraser & Kerr, 1993). The need for affective touch continues throughout life and increases with age (Stanley & Beare, 1999). Nursing home residents perceived that nurses who used comforting touch on the arm of the patient communicated more affection and immediacy than the nurses who did not use touch (Moore & Gilbert, 1995).

Physiological and psychological effects of back massage on anxiety were examined among elderly nursing home residents. Using an experimental design with pre-test/post-test control group conditions, back massage was compared with conversation and no intervention. Results indicated that back massage and conversation were more effective than none, in reducing agitation as evidenced by reduced electromyographic readings, blood pressure, and heart rate and by self-report. These differences, however, did not reach statistical significance. The authors note that despite the fact that the statistical analysis did not clearly answer the research question, there was strong evidence of the positive effect of the interventions (Fraser & Kerr, 1993).

The effect of slow-stroke back massage on agitated behaviors was examined in community dwelling individuals with Alzheimer's disease. Verbal agitation, the most frequently manifested type of agitation in this group was not reduced following back massage. Physical displays of agitation did show a reduction in frequency when back massage was applied (Rowe & Alfred, 1999).

Critically ill, hospitalized older men showed improved sleep as measured electronically, following a six-minute back massage. Subjects receiving back massage slept one hour longer than those who received relaxation training and music at bedtime or those who received no intervention. These results did not reach statistical significance, however, the author did conclude that back massage is useful for promoting sleep in critically ill older men (Richards, 1998).

Using a quasi-experimental design, physiological parameters of relaxation were examined in terminally ill adults being cared for in the home. Results included a reduction in heart rate of 4.2 beats per minute on average. Additionally, reductions in both systolic and diastolic blood pressure (9.17 and 6.14 mmHg respectively) and skin temperature (1.45° Fahrenheit) persisted for five minutes after the intervention. These small reductions in physiological parameters were adequate to demonstrate relaxation in subjects, however they were not sufficient to pose danger of bradycardia, hypotension or hyperthermia (Meek, 1993).

The effectiveness of hand massage therapeutic touch and presence for reducing agitation was examined in 17 residents of an Alzheimer's care unit. Results showed an increase in relaxation and a decrease in anxious behaviors among the subjects who received either treatment. Greater increase in relaxation was observed in the group who received hand massage for ten minutes than the group who received therapeutic touch. No indication of relaxation was observed with presence alone. There was however, no change in the frequency of agitated behaviors. The authors proposed that the relaxation response was too brief to affect the overall levels of agitation (Snyder et al., 1995a). In a subsequent study, the authors examined whether a five-minute hand massage before care activities would reduce the frequency and intensity of agitated behaviors during care in residents of three Alzheimer's care units. Results showed that agitation was decreased during the baseline period with inconsistent results during care activities. It was suggested that decreasing the length of the hand massage from ten minutes in the first study to five minutes in the subsequent study may have accounted for the less significant results in the second study (Snyder et al., 1995b).

Commonalities of the type of touch found in these studies include light pressure, even rhythm and slow strokes. Studies dealing exclusively with therapeutic touch were not considered relevant to this study involving cognitively impaired nursing home residents, as therapeutic touch is described as a reciprocal communication process (Heidt, 1991), and the communication ability of the subjects is likely to be impaired. Additionally, extensive training and practice is necessary to master therapeutic touch. Hand massage was chosen as the form of touch to be used in this study because it is felt to be less threatening in that it is similar to familiar social touch and does not require removal of clothing as is necessary with back massage.

Music

As noted with the touch literature, music had been shown to produce a variety of therapeutic effects in diverse populations. Music was effective in pain control (Schorr, 1993; Whipple & Glynn, 1992), improving sleep in older persons (Mornhinweg & Voignier, 1995), promoting relaxation in mechanically ventilated patients (Chlan, 1995), reducing anxiety in surgical patients (Winter et al., 1995) and in patients who had an acute myocardial infarction (White, 1992), as well as reducing heart rate (Chlan, 1995; White, 1992). Additionally, a music intervention resulted in an increase in positive behaviors and a reduction in restraint use in an acute care setting (Janelli & Kanski, 1997).

Examples specific to agitation in nursing home residents include the descriptive study by Cohen-Mansfield & Werner (1995) in which agitated behaviors were decreased when music was present in the environment in a sample of agitated nursing home residents. Music chosen for calming qualities was shown to reduce agitation on the nursing unit (Tabloski et al., 1995) and during mealtime (Goddaer & Abraham, 1994; Ragneskog et al., 1996). An individualized, preferred music intervention provided during peak agitation periods was consistently effective in reducing the frequency of agitated behaviors in agitated nursing home residents (Gerdner, 2000; Gerdner & Swanson, 1993).

While both calming and individualized music have been shown to reduce agitation, this study used a standardized piece of calming music to eliminate potential confounding of results by memories or emotions that may be evoked by a familiar tune and the possible influence on agitation.

PURPOSE AND HYPOTHESES

Hand massage or calming music each have been shown to reduce agitated behaviors in nursing home residents with dementia. This study investigated the effectiveness of these interventions in reducing agitation, including identifying whether each is equally effective and whether there is an additive or synergistic effect of the combination of interventions on the reduction of agitation in nursing home residents with dementia. The purpose of this study was to compare the effect of hand massage, or calming music, or a combination of hand massage and calming music on the level of agitation in nursing home residents with dementia.

The six hypotheses were that:

1. Agitated nursing home residents with dementia who are exposed to ten minutes of hand massage exhibit fewer manifestations of agitation immediately following intervention than those who receive no intervention.

2. Agitated nursing home residents with dementia who are exposed to ten minutes of calming music exhibit fewer manifestations of agitation immediately following intervention than those who receive no intervention.

3. Agitated nursing home residents with dementia who are exposed to ten minutes of a combination of hand massage and calming music exhibit fewer manifestations of agitation immediately following intervention than those who are exposed to hand massage alone, calming music alone or no intervention.

4. Agitated nursing home residents with dementia experience differential levels of physically aggressive behaviors over time with exposure to hand massage or, calming music or a combination of hand massage and calming music, or no intervention.

5. Agitated nursing home residents with dementia experience differential levels of physically non-aggressive behaviors over time with exposure to hand massage or, calming music or, a combination of hand massage and calming music, or no intervention.

6. Agitated nursing home residents with dementia experience differential levels of verbally agitated behaviors over time with exposure to hand massage, or calming music, or a combination of hand massage and calming music, or no intervention.

METHODS

Design

A four group, repeated measures experimental design was used to test the effect of hand massage and calming music in reducing agitation in nursing home residents with dementia. Agitated nursing home residents were randomly assigned to one of four intervention groups and received a ten minute exposure to either hand massage (HM), calming music (CM) or both hand massage and calming music simultaneously (HMCM), or no intervention. The number of occurrences and types of agitated behaviors were recorded for .ten minute periods, immediately before the intervention, during the intervention, immediately after the intervention, and at one hour.

Sample

To obtain an estimate of the effect size likely to be realized in this study, a pilot study of 24 agitated nursing home residents was conducted and the data used for power analysis. A power calculation was performed for each pair of groups in the sample for which comparisons were to be performed in order to determine the minimum number of subjects needed to detect significant group difference in reduction in agitation. Effect size in the pilot study was 0.55. With the level of significance of 0.05 and power of 0.80, a total sample of 68 subjects with 17 subjects in each of the four treatment groups was predicted to be adequate to detect significant results.

Criteria for inclusion in this study include age of 60 or more years; diagnosis of dementia, exhibition of any agitated behavior occurring an average of one or more times a day during the preceding two weeks as identified by scores on the Cohen-Mansfield Agitation Inventory completed by the charge nurse on the unit; ability to hear; and ability to feel touch on the hands. Subjects who received medication on an as needed basis for agitated behavior within the four hours preceding the intervention were excluded. Informed consent was obtained from the family or legal guardian in writing and verbal assent was obtained from all subjects immediately prior to the intervention.

Instrument

The Cohen-Mansfield Agitation Inventory (CMAI) is a 29 item caregiver rating scale, developed for use in the nursing home, to systematically record the presence and frequency of agitated behaviors in nursing home residents. Each of the 29 items, or agitated behaviors, is rated on a 7-point response format of frequency scaled from 1 (never) to 7 (several times an hour). Ratings refer to behaviors exhibited during the two weeks preceding the test administration. The CMAI may be administered by a caregiver or by interviewing a staff or family caregiver (Cohen-Mansfield, 1991).

Internal consistency of the CMAI has been evaluated in nursing home residents using Cronbach's coefficient alpha and reported to be between 0.74 and 0.91 (Finkel et al., 1993; Miller et al., 1995). Interrater reliability of the CMAI (Pearson's correlation coefficient) has been reported between 0.82 to 0.92 (Cohen-Mansfield et al., 1989; Miller et al., 1995).

Content validity of the CMAI was determined by extensive literature search, concept analysis and nurses' observations and attributions (Cohen-Mansfield, 1986). Convergent validity of the CMAI was examined by correlating responses on the CMAI and the Behavioral and Emotional Activities Manifested in Dementia scale (0.79 to 0.92), the Nursing Home Problem Behavior Scale (0.64 to 0.95) (Miller et al., 1995; Ray et al., 1992), and the Brief Agitation Rating Scale (0.95) (Finkel et al., 1993). Correlations between the CMAI and the Rapid Disability Rating Scale ranged from 0.68 to 0.98 (Chrisman et al., 1991).

Factor analysis revealed three factors, or syndromes of agitated behavior, which were stable across shifts. These were called aggressive behavior, physically non-aggressive behavior, and verbally agitated behavior (Cohen-Mansfield et al., 1989). Subsequent factor analysis revealed a similar factor structure indicating that the factors represent distinct dimensions of agitation (Miller et al., 1995).

The CMAI has been modified from a retrospective data collection instrument to an observer format which is scored for frequency of occurrence of agitated behaviors (Chrisman et al., 1991). A score of '0' indicates that the behavior is not present, '1' indicates that the behavior occurred only once during the observation period, a score of '2' indicates that the behavior occurred two times, etc. The total agitation score is calculated by summing the scores for the individual behaviors. A total score of '0' indicates that the subject is not agitated and the higher the score, the greater the agitation.

Interrater reliability of the modified CMAI has been reported between 0.72 and 0.81 (Chrisman et al., 1991) and 93% agreement (Gerdner, 2000). Interrater reliability for the present ranged between 0.93 and 1 (Pearson correlation). A t-test verified that there was no significant difference ($t = 1.65$, $df = 28$, $p = 0.11$) in ratings of agitated behaviors between the raters.

Convergent validity of the modified CMAI was supported when examined by correlating the responses with the Ward Behavior Inventory and the Confusion Inventory (Chrisman et al., 1991).

Procedure

This study was approved by the Committee for the Protection of Human Subjects in Research. Potential subjects with a medical diagnosis of Alzheimer's disease, multi-infarct dementia or senile dementia were identified by chart review by the principal investigator (PI). The charge nurse was then asked to select from the identified residents, those who exhibit agitation on a regular basis and document this by completion of the CMAI. Informed consent was then obtained in writing from the responsible person listed on the medical record. Prior to data collection, cards were prepared containing a subject number and group assignment and these cards were placed in sealed envelopes. As each subject agreed to participate, an envelope was drawn, providing that subject's number and group assignment. Subjects were thus randomly assigned to one of four groups: HM, CM, HMCM, or control. Each subject was observed for 10 minutes, the modified CMAI completed by a trained research assistant to identify the number of agitated behaviors exhibited immediately before the intervention. If a subject's score was less than 1, which indicates the absence of agitation at the time of the study session, he or she was not assigned to an intervention group for that session.

Subjects assigned to the HM group received ten minutes of hand massage, five minutes on each hand, utilizing the protocol developed by Snyder et al. (1995b) as follows:

1. To the back of the hand
   - using moderate pressure, apply short to medium length straight strokes from the wrist to fingertips followed by large circular strokes from the center to the side of the hand
   - using light pressure, make small circular strokes over the back of the hand.
   - featherlike long strokes from the wrist to fingertips.
2. To the palm of the hand, using moderate pressure, apply
   - short to medium length strokes from the wrist to fingertips
   - gentle milking of tissue of entire palm
   - small circular strokes over entire palm
   - large circular strokes from center to sides.
3. To the fingers, apply gentle squeezing along the length of each finger, followed by gentle range of motion of each finger, ending with gentle pressure on the nailbed.
4. Complete massage by gently drawing your hand over the entire length of the resident's hand and fingers several times on the back then the palm.

Subjects assigned to the CM group were exposed to 10 minutes of Daniel Kobialka's recording of Pachelbel's Canon in D played on a portable compact disc player at a volume between piano and mezzo-forte, a level slightly higher than the environmental noise level but low enough to allow conversation to be heard. This piece was chosen for its slow tempo (52 beats per minute), soft dynamic levels and repetitive themes. Calming music is neutral and does not contain recognizable melodies that may evoke intense emotional responses. Technically, this music is characterized by slow tempo, soft dynamic levels, and irregular, repetitive themes, and absence of sound impulses (Goddaer & Abraham, 1994).

Ten minute duration was selected for the HM intervention based on the work of Snyder et al. (1995a,b) in which a more significant reduction of agitation was achieved with ten minutes of hand massage than with five minutes. Subjects in the HMCM group received both of the above interventions simultaneously and subjects in the control group received no experimental intervention during the ten-minute intervention period. Although it was not possible to blind the data collectors to the intervention, a different data collector conducted the intra-treatment measurement.

All subjects were assessed for level of agitation and the modified CMAI scored during four observation periods of ten minutes each; before the intervention (time 1), during the intervention (time 2), immediately after the intervention (time 3), and at one hour (time 4). Research assistants did not initiate conversation with the subject however, they responded to the subject if requested. Subjects were free to discontinue the intervention at any time; none chose to do so.

In order to minimize the potential influence of other environmental stimuli, the intervention was conducted in the patient's room or familiar lounge area. Times of scheduled activities, meals and routine care administration were avoided to avert stress associated with change in usual routine. Interventions were scheduled for the time of day in which peak agitation occurs, as reported by nursing staff for each resident.

RESULTS

Subjects

Subjects were 68 agitated nursing home residents from four long-term care facilities. They were mostly women (87%), Caucasian (94%), and ranged in age from 62 to 99 years. The mean age was 82.43 (SD 8.09). Level of dementia for these subjects was indicated as moderate to severe. Length of stay in the nursing home ranged from two months to nine years, four months, with 95% residing more than six months. Subjects were dependent or required assistance with activities of daily living (ADL). Level of education in this sample ranged between no formal education for one subject to a PhD for one subject, with a majority having completed less than a high school education (56%).

Baseline levels of agitation

A one-way analysis of variance (ANOVA), comparing baseline levels of agitation in the four treatment groups, indicated the adequacy of randomization. The Levene test for homogeneity of variances indicated equal variance among the four groups ($F = 0.63$, $p = 0.60$). Mean agitation scores for the four intervention groups ranged from 16.47 in the HM group to 22 in the HMCM group, and are summarized in Table 8.1. The overall F test of group differences verified that there were no significant differences among the four group means ($F = 1.09$, $p = 0.36$).

Hypothesis 1, hand massage

A t-test for independent samples was conducted to test Hypothesis 1 that agitated nursing home residents with dementia who are exposed to ten

Table 8.1   Mean agitation scores at baseline

Group	Hand massage	Calming music	Hand massage calming music	Control
Mean	16.47	18.41	22.00	21.76
Standard deviation	9.94	11.18	11.94	9.09
n	17	17	17	17

p-value from one-way ANOVA test of zero group differences = 0.36 (F = 1.09. df = 3, 64).

minutes of hand massage exhibit fewer manifestations of agitation imme-diately following intervention than those who receive no intervention. Scores at Time 3 (after the intervention) were compared for the HM group and the control group. Results indicated that agitation scores in the HM group were significantly different than in the control group ($t = 4.20$, $df = 32$, $p = 0.00$). The mean score at Time 3 was 7.77 (SD 9.55) for the HM group and 20.88 (SD 8.66) for the control group, with a mean difference of 13.12. The control group exhibited on average nearly three times the agitation in the control group after the intervention. Hypothesis 1 was not rejected.

Hypothesis 2, calming music

A t-test for independent samples was conducted to test Hypothesis 2, that agitated nursing home residents with dementia who are exposed to ten minutes of calming music exhibit fewer manifestations of agitation imme-diately following intervention than those who receive no intervention. Scores at Time 3 (after the intervention) from the calming music group and the control group were compared. Results indicated that agitation scores in the CM group were significantly different than in the control group ($t = 4.18$, $df = 32$, $p = 0.00$) at Time 3. The mean score at Time 3 for the CM group was 7.65 (SD 9.79), and for the control group was 20.88 (SD 8.66) with a mean difference of 13.24. On average, subjects who were not exposed to calming music exhibited 13 more agitated behaviors during the ten-minute observation period (nearly three times the agitation) than those who were exposed to calming music. Hypothesis 2 was not rejected.

Hypothesis 3, hand massage and calming music

A one-way ANOVA was conducted to test Hypothesis 3 that agitated nursing home residents with dementia who are exposed to ten minutes of both hand massage and calming music simultaneously exhibit fewer manifestations of agitation immediately following intervention than those who are exposed to hand massage alone, or calming music alone, or no

Table 8.2   Mean agitation scores after intervention

Group	Hand massage	Calming music	Hand massage calming music	Control
Mean	7.76	7.66	7.06	20.88
Standard deviation	9.55	9.78	7.08	8.66
n	17	17	17	17

p-value from one-way ANOVA test of zero group differences $= <0.01$ ($F = 9.79$. $df = 3, 64$).

intervention. Scores from Time 3 (after the intervention) were compared for the four intervention groups. The Levene test for homogeneity of variances was not significant ($p = 0.52$) indicating that the assumption of homogeneity of variance was reasonable. The overall F test was significant ($F = 9.79$, $p = 0.00$) indicating that there was a significant difference in agitation scores among the intervention groups (Table 8.2).

Post hoc analysis using Tukey's HSD test with a level of significance of 0.05 indicated that the control group (mean 20.88; SD 8.66) differed significantly from HM group (mean 7.76; SD 9.55), the CM group (mean 7.65; SD 9.78), and the HMCM group (mean 7.06; SD 7.08). Subjects in the treatment groups exhibited on average between 13.12 and 13.82 fewer agitated behaviors during the ten minute observation period than the control group. These data provide partial support for Hypothesis 3.

Hypothesis 4, change in physically aggressive behaviors over time

Repeated measures analysis of variance was used to test Hypothesis 4 that there is a differential level of reduction of physically aggressive behaviors with hand massage, calming music, and a combination of hand massage and calming music over time. The Mauchly sphericity test was significant, indicating that the sphericity assumption was not met, therefore the Greenhouse-Geisser procedure was used to adjust the degrees of freedom for the F tests. Results showed no significant differences ($F = 1.93$, $p = 0.09$) in physically aggressive behaviors among the four groups. Mean scores are presented in Table 8.3. Hypothesis 4 was rejected.

Hypothesis 5, change in physically non-aggressive behaviors over time

Repeated measures ANOVA was performed on the physically nonaggressive subset of behaviors in all four intervention groups. The Mauchly sphericity test was significant, indicating that the sphericity assumption was not met, therefore the Greenhouse-Geisser procedure was used to

Table 8.3   Mean scores of physically aggressive behaviors over time

	Hand massage	Calming music	Hand massage calming music	Control
Time 1 Mean (SD)	3.71 (4.70)	2.65 (4.12)	3.35 (4.83)	1.18 (1.70)
Time 2 Mean (SD)	2.24 (4.22)	0.94 (2.30)	1.47 (2.62)	1.35 (2.09)
Time 3 Mean (SD)	1.47 (2.50)	0.71 (2.02)	0.82 (1.28)	1.24 (1.75)
Time 4 Mean (SD)	0.71 (1.76)	0.29 (0.99)	0.59 (0.94)	1.06 (1.75)
n	17	17	17	17

$p = 0.09$ from F test from repeated measures ANOVA with Greenhouse-Geisser procedure applied ($df = 5.53, 118$).

Table 8.4   Mean scores of physically non-aggressive behaviors over time

	Hand massage	Calming music	Hand massage calming music	Control
Time 1 Mean (SD)	8.41 (7.13)	9.76 (6.13)	10.88 (6.13)	13.29 (7.64)
Time 2 Mean (SD)	5.35 (6.25)	5.41 (7.21)	4.06 (4.38)	13.94 (8.68)
Time 3 Mean (SD)	4.65 (5.92)	4.41 (5.93)	4.06 (4.34)	13.24 (7.35)
Time 4 Mean (SD)	2.00 (3.81)	3.59 (6.61)	1.76 (3.11)	12.94 (9.20)
n	17	17	17	17

$p < 0.01$ from F test from repeated measures ANOVA with Greenhouse-Geisser procedure applied ($df = 7.36, 157.08$).

adjust the degrees of freedom used to test the F value for significance. Results indicated that there was a significant difference ($F = 3.78, p = 0.00$) among the four groups over time.

Post hoc analysis using Tukey's HSD test with a level of significance of 0.05 showed no difference in physically non-aggressive behavior between groups at the baseline measure (Time 1). During subsequent measurements (Times 2, 3, and 4) agitation scores in the control group were significantly greater than in the three experimental treatment groups. On average, subjects in the control group exhibited nine or more physically non-aggressive behaviors than subjects in any of the experimental intervention groups. Mean scores are shown in Table 8.4. The data provide partial support for Hypothesis 5.

Hypothesis 6, change in verbally agitated behaviors over time

Repeated measures ANOVA conducted on the subset of verbally agitated behaviors in all four groups. The Mauchly sphericity test was significant, indicating that the sphericity assumption was violated, therefore the Greenhouse-Geisser procedure was used to adjust the degrees of freedom

Table 8.5 Mean scores of verbally agitated behaviors over time

	Hand massage	Calming music	Hand massage calming music	Control
Time 1 Mean (SD)	2.41 (5.20)	5.29 (6.08)	5.53 (7.26)	5.65 (5.56)
Time 2 Mean (SD)	0.71 (1.49)	2.41 (4.24)	2.24 (4.31)	5.00 (5.40)
Time 3 Mean (SD)	0.41 (0.94)	2.06 (3.80)	1.71 (3.79)	4.94 (5.18)
Time 4 Mean (SD)	0.12 (0.33)	0.65 (2.42)	1.18 (2.51)	4.88 (5.33)
n	17	17	17	17

$p = 0.10$ from F test from repeated measures ANOVA with Greenhouse-Geisser procedure applied ($df = 4.53, 96.73$).

used to test the F value for significance. The overall F test indicated that there was no significant difference in agitation scores ($F - 1.92$, $p - 0.10$) among the four groups over time.

Post hoc analysis using Tukey's HSD test with a significance level of 0.05 however, revealed a difference between the control group and the HM group at Time 2 and Time 3, and between the control group and the three experimental treatment groups at Time 4. Mean scores are shown in Table 8.5. The hand massage group was less verbally agitated at baseline, however that difference was not statistically significant. Hand massage resulted in a consistently greater reduction in verbally agitated behaviors than that found in the other groups. At Time 4, any intervention resulted in a greater reduction in verbally agitated behavior than no intervention. Hypothesis 6 was not rejected.

ADDITIONAL ANALYSIS

The repeated measures design used in this study allowed for an additional comparison of the effects of the experimental interventions on the frequency of agitated behaviors over time.

Change over time in all four groups

One-way analysis of variance for repeated measures was performed to compare the profiles of agitated behaviors over time among the four treatment groups. Scores from each of the treatment groups (HM, CM, HMCM, control) prior to the intervention, during the intervention, immediately after the intervention and at one hour were compared. Geisser and Greenhouse's procedure was used to adjust the degrees of freedom for all F tests because the Mauchley sphericity test was significant, indicating that the sphericity assumption was violated. The mean levels of agitation over time are shown in Figure 8.1.

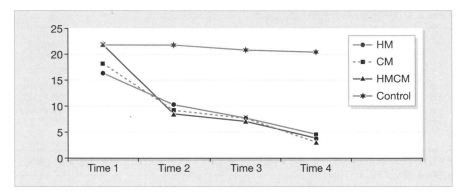

Figure 8.1 Mean agitation scores by treatment group over time.

Table 8.6 Mean agitation scores by treatment group over time

	Hand massage	Calming music	Hand massage calming music	Control
Time 1 Mean (SD)	16.47 (9.94)	18.41 (11.19)	22.00 (11.94)	21.76 (9.09)
Time 2 Mean (SD)	10.35 (11.20)	9.18 (11.11)	8.59 (7.87)	21.88 (10.38)
Time 3 Mean (SD)	7.76 (9.55)	7.65 (9.78)	7.06 (7.08)	20.88 (8.66)
Time 4 Mean (SD)	3.06 (5.44)	4.65 (7.87)	3.76 (4.40)	20.47 (10.90)
n	17	17	17	17

$p < 0.01$ from F test from repeated measures ANOVA ($df = 3, 9$).

A significant difference ($F = 6.47$, $p = 0.00$) in level of agitation over time was found among the four groups. Mean agitation scores are summarized in Table 8.6. Follow-up comparisons using Tukey's HSD procedure with a level of significance of 0.05, showed that the four groups were similar at baseline and that the control group was significantly more agitated than the experimental groups during the intervention, immediately after the intervention and at one hour.

DISCUSSION

Results of this study indicate that hand massage and calming music are easily administered, effective interventions to reduce the level of agitation in agitated nursing home residents with dementia. Subjects who received either of these interventions, alone or in combination, exhibited significantly less agitation than the control group after the intervention. The trend in this investigation was for the level of agitation to decrease considerably during the intervention, with further decrease ten minutes after, and again at one hour. After an initial reduction in agitation several subjects experienced slight increases in agitation upon removal of the intervention. Among the subjects who experienced any increase in agitated behaviors, none returned to baseline levels of agitation during the entire study period.

The receipt of both hand massage and calming music did not appear to result in an additional reduction agitation as originally predicted. Each of the three interventions resulted in significantly greater reduction in agitation than no intervention. However, the reduction in agitation was similar in each of the three experimental intervention groups.

When examined over time, the reduction in agitation among subjects receiving any experimental intervention began during the intervention. Further reduction in agitation was observed during the immediate post-intervention period, with even further reduction observed at one hour. This pattern over the intervention periods differs from that found in previous studies which showed positive effects with the use of music or massage with agitated nursing home residents. In the preliminary study (Tabloski et al., 1995) in which a 15-minute calming music intervention was used, the greatest reduction in agitation occurred during the intervention, followed by a small increase in agitation in the immediate post-intervention period. This suggests that the shorter music intervention used in this study may produce a more sustained effect. Alternately, decreasing a hand massage intervention from ten minutes (Snyder et al., 1995a) to five minutes (Snyder et al., 1995b) resulted in less consistently observed reductions in agitation, suggesting that a five-minute intervention may not be sufficient. Data from this study indicate that a ten-minute intervention of either hand massage or calming music resulted in both a reduction of agitation, as well as a sustained effect.

The music used for the intervention in this study was chosen for its slow tempo, soft dynamic levels, and repetitive themes. A recognizable melody that may evoke intense emotional responses was purposely avoided. Using a piece of music that had personal significance to the subject in earlier years, Gerdner & Swanson (1993) found that there was a lag time in producing an effect of the music intervention. This may be due to the additional cognitive effort required to process memory of a familiar piece of music before a response can occur. Calming music used in this study produced an initial, as well as a progressive response over time.

In summary, either of the interventions investigated in this study produced a reduction in agitation in nursing home residents in this group, and each produced similar results. Moreover, the benefit was sustained and increased over time at levels that were similar with each of the interventions.

None of the experimental interventions produced a significant reduction in physically aggressive behaviors over the four observation periods. This may be due to the fact that the initial level of these behaviors was low and did not allow for variation over time. These results are similar to those found by Goddaer & Abraham (1994) using music during mealtime.

Cohen-Mansfield & Werner (1995) also note a lower prevalence rate of physically aggressive behaviors and propose that these behaviors in a person with dementia may be a response to a perceived noxious stimulus. It may be that calming music or gentle hand massage may have controlled or eliminated the perception of a noxious stimulus, however, initial levels of these behaviors was so low that a significant difference was not detected.

Physically non-aggressive behaviors decreased significantly in the presence of each of the three experimental interventions. Similar results were reported with music (Goddaer & Abraham, 1994) and touch (Cohen-Mansfield & Werner, 1995). These behaviors are the most commonly observed agitated behaviors in the sample nursing home (Cohen-Mansfield & Werner, 1995), as well as in this sample.

Change in verbally agitated behaviors over time was significant in the presence of the experimental interventions. The use of hand massage resulted in less agitation than no intervention at each of the measurement periods, and any intervention resulted in less agitation than no intervention at Time 4 only. Because of the small differences, these results must be interpreted with caution, especially in light of the Cohen-Mansfield & Werner (1995) finding in which verbally agitated behavior increased in the presence of touch.

The findings of this study support the use of either hand massage or calming music for the reduction of agitation in nursing home residents with dementia. Both interventions require little training and are easily administered by both professional and lay caregivers. The cost of providing these interventions is small, especially in comparison with special environmental designs and the administration of medications to control agitation. Time expenditure required by caregivers to provide the interventions is also small. Hand massage as used in this study is a simple intervention that can be used effectively by caregivers. It differs in scope and intensity from that which would be provided by a trained massage therapist.

A limitation of this study pertains to the sample, which was comprised of nursing home residents from middle class communities. A majority of the subjects were white, female, and widowed. This sample may not be representative of all nursing home residents with dementia. Persons with cognitive impairment related to conditions other than dementia of the Alzheimer's type and multi-infarct dementia were not included in the sample. This limits generalizability of the results to the management of agitation in persons with agitation resulting from delirium, depression, brain injury, and other dementias, such as AIDS dementia, Pick's disease and Creutzfeldt-Jakob disease.

No single intervention — pharmacological, environmental or behavioral — is universally effective in reducing agitation. This study demonstrates the effectiveness of two easily administered interventions that may be used as a part of a comprehensive plan to address the specific needs of agitated nursing home residents. Hand massage and calming music represent practical treatment options that can be used alone or augment an individualized therapeutic regimen.

REFERENCES

Barnum, B. S. (1994). *Nursing theory: analysis application evaluation*. Philadelphia: J. B. Lippincott.

Cariga, J., Burgio, L., Flynn, W., & Martin, D. (1991). A controlled study of disruptive vocalizations among geriatric residents in nursing homes. *Journal of the American Geriatrics Society, 39*, 501–507.

Carlson, D. L., Fleming, K. C., Smith, G. E., & Evans, J. M. (1995). Management of dementia-related behavioral disturbances: A nonpharmacological approach. *Mayo Clinic Proceedings, 70*, 1108–1115.

Chafetz, P. K. (1990). Two-dimensional grid is ineffective against demented patient's exiting through glass doors. *Psychology of Aging, 5*(1), 146–147.

Chlan, L. L. (1995). Psychophysiologic responses of mechanically ventilated patients to music: A pilot study. *American Journal of Critical Care, 4*, 233–238.

Chrisman, M., Tabar, D., Whall, A. L., & Booth, D. E. (1991). Agitated behavior in the cognitively impaired elderly. *Journal of Gerontological Nursing, 17*(12), 9–13.

Chutka, D. S. (1997). Medication use in nursing home residents. *Nursing Home Medicine, 5*, 180–187.

Cohen-Mansfield, J. (1986). Agitated behaviors in the elderly II. Preliminary results in the cognitively deteriorated. *Journal of the American Geriatrics Society, 34*, 722–727.

Cohen-Mansfield, J. (1991). *Instruction manual for the Cohen-Mansfield Agitation Inventory*. Washington: Research Institute of the Hebrew Home of Greater Washington.

Cohen-Mansfield, J. (1995). Assessment of disruptive behavior/agitation in the elderly: Function, methods, and difficulties. *Journal of Geriatric Psychiatry and Neurology, 8*, 52–60.

Cohen-Mansfield, J., & Billig, N. (1986). Agitated behaviors in the elderly I. A conceptual review. *Journal of the American Geriatrics Society, 34*, 711–721.

Cohen-Mansfield, J., Marx, M. S., & Rosenthal, A. S. (1989). A description of agitation in a nursing home. *Journal of Gerontology, 44*(3), M77–M84.

Cohen-Mansfield, J., Marx, M. S., & Rosenthal, A. S. (1990). Dementia and agitation in nursing home residents: How are they related? *Psychology and Aging, 5*(1), 3–8.

Cohen-Mansfield, J., & Werner, P. (1995). Environmental influences on agitation: An integrative summary of an observational study. *The American Journal of Alzheimer's Disease and Related Disorders & Research, 10*(1), 32–39.

Cooper, J. K., Mungas, D., & Webber, P. G. (1990). Relation of cognitive status and abnormal behaviors in Alzheimer's disease. *Journal of the American Geriatrics Society, 38*, 867–870.

Corrigan, J. D. (1989). Development of a scale for assessment of agitation following traumatic brain injury. *Journal of Clinical and Experimental Neuropsychology, 1*, 261–277.

Dickinson, J. I., McLain, J. K., & Marshal-Baker, A. (1995). The effects of visual barriers on exiting behavior in a dementia care unit. *Gerontologist, 35*(1), 127–130.

Dossey, B. M., Keegan, L., Guzzetta, C. L., & Kolkmeier, L. G. (1995). *Holistic Nursing: A Handbook for Practice*. Gaithersburg, MD: Aspen.

Evans, L. K., & Strumpf, N. E. (1990). Myths about elder restraint. *Image: Journal of Nursing Scholarship, 22*, 124–128.

Finkel, S. I., Lyons, J. S., & Anderson, R. L. (1993). A Brief Agitation Rating Scale (BARS) for the nursing home elderly. *Journal of the American Geriatrics Society, 41*, 50–52.

Fraser, J., & Kerr, J. R. (1993). Psychophysiological effects of back massage on elderly institutionalized patients. *Journal of Advanced Nursing, 18*, 238–245.

Gagne, D., & Toye, R. C. (1994). The effects of therapeutic touch and relaxation therapy in reducing anxiety. *Archives of Psychiatric Nursing, 3,* 184–189.

Gardner, M. E., & Garrett, R. W. (1997). Review of drug therapy for aggressive behaviors associated with dementia. *Nursing Home Medicine, 5*(6), 199–208.

Gerdner, L. A. (2000). Effects of individualized versus classical 'relaxation' music on the frequency of agitation in elderly persons with Alzheimer's disease and related disorders. *International Psychogeriatrics, 12*(1), 49–65.

Gerdner, L. A., & Swanson, E. A. (1993). Effects of individualized music on confused and agitated elderly patients. *Archives of Psychiatric Nursing, 7,* 284–291.

Goddaer, J., & Abraham, I. L. (1994). Effects of relaxing music on agitation during meals among nursing home residents with severe cognitive impairment. *Archives of Psychiatric Nursing, 8,* 150–158.

Hamel, M., Gold, D. P., Andres, D., et al. (1990). Predictors and consequences of aggressive behavior by community-based dementia patients. *Gerontologist, 30,* 206–211.

Heidt, P. R. (1991). Helping patients to rest: Clinical studies in therapeutic touch. *Holistic Nursing Practice, 5*(4), 57–66.

Hussian, R. A., & Brown, D. C. (1987). Use of two dimensional grid patterns to limit hazardous ambulation in demented patients. *Journal of Gerontology, 42,* 558–560.

Janelli, L. M., & Kanski, G. W. (1997). Music intervention with physically restrained patients. *Rehabilitation Nursing, 22*(1), 14–19.

Knopman, P. S., & Sawyer-Demaris, S. (1990). Practical approach to managing problems in dementia patients. *Geriatrics, 45,* 27–35.

Lipowski, Z. J. (1992). Update on delirium. *Psychiatric Clinics of North America, 15,* 335–345.

Marx, M. S., Werner, P., & Cohen-Mansfield, J. (1989). Agitation and touch in the nursing home. *Psychological Reports, 64,* 1019–1026.

Meek, S. S. (1993). Effects of slow stroke back massage on relaxation in hospice clients. *Image: Journal of Nursing Scholarship, 25,* 17–21.

Meyer, R. M., Kraenzle, R. N., Gerrman, J., & Morely, M. B. (1994). The effect of reduction in restraint use on falls and injuries in two nursing homes. *Nursing Home Medicine, 2*(6), 23–26.

Miller, R. J., Snowdon, J., & Vaughan, R. (1995). The use of the Cohen-Mansfield Agitation Inventory in the assessment of behavioral disorders in nursing homes. *Journal of the American Geriatrics Society, 43,* 546–549.

Moore, J. R., & Gilbert, D. A. (1995). Elderly residents: Perception of nurses' comforting touch. *Journal of Gerontological Nursing, 21*(1), 6–13.

Moorse, J. M., & McHutchion, E. (1991). Releasing restraints: Providing safe care for the elderly. *Research in Nursing and Health, 14,* 187–196.

Mornhinweg, G. C., & Voignier, R. R. (1995). Music for sleep disturbance in the elderly. *Journal of Holistic Nursing, 13,* 248–254.

Negley, E. N., Molla, P. M., & Obenchain, J. (1990). No exit: The effects of an electronic security system on confused patients. *Journal of Gerontological Nursing, 16,* 21–24.

Omnibus Budget Reconciliation Act. (1987). House of Representatives, 100th Congress, First session. Washington, DC: US Government Printing Office.

Ragneskog, H., Kilgren, M., Karlsson, I., & Norberg, A. (1996). Dinner music for demented patients. *Clinical Nursing Research, 5*(3), 262–277.

Ray, W. A., Taylor, J. A., Lichtenstein, M. J., & Meador, K. G. (1992). The Nursing Home Behavior Problem Scale. *Journal of Gerontology: Medical Sciences, 47*(1), M9–M16.

Richards, K. C. (1998). Effect of back massage and relaxation intervention on sleep in critically ill patients. *American Journal of Critical Care, 7,* 288–299.

Rowe, M., & Alfred, D. (1999). The effectiveness of slow-stroke massage in diffusing agitated behaviors in individuals with Alzheimer's disease. *Journal of Gerontological Nursing, 25,* 222–234.

Schorr, J. A. (1993). Music and pattern change in chronic pain. *Advances in Nursing Science, 15,* 27–36.

Snyder, M., Egan, E. C., & Burns, K. R. (1995a). Interventions for decreasing agitation behaviors in persons with dementia. *Journal of Gerontological Nursing, 21*(7), 34–40.

Snyder, M., Egan, E. C., & Burns, K. R. (1995b). Efficacy of hand massage in decreasing agitation behaviors associated with care activities in persons with dementia. *Geriatric Nursing, 16,* 60–63.

Stanley, M., & Beare, P/G. (1999). *Gerontological nursing.* Philadelphia: F.A. Davis.

Swearer, J. M., Drachman, D. A., O'Donnell, B. F., & Mitchell, A. L. (1988). Troublesome and disruptive behaviors in dementia: Relationships to diagnosis and disease severity. *Journal of the American Geriatrics Society, 36,* 784–790.

Tabloski, P. A., McKinnon-Howe, L., & Remington, R. (1995). Effects of calming music on level of agitation in cognitively impaired nursing home residents. *American Journal of Alzheimer's Care and Related Disorders & Research, 10*(1), 10–15.

Teri, L., Rabins, P., Whitehouse, P., et al. (1992). Management of behavior disturbance in Alzheimer Disease: Current knowledge and future directions. *Alzheimer Disease and Associated Disorders, 6,* 77–88.

Tinetti, M. E., Liu, W., Marottoli, R. A., & Gentner, S. F. (1991). Mechanical restraint use among residents of skilled nursing facilities: Prevalence, patterns and predictors. *Journal of the American Medical Association, 265,* 468–471.

Werner, P., Cohen-Mansfield, J., Braun, J., & Marx, M. (1989). Physical restraints and agitation in nursing home residents. *Journal of the American Geriatrics Society, 37,* 1122 1126.

Whipple, B., & Glynn, N. J. (1992). Quantification of the effects of listening to music as a noninvasive method of pain control. *Scholarly Inquiry for Nursing Practice, 6*(1), 43–58.

White, J. M. (1992). Music therapy: An intervention to reduce anxiety in the myocardial infarction patient. *Clinical Nurse Specialist, 6*(2), 58–63.

Williams-Burgess, C., Ugarriza, D., & Gabbai, M. (1996). Agitation in older persons with dementia: A research systheses. *Online Journal of Knowledge Synthesis for Nursing, 3*(37).

Winter, M. J., Paskin, S., & Baker, T. (1995). Music reduces stress and anxiety of patients in the surgical holding area. *Journal of Post Anesthesia Nursing, 9,* 340–343.

Zimmer, J. G., Watson, N., & Treat, A. (1984). Behavior problems among patients in skilled nursing facilities. *American Journal of Public Health, 74,* 1118–1121.

Massage and the workplace

SECTION CONTENTS

INTRODUCTION TO SECTION 4

The final chapter in this book examines work-site massage. The possibility of using massage in the workplace is exciting and health psychologists have frequently used work sites for community intervention programs in the past (Kaplan et al., 1993). Health psychologists consider such settings important in part because 'most adults are employed, people spend a great amount of time at work, there are existing communication channels that can be used for health education, and companies are motivated to keep employees healthy and productive' (Kaplan et al., 1993, p. 452).

Much research has examined workplace stress and numerous studies describe such effects as psychological distress and physical illness (Taylor, 1999). Evidence suggests that workplace stress may be largely preventable, an important consideration since disability payments to workers for stress-related ailments are numerous and expensive (Taylor, 1999). Previous studies indicate that work-site stress can be alleviated in part by rewarding workers for jobs well done and by making the workplace interesting (Taylor, 1999). Studies also indicate that job stress may lead to increased illness and tardiness (Taylor, 1999), outcomes that employers would certainly prefer to avoid. Perhaps massage therapy could provide part of the answer to this widespread and costly social issue.

In the following chapter, Margaret Hodge and her colleagues suggest that massage can indeed benefit workers. Hodge and colleagues examine 100 male and female health care workers between the ages of 25 and 60. The group receiving massage received massage twice each week for 20 minutes. Certified massage therapists followed a standard protocol and continued treatment for eight weeks. Hodge and colleagues demonstrate decreased anxiety and depression, and a decrease in perceived sleep disturbance among workers who received worksite massage. Such results have important and exciting implications for work-site stress reduction programs.

Hodge and colleagues' results mirror the results of other studies of massage that use the State-Trait Anxiety Inventory, such as numerous studies reviewed by Field (2000). Specifically, Field (2000) reviews a study she conducted with her colleagues on job stress and performance among a sample of somewhat different health care professionals, fifty medical faculty and staff members. The group receiving massage received chair massage 15 minutes a day, twice weekly for five weeks (Field, 2000, p. 107). Massaged subjects reported decreased anxiety and depression, and decreased job stress. As in Hodge and colleagues' study, Field's group also found improved cognition scores. Given the potential cost savings of massage in the workplace, future studies should specifically examine potential cost savings of including work-site chair massage in stress reduction programs.

REFERENCES

Field, T. (2000). *Touch therapy*. Edinburgh: Churchill Livingstone.
Kaplan, R., Sallis, J., & Patterson, T. (1993). *Health and human behavior*. New York: McGraw Hill.
Taylor, S. (1999). *Health psychology*. Boston: McGraw Hill.

9

Employee outcomes following work-site acupressure and massage*

Margaret Hodge, Carol Robinson, Judie Boehmer, Sally Klein

INTRODUCTION

Fast-paced work environments with high demands, little chance of relief and limited control, characterize high stress occupations. Recent studies have reported work related stress rates as high as 30–46% (Lusk, 1997; Murphy, 1996). In a study of 28,000 workers in 215 different organizations, Kohler & Kamp (1992) reported that stress at work was associated with employee burnout, acute and chronic health problems, and poor work performance. In addition, a study of 130 occupations conducted by the National Institute for Occupational Safety and Health, found that 40 occupations had a higher than expected incidence of stress-related disorders or stress responses (Seago & Faucett, 1997). Seven of these high stress occupations were in the health care field.

Health care workers have identified occupational issues such as poor staffing, shift work, increased work load, death and dying, and conflicts with other health care providers as leading to increased work stress (Field et al., 1997; Jenkins & Rogers, 1997). Stress can result in low morale, increased anxiety and depression, as well as other health related concerns (Jenkins & Rogers). Studies have shown that job stress can lead to increases in blood pressure and heart rate as well as decreasing cognitive functioning (Field et al., 1996; Murphy, 1996). As a result, health care workers are at risk for significant untoward physiological effects including hypertension and cardiovascular disease. For the organization, there are significant financial costs associated with job stress, including increased errors, absenteeism, and work related injuries in addition to decreased

*This chapter was first published as a paper in *Massage Therapy Journal* 2000, *39(3)*, 48–64; *39(4)*, 40–47.

productivity as the result of poor job satisfaction. Therefore, the development and investigation of work site strategies to decrease stress are relevant and critical in the current health care environment.

The purpose of this study was to systematically investigate the physiological, psychological/cognitive, and organizational effects of a stress reduction strategy, work-site acupressure/massage (WSAM), for employees in high stress health care occupations. This study is important because it represents a potentially cost effective strategy for decreasing perceptions of stress in employees in high stress occupations.

BACKGROUND

While a growing number of institutions, including the US Department of Justice, offer massage in the workplace, there are limited data reported on the benefits of massage in high stress work environments. Health care environments have traditionally been associated with high occupational stress and recent changes in the health care environment have resulted in increased job stress, placing health care workers at risk for significant untoward physiological and psychological effects.

Health care organizations, in the face of frequent changes, widespread uncertainty, and increased competitiveness, need to consider the impact of these changes on employee work stress and foster the development of strategies to promote employee wellness (Erbin-Roesemann & Simms, 1997; Jenkins & Rogers, 1997; Kennedy & Grey, 1997). This study is of importance to both health care employees and health care organizations because it represents a potentially low risk strategy for coping with the effects of job stress.

Literature review

Mind–body connection

The use of alternative therapies, such as acupressure and massage, has re-emerged in recent years as a strategy leading to multiple favorable health outcomes. In the late 1970s, George Engel (Engel, 1974), introduced a bio-psycho-social model of health and illness. This model states that health is an outcome with multiple integrated components such as genetics, lifestyle, attitude, environment, and social relationships. The stress response is one example of how the integration of biological, psychological and social factors affect health. When faced with an acute challenge or threatening situation, the body responds by initiating the fight or flight reaction which prepares the body to function at a higher level of efficiency. As a result, the body initiates a complex physiological response which includes an increase in blood pressure and heart rate, increased oxygen consumption, and increased muscle tension (Jenkins & Rogers, 1997; Murphy, 1996). While each of these responses is intended to protect the body, prolonged exposure to stress can result in physiological and psychological problems.

Conversely, in 1976, Benson demonstrated a pattern of changes known as the relaxation response. Physiologic changes included in the relaxation response show reversal of the acute stress response with corresponding reductions in blood pressure and heart rate, decreased oxygen consumption and reduced muscle tension. This response provides a framework for examining the effect of various relaxation therapies such as, massage, acupressure and reflexology, on work related stress.

A variety of psychologically related measures such as anxiety, depression, and coping skills have been associated with job stress (Cady & Jones, 1997; Jenkins & Rogers, 1997). Fatigue has also been linked to job stress as the result of high demands or workload (Labyak & Metzger, 1997). In a study of over 11,000 health care workers Hardy et al. (1997) found significantly higher levels of fatigue than expected and found that work demands predicted additional general fatigue.

Responses to massage

Although there are a wide variety of massage therapy techniques, each with their own cultural and theoretical perspectives, proponents suggest that beneficial outcomes in response to most, if not all types of massage include: improved blood flow, release of muscle tension, improved musculoskeletal structure and function, and a reduction in the perception of stress (Benson, 1976; Jacobs, 1996). While there are anecdotal reports of the aforementioned benefits, there are few systematic investigations to determine the effects of massage on physiological, psychological and organizational outcomes. A meta-analysis of previous studies of the physiological benefits of massage showed reductions in blood pressure and heart rate (Cady & Jones, 1997). One study of 50 healthy adults demonstrated that massage therapy leads to improved concentration and mood, lower anxiety and depression, increased alertness as measured by electroencephalogram, and decreased salivary cortisol levels (Field et al., 1997).

Musculoskeletal injuries, one of the most frequent work related injuries reported by nurses, may be caused by fatigue, lifting or work overload (Seago & Faucett, 1997). Massage reduces muscle tension and tonic contraction, decreasing both postural and muscle imbalances that can lead to muscle fatigue and injury. Massage therapy is purported to affect both the structure and function of the musculoskeletal system by promoting the relaxation response and reducing muscle tension and fatigue while improving posture (Benson, 1976). The integration of these improvements in the musculoskeletal system, in turn, may lead to greater ease of body movement, wider range of motion, and greater flexibility, resulting in decreased musculoskeletal injuries.

Given this theoretical framework, the research hypotheses of this study were:

1. Employees who receive WSAM (work-site acupressure massage) will exhibit decreased absenteeism, work related injuries, sleep disturbances, perceptions of fatigue and anxiety when compared with a control group.
2. Employees who receive WSAM will exhibit decreased blood pressure, heart rate and somatic complaints when compared with a control group.
3. Employees who receive WSAM will have improved cognition, mood, well-being, and job satisfaction when compared with a control group.

METHODS

While there are limited data on the effect of massage on selected physiological and psychological outcomes, the effect of massage on organizational factors, such as job satisfaction and work-related injuries, has not been reported. For purposes of this study, the psychological variables of interest included measures of the perceptions of mood, anxiety, fatigue, sleep disturbances as well as measures of cognitive function. The physiologic variables of interest included blood pressure, both systolic and diastolic, as well as heart rate and measures of somatic complaints such as fatigue and muscle tension. Organizational outcomes were addressed in measures of employee job satisfaction, work-related injuries and absenteeism.

Design/sample

The study design was a randomized, controlled experimental investigation. Male and female health care workers ($n = 100$) between the ages of 25 and 60 years were recruited to participate in this study. Anticipating a moderate effect size, power analysis (power $= 0.8$, $p = 0.05$) confirms this was an adequate sample for a clinically relevant effect (Cohen, 1988). In order to control for the effect differences in management style might have, subjects were recruited from purposively chosen units within the organization. Health care personnel in units supervised by the same manager, were randomized by unit to participate in either the treatment or control group. The massage therapy group ($n = 50$) received WSAM, twice weekly for 20 minutes, while the control group ($n = 50$) did not receive any specific intervention during break times of equal duration.

Procedures

Approval for the study was obtained from the hospital's institutional review board. All participants gave written, informed consent prior to entering the study. Staff were recruited after meeting with members of this research team. The gender and ethnic composition of the sample reflected a diverse population.

Subject inclusion criteria were: (1) agreement to no change in life style during the eight-week period of the protocol. This included no changes in normal patterns of exercise, diet, rest, or alternative therapies. Subject exclusion criteria were: (1) presence of an infection during the previous two weeks and (2) employees who receive regularly scheduled massage therapy. In order to control for hormonal effects associated with menstruation, all pre-menopausal women in the control and treatment group began the study between menstrual cycle days 5 and 11.

Treatment

The WSAM procedure was provided by certified massage therapists, who were trained in the specific protocol. Each subject in the experimental group received a 20-minute massage, twice weekly for a period of eight weeks. The massage was scheduled in the later half of the employee's shift. Subjects were fully clothed and the massage consisted of a blend of traditional massage, acupressure, and reflexology.

The massage protocol included bodywork on the upper to middle back, back of the neck, the face, upper chest, shoulders and feet. Deep tissue massage was not used during any part of this protocol. The first area to be worked was the back of the neck, the shoulders, and the region below the shoulder blades. Treatment consisted of applying light to medium pressure in each area for one minute in a circular motion. The face and upper chest area were worked using acupressure, which consisted of light finger and thumb pressure. Each point was worked for a slow count of 10. Foot reflexology was used to reduce stress by applying medium pressure in an alternating pattern starting just below the toes and working down to the heel and back to the base of the toes. In addition, each toe was worked, again using medium pressure.

Subjects in the control group were expected to take a 20-minute break twice weekly without WSAM treatments. A quiet room was provided where subjects in the control group could remove themselves from the work environment. Investigators met with the control group at least every other week to monitor subjects for compliance with study procedures.

Outcome measures

Baseline demographic and health history data for each subject was obtained prior to initiating the treatment. In addition, at the beginning of the study, and on completion of the study, subjects completed the General Well-Being Scale, Profile of Mood States, State-Trait Anxiety Inventory, Multidimensional Fatigue Inventory, General Sleep Disturbance Scale and Index of Work Satisfaction questionnaires. Data were also collected on work related injuries and absenteeism.

Psychological measures

The General Well-Being Scale (GWBS) was used as a measure of subject mood before and after the eight week study intervention. The GWBS contains subscale measures of depression, emotional control, emotional ties, affect, and anxiety. Adequate concurrent validity and internal consistency has been reported ($r = 0.90$).

The State-Trait Anxiety Inventory (STAI) was used to measure the subject's perception of anxiety, pre and post eight week treatment intervention (Spielberger, 1983). The STAI is one of the most frequently used instruments for measuring anxiety. Both components of the STAI have demonstrated good reliability. Concurrent validity has been demonstrated through correlation with another anxiety index ($r = 0.85$) and the adjective checklist ($r = -0.54$).

The Multidimensional Fatigue Inventory (MFI-20) was used to evaluate the perception of fatigue pre and post eight-week treatment intervention. This 20-item questionnaire provides scores for general fatigue, physical fatigue, reduced activity, reduced motivation and mental fatigue. The MFI-20 has demonstrated both construct and convergent validity and shows good internal consistency (Smets et al., 1995).

The General Sleep Disturbance Scale (GSDS) was used to evaluate sleep patterns pre and post eight week treatment intervention. The GSDS is a 21-item questionnaire which measures the use of substances to aid sleep, sleep quality, sleep quantity, frequency of awakening, and sleepiness. The GSDS shows good internal consistency (Chronbach's alpha $= 0.88$) (Lee, 1992).

The Symbol Digit Modalities Test (SMDT) was used to measure cognition in both the control and treatment group. The SMDT is a 90-second timed instrument which provides useful indices of normal capacities in testings of adults as well as improvement resulting from specific therapeutic interventions. The treatment group completed the SMDT prior to and immediately following massage in weeks one, four, and eight. Construct validity has been demonstrated with selected factors of the Weschler Performance and Verbal IQ tests.

Physiological measures

Physiological outcomes of interest included blood pressure, heart rate, and somatic complaints such as headache, backache, etc. Before and after each massage therapy session for the treatment group, and every other week for the control group, systolic and diastolic blood pressure as well as heart rate were measured using a Dyna-Map. The Dyna-Map is a non-invasive instrument which can be used to obtain each of these readings with minimum operator error. Prior to the start of the study each Dyna-Map was calibrated per manufacturer's recommendations. The massage therapists were trained in the use of the Dyna-Map, thus controlling for measurement errors as the result of discrepancies in the skill level of those obtaining these measures. In addition to the objective measures of blood pressure and heart rate described above, subjects were asked to rate symptoms or feelings he/she had, such as fatigue and anxiety as well as somatic complaints such as headache and backache immediately prior to and following each WSAM treatment, as well as weekly in the control group.

Somatic complaints were assessed before and after treatment using a 10-point Likert scale. Subjects were asked to rank their level of fatigue, muscle tightness, and overall health on a scale of 0 to 10, with 0 indicating absence of the attribute and 10 indicating the maximum level of the attribute.

Organizational measures

The Index of Work Satisfaction (IWS) is a two-part questionnaire developed to evaluate job satisfaction in nurses pre and post eight-week treatment intervention. Alpha reliability for the Index of Work Satisfaction is reported as 0.85 (Stamps, 1997).

RESULTS

Data analysis was carried out using SPSS, version 9.0 (for computerized statistical analysis). Descriptive statistics, including frequencies, means, and standard deviations were analyzed. Inferential statistics included one-tailed *t*-tests to determine pre and post study differences. For purposes of this study, a *p* value less than 0.05 was considered significant.

Demographic data

Table 9.1 shows the demographic and health data for the study participants in the experimental and control groups. A total of 100 subjects initially participated in the study, but not all post-study instruments were completed. There were 89 subjects who completed all of the pre and post study instruments. Reasons given for non-compliance included being too

Table 9.1 Demographic data

Demographics	Control group	Treatment
Age	Mean = 41.5 ± 8.7	Mean = 41.6 ± 7.7
Gender	Males = 8	Males = 7
	Females = 24	Females = 48
Ethnicity	White = 24	White = 43
	African American = 1	African American = 1
	Hispanic = 3	Hispanic = 4
	Asian = 4	Asian = 4
	Other = 1	Other = 3
Overall health rating (1–3)	Mean = 1.8 ± 0.70	Mean = 1.7 ± 0.52
Smoking history	Yes = 3	Yes = 7
	No = 30	No = 49
Personal use of alternative therapies	Yes = 19	Yes = 27
	No = 14	No = 29

busy, forgetting, or misplacing some of the instruments. Compliance was poorest among those subjects in the control group, even though, as an incentive, a one-hour massage was offered to the control group upon completion of the study.

The mean age for the sample was 41.6 ± 8.1 years. Ten of the 89 subjects were smokers. Sixty-five subjects reported that they regularly exercised. Chi-square analysis showed no significant differences between the control group and treatment group for gender ($p = 0.15$), marital status ($p = 0.80$), ethnicity ($p = 0.27$), overall health ($p = 0.26$), smoking ($p = 0.45$) or personal use of alternative therapies ($p = 0.26$). No significant differences in demographic data were noted in subjects who did not complete the study.

Health care workers at this institution generally work a 12-hour shift. Forty-four of the participants worked a 12-hour day shift, while 31 participants worked a 12-hour night shift. Fourteen of the subjects worked an 8-hour day shift. For subjects working a 12-hour shift, the treatment occurred between the 7th and 9th hours of their shift. For subjects working an 8-hour shift, the treatment occurred during the later half of their shift. All participants in the experimental group completed a minimum of 14 of the 16 scheduled massage therapy sessions.

In relation to the first hypothesis (Table 9.2), which looked at perceptions of mood, the treatment group demonstrated significant decreases in both state anxiety ($t = 2.4$, $p = 0.009$) and trait anxiety ($t = 1.7$, $p = 0.04$). The General Well-Being Scale was used to measure subject's perception of overall health. Subjects in the treatment group reported significantly decreased levels of anxiety ($t = 2.8$, $p = 0.003$) and depression ($t = 2.0$, $p = 0.024$), as well as significantly increased feelings of emotional control ($t = 1.9$, $p = 0.029$) and positive affect ($t = 1.9$, $p = 0.029$) when compared

Table 9.2 Comparison of differences in pre- and post-treatment scores between the control group and the treatment group (pre-test score minus post-test score)

Variable	Control group Mean ± SD	Treatment group Mean ± SD	Significance (1-tailed)
State anxiety (high score = high anxiety)	0.93 ± 12.1	7.7 ± 11.9	$t = 2.4$ $df = 78$ $p = 0.009$
Trait anxiety (high score = high anxiety)	3.2 ± 13.7	8.4 ± 11.3	$t = 1.8$ $df = 74$ $p = 0.04$
GWB anxiety (high score = high anxiety)	−0.15 ± 5.1	2.7 ± 4.4	$t = 2.8$ $df = 85$ $p = 0.003$
GWB depression (high score = low depression)	0.33 ± 2.5	1.3 ± 2.6	$t = 1.7$ $df = 85$ $p = 0.05$
GWB emotional control (high score = high emotional control)	0.84 ± 4.2	−2.3 ± 4.2	$t = 1.61$ $df = 85$ $p = 0.05$
General sleep disturbance? (high score = high sleep disturbances)	−1.9 ± 11.7	7.3 ± 11.9	$t = 2.9$ $df = 60$ $p = 0.02$

with the control group. No significant differences were observed for the subscales of anger, confusion, or fatigue.

A significant decrease in perceived sleep disturbances was noted for subjects in the treatment group, working 12-hour shifts ($t = 2.9$, $p = 0.005$); while no differences in perceptions of sleep disturbances were noted in subjects working 8-hour shifts.

The Multidimensional Fatigue Inventory was used as a measure of the dimensions of general fatigue, physical fatigue, mental fatigue, reduced motivation, and reduced activity. For each of these subscales, no significant differences were noted between the control and treatment groups.

The massage treatment group exhibited a significant decrease between pre- and post-treatment systolic blood pressure ($t = 2.7$, $p = 0.014$) and pre- and post-treatment diastolic blood pressure ($t = 4.0$, $p = 0.000$) when compared with the control group. No pre- and post-treatment differences were noted in subject's heart rate. In addition significant differences were noted between the pre-treatment and post-treatment systolic blood pressure ($t = 68.4$, $p = 0.002$) and between the pre-treatment and post-treatment heart rate ($t = 142.3$, $p = 0.000$) of subjects in the massage treatment group. No significant differences were noted between the pre-treatment and post-treatment diastolic blood pressure for this group ($t = 24.7$, $p = 0.39$). In other words, subjects in the treatment group had a greater decrease in blood pressure readings between the blood pressure taken before massage and that taken after massage, than did the subjects in the control group who had their blood pressure taken before and after a rest break. The subjects in the treatment group also had a greater change when comparing each subject's blood pressure and heart rate from before massage or break with after massage or break.

The massage treatment group exhibited significantly improved differences in cognition scores, as measured by the SDMT, when compared with the control group ($t = 3.8$, $p = 0.000$). In addition, significant improvement in cognition occurred between pre-treatment and post-treatment ($t = 144.8$, $p = 0.000$) for subjects in the massage treatment group.

Significant improvements in overall health rating ($t = 326.4$, $p = 0.000$) were noted for subjects in the treatment group. In addition, for this group, significant decreases in subject's perception of muscle tightness ($t = 914.3$, $p = 0.000$) and overall fatigue ($t = 227.8$, $p = 0.000$) were noted between the pre-treatment and post-treatment measures. No differences were noted for other somatic complaints.

In relation to job satisfaction, subjects completed the Index of Work Satisfaction (IWS) prior to and at the end of the study. Results demonstrate that prior to beginning the study, IWS scores were lower for the treatment group (IWS = 13.1) than for the control group (IWS = 14.4). Upon completion of the study, IWS scores remained consistent for the treatment group (IWS = 13.4), while the control group demonstrated a decrease in scores (IWS = 12.7). Chi-square analysis of absenteeism showed no differences between the treatment group and control group ($p = 0.7$).

During the three months in which the study was conducted, there was only one work related injury reported among the subjects enrolled. Therefore, it is not possible to draw inferences on the effect of WSAM on work-related injuries.

Limitations

Limitations in the study design are related to (a) generalizability, and (b) sampling. A convenience sample of subjects from a large university teaching hospital located on the west coast was used. Results from a Robert Woods Johnson Foundation survey found that subjects in the west were more likely to utilize alternative therapies (Paramore, 1997). Therefore, these results may not be generalizable to employees in areas less accepting of alternative therapies. In addition, increased managed care leading to changes in the health care environment may have contributed to a degree of stress that is greater than elsewhere. This, too, may affect the generalizability of the study findings to other health care environments.

In order to control for the effect differences in management style might have, subjects were recruited from units managed by the same supervisor.

As a result, there may be differences between the general population and the sample population, which may affect the findings.

DISCUSSION

The purpose of this study was to investigate the effect of work-site acupressure massage (WSAM) on selected physiological, psychological/cognitive, and organizational outcomes. Previous research has shown that employees in high stress occupations are at risk for untoward psychological problems related to anxiety and depression, physiological problems such as hypertension and heart disease, and musculoskeletal problems, which may result in work related injuries. Downsizing, shorter patient stays, restructuring and layoffs add to the stress in health care environments. Employees responsible for providing health care are, therefore, at a greater risk for illness while health care organizations face problems of reduced productivity, absenteeism, accidents and injuries.

Results of this study demonstrate the benefits of work-site acupressure massage. Subjects in the experimental group exhibited decreased systolic and diastolic blood pressure. In addition, subjects in the experimental group exhibited decreased post-treatment systolic blood pressure and heart rate when compared with their pre-treatment systolic blood pressure and heart rate.

Subjects in the experimental group exhibited improved cognitive function, general well-being, as evidenced by decreased anxiety and depression, as well as increased emotional control and overall well being. In addition, participants reported a decrease in general sleep disturbances.

Although no improvement in employee job satisfaction was noted, subjects in the treatment group maintained their pre-study level of job satisfaction, while subjects in the control group demonstrated a decrease in their level of job satisfaction. This may be explained in part by increases in patient acuity and hospital census, as well as decreases in staffing which occurred during the course of this study. An increase in job stress, as well as a decrease in job satisfaction is consistent with these changes. Subjects in the treatment group may have perceived less job stress as a result of WSAM and, therefore, did not exhibit a decrease in job satisfaction.

The effects of WSAM, as defined in this present study, are multiple, providing benefits to both the employee and the organization. Implications for future research include the need to look at the effect of WSAM on absenteeism and work-related injuries over a longer period of time and with a larger sample size. Additional research is also necessary to examine the association between health care workers, WSAM, and patient care delivery. Given the beneficial responses found, it is possible that these favorable outcomes might lead to improved patient care and patient care outcomes.

ACKNOWLEDGEMENTS

Partial funding for this study was received from the American Massage Therapy Association and Sigma Theta Tau, Zeta Eta Chapter.

REFERENCES

Benson, H. (1976). *The relaxation response.* New York: Avon.

Cady, S. H., & Jones, G. E. (1997). Massage therapy as a workplace intervention for reduction of stress. *Perceptual and Motor Skills, 84,* 157–158.

Cohen, J. (1988). *Statistical power analysis for the behavioral sciences.* London: Lawrence Erlbaum Association.

Engel, G. (1974). Memorial lecture: The psychosomatic approach to individual susceptibility to disease. *Gastroenterology, 67*(6), 1085–1093.

Erbin-Roesemann, M. A., & Simms, L. M. (1997). Work locus of control: the intrinsic factor behind empowerment and work excitement. *Nursing Economics, 15*(4), 183–190.

Field, T., Ironson, G., Scafidi, F., et al. (1996). Massage therapy reduces anxiety and enhances EEG pattern of alertness and math computations. *The International Journal of Neuroscience, 86,* 197–205.

Field, T., Quintino, O., Henteleff, T., et al. (1997). Job stress reduction therapies. *Alternative Therapies, 3*(4), 54–56.

Goats, G. C. (1994). Massage — the scientific basis of an ancient art: Part 1. The techniques. *British Journal of Sports Medicine, 28*(3), 149–152.

Hardy, G. E., Shapiro, D. A., & Borrill, C. S. (1997). Fatigue in the workforce of national health service trusts: Levels of symptomatology and links with minor psychiatric disorder, demographic, occupation and work. *Journal of Psychosomatic Research, 43*(1), 83–92.

Jacobs, J. (1996). *The encyclopedia of alternative medicine: A complete family guide to complementary therapies.* Boston: Journey Editions.

Jenkins, R., & Rogers, A. (1997). Managing stress at work: An alternative approach. *Nursing Standard, 11*(29), 41–44.

Jones, E. (1997). Creating healthy work: Stress in the nursing workplace. *Revolution — The Journal of Nurse Empowerment,* Summer, 56–58.

Kennedy, P., & Grey, N. (1997). High pressure areas. *Nursing Times, 93*(29), 26–32.

Kohler, S., & Kamp, J. (1992). *American workers under pressure.* Technical report. St. Paul Fire and Marine Insurance Company.

Labyak, S. E., & Metzger, B. L. (1997). The effects of effleurage backrub on the psychological components of relaxation: A meta-analysis. *Nursing Research, 46*(1), 59–62.

Lee, K. (1992). Self-reported sleep disturbances in employed women. *Sleep, 15*(6), 493–498.

Lusk, S. L. (1997). Health effects of stress management in the worksite. *American Association of Occupational Health Nurses, 45*(3), 149–152.

Murphy, L. R. (1996). Stress management in work settings: A critical review of the health effects. *American Journal of Health Promotion, 11*(2), 112–135.

Paramore, L. C. (1997). Use of alternative therapies: Estimates from the 1994 Robert Wood Johnson Foundation National Access to Care Survey. *Journal of Pain and Symptom Management, 13*(2), 83–89.

Seago, J. A., & Faucett, J. (1997). Job strain among registered nurses and other hospital workers. *The Journal of Nursing Administration, 27*(5), 19–25.

Smets, E. M. A., Garsen, B., & Bonke, B. (1995). *Multidimensional fatigue index.* Amsterdam: Academisch Medisch Centrum.

Speilberger, C. D. (1983). *State-trait anxiety inventory.* Consulting Psychologists Press, Inc.

Stamps, P. L. (1997). *Nurses and work satisfaction: An index for measurement.* Chicago: Health Administration Press.

Index

CONQUERING
INFERTILITY

CONQUERING INFERTILITY

A GUIDE FOR COUPLES

FOURTH EDITION

Stephen L. Corson, M.D.

Notice: Our knowledge in the clinical sciences is constantly changing. As new information becomes available, changes in treatment and the use of drugs become necessary. The author and the publisher of this volume have, as far as it is possible to do so, taken care to make certain that the doses of drugs and schedules of treatment are correct and compatible with the standards generally accepted at the time of publication. The reader is advised to consult carefully the instruction and information material included in the package insert of each drug or therapeutic agent before administration in order to make certain that the recommended dosage is correct and that there have been no changes in the recommended dose of the drug or in the indications or contraindications in its utilization. This advice is especially important when using new or infrequently used drugs.

EMIS-Canada
P.O. Box 47026
19-555 West 12th Ave.
Vancouver, B.C. V5Z 4L6

First Edition 1983
© 1983 by Appleton-Century-Crofts
Revised Edition 1990
© 1990 Revised text by Stephen L. Corson, M.D.
Third Edition 1995
© 1995 by Stephen L. Corson, M.D.
Fourth Edition 1998
© 1999 by Stephen L. Corson, M.D.

ISBN 1-895213-24-X

Printed in Canada

COVER PHOTO:
Intracytoplasmic sperm injection – ICSI.
Placing a single sperm into an egg under microscopic guidance.

Dedication

In 1982 Mary English was working as an emergency room nurse at Pennsylvania hospital. I told her that there was a job opportunity opening as the nurse for our soon to be launched in vitro fertilization program, and that the only promise that I could make was that she would never be bored. Today as the Clinical Coordinator of the program (translation: the real boss) she oversees a program that has grown to include ancillary services such as egg donation and gestational carrier pregnancy and which has 2,000 babies to its credit.

Kathryn Go, Ph. D. has been the laboratory director of our program for the past 15 years. She has implemented new advances in IVF such as embryo freezing (we have a successful delivery eight years after cryopreservation) embryo co-culture, and of course, direct insertion of a single sperm into an egg – intracytoplasmic sperm injection (ICSI). We are entering the era of pre-implantational genetics with high hopes that these technologies can be used to help our patients have children who can lead normal, productive and happy lives, free from the effects of major life-altering abnormalities. She and her crew of laboratory biologists are the indefatigable guardians and nurturers of our embryonic patients.

Mary and Kathy, the nurses and the labsters, as we call them, are the soul of our program, the engines that make it run. This book is dedicated to their unstinting efforts and devotion.

Stephen L. Corson, M.D.

Contents

About the Author

STEPHEN L. CORSON, M.D., is the director of the Women's Institute and the in vitro fertilization program at Thomas Jefferson University in Philadelphia where he is a professor and section head in reproductive endocrinology and infertility in the department of obstetrics and gynecology. He is the editor-in-chief of the International Journal of Fertility and Women's Medicine, a past president of the American Association of Gynecologic Laparoscopists and has been an officer and board member in many infertility societies. He has over 200 published papers in peer reviewed journals and 50 book or chapter contributions.

PREFACE

In this, the fourth edition of Conquering Infertility, the goal of bringing useful information to the reader is the same as in the previous editions. Vignettes of success stories are sometimes inspirational, but today, more than ever, patients who realistically have therapeutic choices, often expensive and complicated, want as much factual material as possible on which to base their decisions. The first four chapters of this book constitute an effort to give you a crash course in the basics of reproduction so that you can better understand the foundations on which the therapies discussed in the later chapters are based.

As was the case in the previous revisions, the new text was written as developments in the field of fertility management and care necessitated updating and change. Additionally, two separate but parallel forces were at play. The first was the development of HMO programs which sharply define the services covered, and put a tight rein on the reimbursement package. The second was the concomitant trend in all fields of medicine to practice what has been called "evidence based medicine". Many favorite and time honored protocols of treatment were never exposed to close scrutiny as to how well they worked, at what point the treatment should be changed, and what the costs really were. Few practices keep accurate statistics for success rates associated with each type of therapy, although the development of sophisticated medical office computer systems is changing that. Historically, physicians have relied on meetings and the literature to guide them. Initial results achieved in preliminary studies frequently are not matched in mainstream practice. The statistical method of meta analysis has allowed for rapid evaluation of new therapies by combining results of independent but well designed studies.

The medical literature sometimes can become quite complicated to interpret. In vitro fertilization results, for instance, are often expressed as cost per baby. Related costs such as hospital expenses caring for hyperstimulated patients, and for premature delivery and nursery costs for the multiple pregnancies which are so common in these programs, also must be factored in.

We—patients and doctors— fall in love with the new, which invariably is more expensive than what it replaces. Fertility evaluation and treatment should be conducted in a logical step-wise fashion—not every couple needs a high tech approach such as in vitro fertilization. Therefore, in this edition, an effort will be made to define how long a particular therapy should be employed before a change is made and what the reasonable expectation for success is.

Without question, the most exciting recent advance which has become employed on a daily basis is that of intra-cytoplasmic sperm injection(ICSI). This is an in vitro fertilization (IVF) technique in which under the microscope a small hole is created in the outer membranes of the egg so that a single sperm can be placed within the substance of the egg in order for fertilization and embryo development to occur. This has produced many pregnancies in cases of severe seminal problems that previously could only have been achieved with the use of donor sperm. Even immature sperm obtained directly from the testis with a needle aspiration under local anesthesia can bring about a normal pregnancy.

Pre treatment assessment of the female partner with dynamic ovarian testing is becoming more common. It is well known that starting in the middle 30s a woman becomes less fertile and is subject to a higher abortion rate as well. Both of these facts are related to egg quality rather than quantity. Although men produce sperm daily, a woman is born with the most eggs that she will ever have. Thus, the aging effect is less kind to women than men so far as reproduction is concerned. Results from egg donor - recipient programs clearly prove that the uterus is not the limiting feature; women in their 40s and even beyond have pregnancy rates and miscarriage rates which reflect the age of the egg donor rather than the recipient. Many cases of so-called unexplained infertility are really egg quality problems for which there is little direct treatment. Nevertheless, early diagnosis of the situation will save the couple a great deal of expense and frustration by avoiding fruitless therapy.

Although freezing (cryopreservation) of sperm and embryos has been successfully practiced for some years, the quest for a reliable method of freezing human eggs remains one of the holy grails of reproductive endocrinology. The egg (oocyte) initiates a meiotic division in embryonic life which is only completed many years later as part of the ovulation process. This certainly makes it more vulnerable to errors of chromosome content and additionally compounds the difficulty in freezing, thawing and maturing in tissue culture while preserving normal potential for development. A few scattered reports on early success with human frozen — thawed eggs have appeared, and the hope is that a standardized method which could be employed by any competent IVF laboratory will evolve. If this comes to pass, women could bank eggs prior to receiving chemotherapy which might permanently damage their eggs, salvage eggs for freezing at the time of ovarian surgery, and protect against the effect of age on reproduction by electively storing eggs.

New technologies bring real hope for couples previously untreatable. We still have far to go. It is my hope that you'll find this book helpful in giving you the background to understand the nature of the problem and the various choices of therapies which can be applied. Don't be afraid to ask questions. Most fertility programs encourage you to be part of the decision-making process. Armed with the proper facts you can make these difficult choices in an intelligent fashion.

We are truly graced by the chapter written by Dr. Andrea Braverman on psychologic aspects of infertility. She has chaired the special interest group on psychology of the American Society of Reproductive Medicine and has written extensively in the psychologic literature on the dynamics of the infertile couple and the effects of various therapeutic measures including an analysis of the family unit following IVF.

1

An Overview

An alien space ship sends two observers to Earth in order to sample the population. They land in Manhattan, enter a hotel and separate. The first slips into the corner of a conference room in which there is a convention of the Little People of America. Using its bionic telemetry systems the alien takes measurements of height, weight, and other features. The other alien manages to enter a room in which the men's National Basketball Association members are having a meeting. Similar measurements are taken. When the data are compared, the first alien suggests that the second needs to have a tune-up of its circuitry. This analogy is meant to illustrate the problem of sampling errors when a population is studied. Less dramatic, but more important for our purposes, are the responses of Dr. Smith and Dr. Jones to the question of what are the major causes of infertility. Dr. Smith, known for her expertise in treating endometriosis would give you one answer, while Dr. Jones, a renowned tubal surgeon would give another, thus illustrating the bias in patient selection. If asked in a survey, 14%-16% of all couples will respond yes to the question "have you ever been infertile?" But the real population of patients considered to be infertile is probably 8%-12%. Figure 1.1 shows the **cumulative pregnancy rate** in an unselected or randomly picked population. The most fertile couples conceive with a rate of about 20%-25% during the first three months, which then dramatically falls so that by 12 months about 85% in all have conceived. For instance, if 25% conceived in the first month, that would leave 75; 25% of that remainder would be 19 and 25% of the remaining 56 in the

1

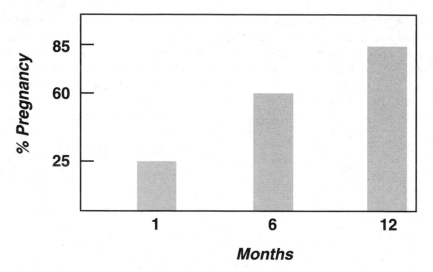

FIGURE 1.1 Cumulative pregnancy rate in an unselected population.

third month would add up to 59% pregnant by the end of the third month.

About one in ten left at the end of one year will conceive during the next year without any therapy. This method of quantifying fertility per cycle is the yardstick by which most therapies are measured and is known as **fecundity.**

Sometimes infertility is simply a matter of age, particularly in the female; but it may be caused by medications, drugs, various diseases, or by conditions present at birth. Nevertheless, over 70% of all couples undergoing treatment for infertility will eventually be successful in having a baby if they're able to complete the treatment protocols. The goal of this book is to give you an understanding of the various therapies which are available, since often there are legitimate choices to be made. You cannot be part of this decision-making process unless you understand the pros and cons of each of these paths. You need to know how each procedure works, what the expected yield in terms of pregnancy should be, and for how long each choice should be pursued before moving on to the next level.

It is important in any discussion to distinguish between **sterility** and **infertility.** Sterility is an absolute term which means that conception is not possible. In a man this occurs when the testes no longer produce sperm. In that case, donor sperm can be used. In a woman, sterility occurs when the ovaries no longer contain eggs and menopause begins. With today's new technologies, a woman can accept donor eggs from another woman and carry a normal pregnancy. Thus, even sterile people can parent. As a couple, you may be infertile if the man has a low sperm count, or if the woman is approaching her 40s, if ovulation occurs infrequently, or if the fallopian tubes are damaged. Under any of these circumstances you may conceive without any special medical treatment, but your chances of doing so are not as good as normally functioning younger couples. Doctors often define infertility as primary and secondary. The first refers to failure of conception after one year for couples who have never before been pregnant, while the second term is reserved for failure to conceive after six months for previously fertile couples. The definitions blur, for example, when one of the partners has been fertile in a previous relationship. Both definitions assume adequate sexual contact having to do both with frequency of intercourse and the ability to deposit sperm into the vagina. Some couples conceive less quickly than others but without the need for any medical intervention. Calling them infertile according to an arbitrary definition is less than accurate; perhaps the term **subfertile** would be more correct.

Adequate Sexual Contact

To have adequate sexual contact semen must be deposited within the vagina during sexual intercourse. This may seem to be an obvious point, but there are many ways in which people express themselves sexually, and not all of them end with semen in the vagina. In this context adequacy refers only to the initiation of pregnancy and ignores all of the social and emotional factors associated with sexual function. Moreover, certain anatomical conditions and abnormalities may make it difficult to achieve adequate sexual contact. For example, some men are born with a congenital condition known as **hypospadias**, in which the opening of the urethra, the channel through which both urine and semen pass, is located on the underside of the penis, instead of at the tip. Many men with this problem fail to achieve adequate sexual contact because semen is ejaculated outside the vagina. Most cases of hypospadias can be surgically corrected. For those other cases, the semen can be collected by masturbation and placed into the vagina or cervix with artificial insemination, which is a simple solution. Extreme obesity can also interfere with adequate vaginal penetration. Insemination is the answer to this problem as well.

Frequency of Intercourse

The more frequent sexual intercourse you have, the greater the chances for conception—up to a point. Most couples report intercourse two or three times weekly, but the range is great. Sexual frequency usually declines with the duration of marriage and with the age of the male. The frequency of intercourse in the early stages of the relationship determines the pattern in later years. Although most men regenerate a normal sperm concentration within a day or two after ejaculation, this may not always be the case in an older individual, one who is taking medication, or a man in any age group who has a low sperm count. Frequent intercourse for him may be counterproductive.

Stress and fatigue in the workplace may be brought home and under those circumstances interfere with the initiation of intercourse. Working couples tend to cluster sexual activity on weekends and vacations. Urinary ovulation detection kits are helpful in pinpointing the best time for intercourse to occur when pregnancy is desired. Infrequent sexual activity may be the sole reason for subfertility.

The Age Factor

When I started to practice reproductive medicine, the average age of the female patient that I saw was 28; it is now about 36. This represents the result of changes in the population with later marriage and postponement of childbirth. Indeed, the rate of first births in women over 35 has tripled in the last 15 years. On the other hand, one-third of all women who have previously conceived can no longer do so over the age of 35. The chief reason for this has to do with egg quality. This delaying trend may make sense professionally, economically, and psychologically, but it also means that women are not having children during the best biologic time of their lives, which is between the ages of 18 and 26. Beginning in the early 30s women become less fertile. For some this means that it may take longer to conceive; for others, it might mean loss of reproductive potential entirely. At menopause, regardless of age, all women lose the ability to become pregnant. With increased age also comes an increase in miscarriage rate. The issue of sampling is at play here as well. Women who were very fertile in their younger years tend to remain so well into their 40s.

In general, age is reproductively kinder to men than women. Initiation of pregnancy by men in their 60s and 70s is not unusual, but it is quite rare for a woman over 50 to conceive (without an egg donor). Therefore, a fertility investigation should be conducted if pregnancy has not occurred within six months in a couple in which the female partner is 35 or over. Fortunately, we now have a method of analyzing both the quality and quantity of eggs within the ovary which involves blood testing before and after taking pills for five days as an ovarian stimulant. This screening test is readily available , and in my opinion it should be performed in all women over 35 seeking infertility therapy and in younger women whose history is suggestive of problems with ovarian function.

Miscarriage

Not all fertility problems have to do with conception. The word **fertility** in its fullest sense means the ability to carry a pregnancy successfully and to deliver a healthy newborn. Pregnancies end in miscarriage or spontaneous abortion more often than most people realize. Many women who are a few days or a week late with menses actually have had an early abortion. The rate of abortion is age sensitive with a 16% rate up to the early 30s rising to over 50% for women in their 40s. The new pregnancy tests are very sensitive, and can be positive even before the missed menses . Therefore, we return to our original issue of sampling errors. If testing is done very early as with an infertile population eager to know if pregnancy has occurred, the abortion rate will be perceived to be higher than in a general population in which the testing is done in a more leisurely fashion a few weeks after a missed period. Most early pregnancy loss results from either poor implantation of the fertilized egg (a blastocyst) in the wall of the uterus or faulty chromosomal division of cells in the embryo. Analysis of chromosomes in tissue taken from spontaneous abortions shows that the fetal genetic material is abnormal in 50% to 60% of cases, and that nature is quite efficient in producing a natural cure for the situation.

The Right Doctor

Every couple is unique, and therefore there is more than one correct approach to the problem of infertility. Algorithms of the fertility investigation and treatment , however, have become popular in recent years. There's no question that a standardized step-wise approach is helpful as a teaching aid. The medical insurance companies, particularly the HMO's, also favor this approach because it allows them to dictate the type of treatment which they believe to be most cost-effective, and facilitates record-keeping and cost analysis. The individual therapist should be one who has experience, insight and sensitivity sufficient enough to get to the heart of the problem quickly and without the burden of unnecessary tests, some of which may be both expensive and uncomfortable. Today, many fertility practices have more than one physician, and you may be seen by various members of the team. Under these circumstances communication between the patient and physicians and especially among physicians themselves is important. Any competent physician should not mind if you seek a second opinion, if for no other reason than to be reassured that the course taken is a proper one. How to find the right physician or practice is not always easy. Certainly recommendations from friends who have gone through this type of care should be helpful. Referral from your family physician or general gynecologist is a good way of reaching a fertility specialist. RESOLVE, which is a national organization of infertile couples, with local chapters in or near most large cities is an excellent referral source. The American Society for Reproductive Medicine web site (www.asrm.com) has a listing of members by state locale. There are other links on the web which may be helpful, but be careful because many of them are unregulated and may give information of dubious value.

The Psyche

Coping with the pressures of infertility treatment can be all encompassing. We live in a society of instant gratification; if we want something all we need to do is pull out our credit card. We tend to be goal-oriented and want results **NOW!** It's a world where contraception is easily used and quite efficient. People naturally expect that pregnancy will occur just as easily as contraception kept it away. It comes as a painful surprise that becoming pregnant for some is not easy. This disappointment leads to anxiety often followed by frustration. During the infertility work-up and treatment phase it is important for the couple to pace themselves. Try not to spend too much emotional currency on a single loss or misfire. A clinical psychologist with special interest and expertise in caring for infertile couples can help you maintain your equilibrium and a proper perspective on the problem.

2

The Female Reproductive System

The Vulva

The major parts of the female reproductive system are illustrated in figures 2.1 and 2.2. The external genital organs include the outer lips, the **labia majora**, the inner lips known as the **labia minora,** and the **clitoris.** Collectively they are known as the **vulva.** The hairy outer lips contain fatty tissue which acts as a cushion. The two inner lips meet in front of the **urethra** where they partially cover the clitoris as a hood. During sexual arousal the clitoris becomes engorged with blood and erects, like a man's penis. Stimulation of the clitoris produces orgasm, although orgasm can occur in the absence of direct clitoral stimulation. You may have heard or read that rhythmic contractions of pelvic muscles during orgasm help propel sperm upward toward the uterus during intercourse. This sounds great for many reasons, but there is no proof that this is true or that orgasm has any positive effect on becoming pregnant.

The Vagina

The vulva opens into the **vagina,** a muscular tube or cylinder through which menstrual flow (menses) passes down from the uterus and through which sperm migrate upwards. A membrane called the **hymen** lies across the vaginal opening behind the vulva. The hymen usually has more than one opening that allows menstrual blood to pass. Traditionally an intact hymen

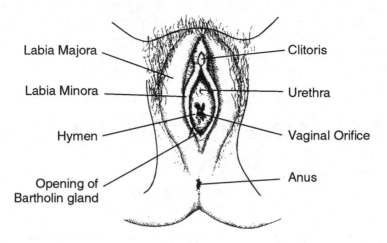

FIGURE 2.1 External female genital anatomy.

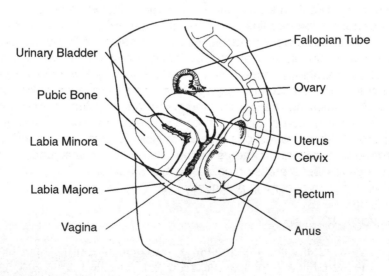

FIGURE 2.2 Cross section of the female pelvis.

was considered as the only real test of virginity. This is medically incorrect, since strenuous physical activity and/or early use of tampons can enlarge the opening in the absence of sexual activity. Near the bottom of the vaginal canal just behind the opening of the vulva are two glands called Bartholin's glands, which produce (secrete) mucus to lubricate the vagina during sexual arousal.

PHEROMONES

The cells of the vaginal lining contain large amounts of starch called glycogen. Bacteria normally present in a healthy vagina ferment the glycogen, causing the vagina to become acidic. This process also leads to production of chemicals known as **pheromones.**

These organic acids have a distinct pungent odor and appear to be most prevalent around the time of ovulation. Pheromones play an important role in reproduction in animals. In monkeys, for example, the odor identifies to the male those females who have entered the fertile interval. Experiments have shown that when castrated male monkeys are painted with secretions taken from the vagina of females at the time of ovulation, other male monkeys will attempt to mount them. Pheromones also seem to explain why women living together tend to develop synchronized menstrual cycles as a consequence of the hypothalamus becoming "in phase". This might be a vestige of a primitive way of regulating reproduction within a tribal society to occur as a group phenomenon. It is thought that chemical signals are transmitted through the olfactory nerves to the brain which eventually regulates ovarian function. The sense of smell may play some role in human reproduction even now, since there is some evidence that human males become sexually aroused by pheromones. The perfume industry has recently latched onto this, but I don't know of any scientific study which has addressed the issue of whether or not women who use these products have any change in their sex lives.

VAGINAL HEALTH

Various bacterial infections can alter the normal acidity of the vaginal lining, so too can douches, artificial lubricants, and antibiotics, none of which should be used without good reason. Under normal conditions many different kinds of bacteria flourish in the vagina. Infection is said to occur when some of these bacteria become dominant, or if new hostile bacteria invade. Infections require treatment usually because of symptoms such as burning or itching coupled with an annoying vaginal discharge. Additionally, certain bacteria and other organisms can kill or immobilize sperm. The responsible organism can usually be identified during a vaginal examination when a microscopic smear is examined. Sometimes it is necessary to get a laboratory culture to settle the issue. The appropriate medication can then be given, either orally or directly into the vagina, as a suppository, gel, or cream.

Some couples routinely use artificial lubricants during intercourse. Sexual foreplay is almost always sufficient to bring about adequate vaginal lubrication if performed in a reasonable fashion. Most fertility therapists discourage use of artificial agents around the time of ovulation, because they may act as impediments to sperm passage from the vagina into the cervix. Under no circumstances should petroleum based jellies such as Vaseline be used in the vagina because they may irritate the lining and kill the sperm. Douching with bicarbonate of soda has been recommended as a remedy for poor postcoital survival of sperm thought to be related to acid secretions of the vagina and cervical mucus. Since water and mucus do not mix, the cervical mucus is unaffected by douching and this form of therapy while easy and inexpensive, is also ineffective.

The Cervix

THE ROLE OF CERVICAL MUCUS

The cervix telescopes into the top of vagina. It has a channel which leads to the interior of the uterus. It is through this canal that menstrual blood flows, sperm ascend into the tubes, and eventually a baby is delivered. The cervix produces alkaline mucus which protects the sperm from the acidity of vaginal secretions. Sperm reach the cervix moments after ejaculation takes place in the vagina and are thus protected in this fashion. Examination of the mucus microscopically documents that sperm can survive for as long as three days following intercourse. This forms the foundation for the postcoital test, which is part of the basic fertility investigation, by addressing the issue of whether or not sperm will survive in cervical mucus around the time of ovulation. Although this test is frequently performed within an hour or so following coitus by many practitioners, this is obviously not physiologic with respect to what normally happens; the evaluation should be conducted 8 to 14 hours after intercourse, and should be timed according to an ovulation detection kit.

The mucus is produced in small sacs called **crypts,** which line the walls of the cervix (figure 2.3). These small sacs serve as reservoirs for the sperm. Packets of sperm are released at intervals many hours after

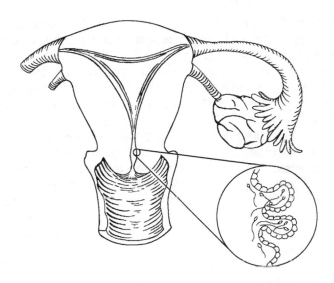

FIGURE 2.3 Cervical crypts that secrete mucus and serve as reservoirs for sperm.

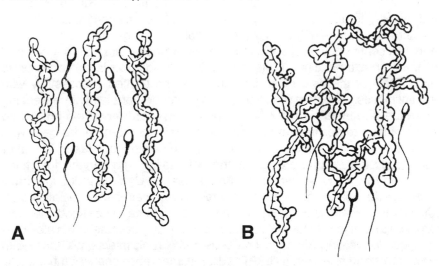

FIGURE 2.4 Microscopic appearance of protein strands in cervical mucus. (A) Appearance at the time of ovulation with channels favoring efficient sperm penetration and migration upward, (B) Unfavorable maze-like configuration found at other times during the menstrual cycle.

intercourse. Both the quantity and composition of cervical mucus change during the menstrual cycle. Early in the cycle, just after menstruation, there is a relatively small amount of rather thick mucus which actually acts as a barrier to sperm migration. As ovulation approaches estrogen levels become higher and greater amounts of mucus are produced with a consistency which is more watery, quite elastic, and with a high salt content. This elastic quality is frequently known by the German word **spinnbarkeit.** Around the time of ovulation, when mucus has just the right proportion of water and salt, the molecules line up in such a way as to form channels known as **micelles,** through which sperm can easily pass (figure 2.4). Following ovulation, estrogen levels decline and progesterone levels increase, causing the mucus once again to thicken and to decrease in quantity. It is not unusual for a woman to be able to accurately predict impending ovulation according to the changes in her vaginal secretions which actually emanate from the cervix.

CERVICAL INFECTIONS

Some women never seem able to produce mucus of sufficient quality and quantity to allow pregnancy to occur easily. Sometimes this is related to a chronic infection of the crypts, a parallel to chronic tonsillitis. Frequently there is a continuous discharge, and the cervix appears to be reddened and inflamed on examination. If this is the case, the diagnosis of "cervicitis" is made. Most of the time these infections can be treated successfully with oral antibiotics. Resistant infections usually can be handled with a freezing technique performed in the office known as **cryocautery.** This procedure does not lead to permanent damage to the cervix as can be the case with use of either a electrical instrument known as a cautery, or a laser. The latter was initially touted as a precise method of dealing with cervical infections and abnormal cells (detected in Pap smears). Unfortunately, we have learned that use of the laser on the cervix may be associated with considerable scarring, causing the canal to become constricted (cervical stenosis) and also with loss of the mucus producing cells. A newer electrical technique for dealing with abnormal cells and chronic infection is "large loop excision" often known as a "LEEP" . Sometimes poor cervical mucus is a result of medical intervention as may be the case with cervical biopsies or cautery procedures. When indicated, these cervical surgeries should be done with the least amount of cervix possible subjected to alteration or destruction. **Cervical eversion** is a term used to describe an outrolling of the cervical lining in the canal onto the face of the cervix in a manner similar to what happens when someone rolls up the cuff on a pair of jeans and exposes the underside of the material. This is not a pathologic condition, and in fact, is fairly common in women using oral contraceptives and in those who have recently delivered. This is often mistaken for a **cervical erosion** also known as a cervical ulcer.

In perhaps three percent of infertile women, the mucus may actually act contraceptively because it contains sperm-specific antibodies. These antibodies can cause sperm to stick together (agglutinate) and lose motility. We'll cover diagnosis and treatment of this condition in a subsequent chapter.

The Uterus

Above and contiguous with the cervix is the body of the **uterus.** This hollow muscle normally weighs about two ounces. But during pregnancy the uterus undergoes amazing growth and develops a special arrangement of blood vessels that allows nutrients to pass through the placenta to the fetus with minimal mixing of the blood of the mother and fetus. During labor, the full muscle power of the uterus comes into play as it pushes the baby into the birth canal and out into the external world.

UTERINE STRUCTURAL ABNORMALITIES

In the developing fetus, the uterus begins formation as two rudimentary pouches, one on either side of the pelvis. The segments gradually migrate toward each other and begin to fuse. Under normal circumstances the common wall between them is absorbed and a single cavity is formed as shown in figure 2.5. Some women are born without a uterus and without a fully formed vagina. This is known as the **Rokitansky** syndrome in which pregnancy is obviously impossible. A functioning vagina can be created with self treatment using dilators or with surgical construction of a vagina allowing for satisfactory sexual function. The technology exists to allow a woman with this condition to have her eggs taken from her ovaries and fertilized in an in vitro fertilization (IVF) procedure with the embryo carried by a genetically inert woman. This is known as a "carrier gestation". Although it is technically possible to transplant a uterus just as is the case with heart, liver, kidney and lungs, there is a significant risk to the patient, and the need to give powerful immunosuppresive drugs in order to avoid rejection of the implant makes this operation completely impractical.

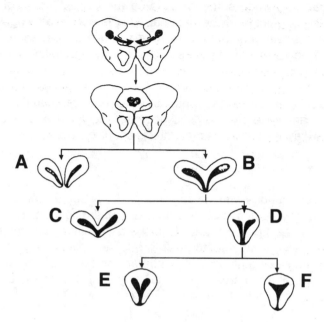

FIGURE 2.5 Steps in formation of the embryonic uterus. Top, migration of each half from a lateral position to the midline. (A) Two separate uteri and cervices as a result of failure to fuse, (B) Normal fusion beginning from bottom to top, (C) Bicornuate uterus from partial failure of fusion, (D) Proper complete fusion, (E) Septate uterus resulting from persistence of septum, (F) Normal uterus.

Two lesser disorders involving the migration and fusion of the rudimentary portions of the uterus are the **bicornate** and **septate** malformations , both illustrated in figure 2.5. In both types there are two cavities at the top which usually come together near the cervix. Approximately two percent of all women will have a two - chambered uterus. This does not necessarily mean that the individual will have difficulty in carrying a pregnancy. And this has nothing to do with the ability to conceive. In fact, the vast majority of these women will have no reproductive problems at all. In some cases, however there is repetitive abortion. Surgical correction is usually easy and quite effective but should be done only when there is evidence of reproductive wastage and with no other cause identifiable. A woman with a bicornate uterus usually has premature labor and delivery not only because of the uterine structural change but also because the cervix dilates many weeks prior to labor. Once detected, a simple cervical banding procedure known as a **cervical cerclage** can be performed. This is essentially placing a thick suture around the cervix in the manner of a pursestring. The patient with the septate uterus is more likely to experience a problem much earlier in pregnancy with losses occurring near the end of the first trimester (by 13 weeks). While the bicornate uterus needs to be repaired with an open procedure (laparotomy), the septate uterus can be repaired on an outpatient basis via hysteroscopy with subsequent vaginal delivery. The bicornate uterus is a failure of fusion while the septate uterus represents a failure of absorption. Some patients have two separate uteri with two cervices and often a vaginal septum. These patients actually do well reproductively. When one of the rudimentary pouches fails to develop the end result is a half uterus, known as a **unicollate** uterus. This may occur in conjunction with failure of the kidney to develop on the side where uterine development ceased. These women can usually be brought through pregnancy with a combination of reduced activity (sometimes bed rest) and medications to keep them out of premature labor.

DES SYNDROME

Exposure of the fetus to large doses of synthetic estrogens may lead to malformations of the vagina, cervix, uterus, and fallopian tubes. It also should be noted that the same anatomic changes can occur in cases where the mother took no such drugs. The well-publicized diethylstilbestrol (DES) syndrome is caused not only by DES but can occur after exposure of the fetus to other synthetic estrogens that used to be administered early in pregnancy in the belief that this treatment was helpful to prevent miscarriage. Women whose mothers used DES may have small, irregular uterine cavities, often in the shape of a "T". The cervical canal is disproportionately long compared with the uterine cavity, and often the cervix dilates during pregnancy, necessitating cerclage in order to protect against extreme premature delivery. Women with obvious DES-related cervical changes have a threefold increase in pregnancy loss compared with other women. Because there are also changes in the fallopian tubes, the risk of ectopic pregnancy may be as high as 10%. These women may have greater difficulty in conceiving because the cervix acts as a barrier to sperm migration.

THE ENDOMETRIUM

The lining of the uterine cavity is called the **endometrium**. After conception the fertilized egg, now known as a blastocyst, implants in the wall of the uterus where there are many blood vessels and glands to supply nourishment. Early in the menstrual cycle the endometrium is thin and the blood supply sparse. As the menstrual cycle continues, rising levels of estrogen made by the ovary cause the endometrium to become lush and thick with increased vascularity, a process called proliferation. The blood vessels increase both in size and number, and glands begin to develop. Following ovulation progesterone is manufactured by the ovary, and this causes the glands to release their nutrients, and the endometrium is now described as "secretory". If pregnancy does not occur, progesterone production ceases and the thickened endometrium can no longer be sustained. This sloughing is the menstrual flow. The endometrium returns to its previous basal state and the cycle begins anew. The uterus is quite capable of a normal response to hormonal stimulation well into the 60s as has been proven by the experience with egg recipients whose uterus functions well under these circumstances.

The Fallopian Tubes

Near the top of the uterus on each side is an oviduct, called the fallopian tube (see figures 2.6 and 2.7). Through the tube sperm pass from the uterus on their way to contact and fertilize the egg. The egg is conveyed by the tube (whether fertilized or not) to the uterus. Hence, the tube is a two-way street with traffic in both directions. The portion closest to the uterus has a thick wall with a very small opening (lumen) that is just wide enough for a fertilized egg to pass into the uterus. This part is called the **isthmus.** About halfway along its length of four to six inches the lumen widens into the **ampulla.** At the very end of the tube can be found small tentacle-like projections called **fimbria.** These sweep over the surface of the ovary especially during ovulation and are actually incredibly efficient in the process of egg capture. These structures are very delicate and are easily damaged by infection.

Inside each tube is a lining of folded tissue known as the **endosalpinx.** Special cells secrete a fluid that both nourishes and helps to transport sperm and eggs. The fluid also has the effect of activating the sperm making them capable of fertilization in a process called **capacitation.** This endosalpinx also contains numerous special cells which grow thin, hair-like filaments

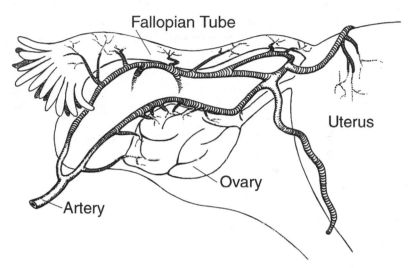

Fallopian Tube

Uterus

Ovary

Artery

FIGURE 2.6   The fallopian tube, its blood supply, and its relationship to uterus and ovary.

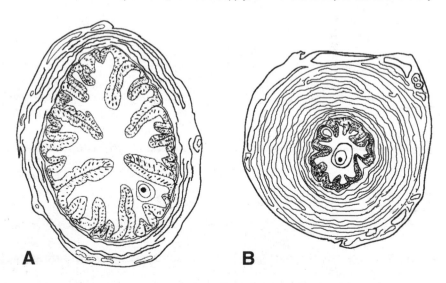

A

B

FIGURE 2.7   Cross-section of a fallopian tube. (A) An egg in the ampulla which has a large, multifolded lumen, (B) The narrower isthmic portion of the tube.

which protrude into the lumen. These little hairs, called **cilia,** beat in a coordinated wave toward the uterus. This action, coupled with the contraction of the muscles in the tube serves to propel the egg toward the uterus. The sperm, however, are always swimming against the current.

TUBAL INFECTIONS

Tubal infections may impair fertility in a number of ways. At the first level the cells which produce the fluid necessary for nourishment and transport may be destroyed. The cilia may be damaged and destroyed; these cells regenerate poorly, if at all. Under these circumstances egg transport becomes problematic. Even if the tube is open, loss of cilia, especially when coupled with formation of scar tissue within the lumen, can lead to the fertilized egg being trapped in the tube, thus creating an ectopic pregnancy. If the damage from the infection is more severe, the tube becomes closed either at the uterine end or distally at the fimbriated ovarian junction. The first bout of tubal infection sufficient to cause fever and pain will leave 15% of victims with closed tubes, and that figure doubles with each additional episode even in the face of vigorous intravenous antibiotic treatment.

Years ago gonorrhea was the most common sexually transmitted infection capable of causing tubal damage. But chlamydial infections have taken over that position. The latter is more insidious clinically, since in many cases the infection has been silent, producing no symptoms, and is only recognized years later by blood tests which demonstrate contact with the organism at some time in the distant past. Tubal infections can also be caused by organisms normally found in the gastrointestinal tract. Poor bathroom hygiene and sexual behavior involving anal penetration with subsequent vaginal contamination can lead to this result. Both Streptococcus and Staphylococcus, commonly found organisms, are capable of causing tubal damage, especially as part of the process of delivery.

The Ovaries and the Hormonal Cycle

The ovary has a dual role of providing the hormones which bring about sexual maturation and distinguish women from men, coupled with its function as the storehouse for the gametes (eggs) necessary to produce the next generation.

The ovaries are located behind and to the side of the uterus to which they are attached by a ligament. The tube is in close contact with the ovary, and the fimbriated end actually sweeps over the ovarian surface in order to capture the egg at the time of ovulation. Each egg is encased in its own sac of fluid known as a **follicle**. Women are born with a finite number of eggs, about 400,000 in each ovary. This is in contradistinction to men who produce sperm daily from the onset of puberty until death. The egg supply diminishes naturally over time, with the decrease actually beginning during embryonic life. Most women exhaust the reservoir near the age of 50, and at that point menstruation ceases and menopause begins. Normally, a cluster of eggs is "recruited" during each menstrual cycle, and from these one is chosen as the dominant follicle destined to continue development and to reach ovulation. But the eggs are used up whether patients ovulate or not by the process known as **atresia**. The use of birth control pills neither stores nor accelerates egg loss.

ESTROGEN AND OVULATION

Hormones are chemicals which regulate the body's internal activities. There are many different hormones, each controlling one or several specific activities. Insulin, for example, controls the rate at which the body metabolizes sugar, but it also has actions in other places including influencing the mix of hormones made by the ovary. A hormone is released (secreted) by a gland and carried by the bloodstream to the appropriate target cells upon which it acts. The cells are covered with **receptors,** which have a specific surface structure designed to capture the hormone molecule and bind it to the cell surface after which it can enter the cell. A hormone will attach only to a receptor that has exactly the right chemical and physical structure as illustrated by the lock and key analogy in figure 2.8.

Estrogen is a term used to describe many similar hormones, the most important of which is estradiol. It is estrogen which brings about the changes in a woman at the time of menarche. The physical contour changes dramatically with continued development of breasts and changes in the hips and buttocks. At this time the part of the brain which controls the menstrual cycle begins to function in a regular and rhythmic fashion. The hypothalamus which sits right over the pituitary gland produces a hormone known as **gonadotropin releasing hormone,** (GnRH) which in turn stimulates the pituitary to release **follicle stimulating hormone** (FSH) and **luteinizing hormone** (LH). Reference to figures 2.9 and 2.10 will help you to understand the hormonal control of ovulation. FSH and LH are known as "gonadotropins", meaning gonad stimulators, and that is exactly what they do. In response to GnRH the pituitary begins to store FSH which it

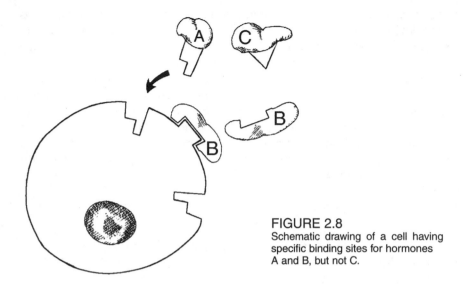

FIGURE 2.8
Schematic drawing of a cell having
specific binding sites for hormones
A and B, but not C.

releases in slowly increasing amounts. All of the hormone systems in the body have feedback mechanisms in order to regulate how much hormone is released over a period of time. **Inhibin** is a hormone made by the granulosa cells, which are essentially the nurse cells around the follicle that bring nutrients and hormones to the developing egg. Inhibin actually can be divided into two separate forms, each of which has its own action and pattern throughout the cycle. Inhibin B acts to keep FSH levels under control. The action of estrogen on the pituitary gland is quite interesting in that early in the cycle estrogen levels inhibit FSH release, but later in the cycle, in the late follicular phase just before ovulation, quickly rising levels of estradiol serve to stimulate not only a small rise in FSH but additionally provoke the major surge in LH release which brings about the actual ovulatory event.

THE CORPUS LUTEUM: A PROGESTERONE FACTORY

If estrogen is the hormone of femininity, then progesterone is the hormone of pregnancy. The area on the ovary at the site of the recently ruptured follicle begins to turn yellow as a consequence of steroids in high concentration being used to make progesterone. This structure is called the **corpus luteum** which literally translated means "yellow body". Actually, the ovary starts to shift from an estrogen producer to a progesterone maker just

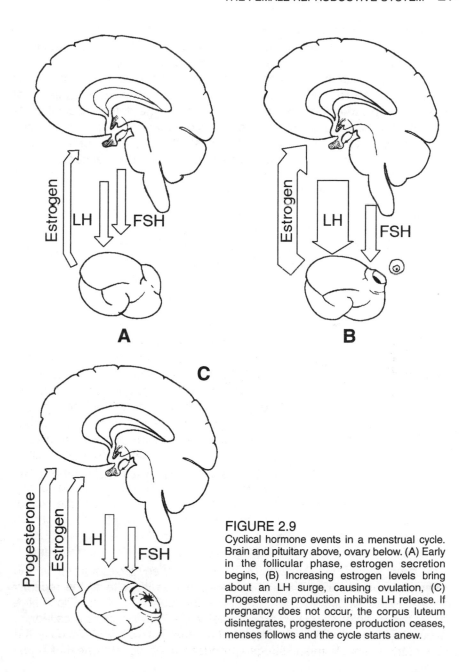

FIGURE 2.9
Cyclical hormone events in a menstrual cycle.
Brain and pituitary above, ovary below. (A) Early
in the follicular phase, estrogen secretion
begins, (B) Increasing estrogen levels bring
about an LH surge, causing ovulation, (C)
Progesterone production inhibits LH release. If
pregnancy does not occur, the corpus luteum
disintegrates, progesterone production ceases,
menses follows and the cycle starts anew.

before ovulation as a consequence of the sudden release of LH. The main purpose of progesterone reproductively is to prepare the endometrium for implantation of the blastocyst by increasing blood supply and glandular development. If conception occurs, the cells surrounding the fetus will secrete a special hormone that keeps a corpus luteum active; this is, of course, **human chorionic gonadotropin**, (hCG), the detection of which is the basis for the pregnancy test. If conception does not occur, the corpus luteum ceases to be active about 14 days after ovulation; progesterone levels fall, the endometrial lining breaks down and menses ensues.

DETECTION OF OVULATION

Because rising estrogen levels influence the cervical cells to secrete more mucus with an increasing water content and elasticity, some women can accurately predict ovulation by the changes which occur in vaginal fluids. This is true for a minority of women, and the pattern may be altered by medications used to promote fertility such as clomiphene citrate (reduction of mucus) or gonadotropins (increased mucus). Some women have pain around the time of ovulation, known by its original German description as **mittelschmerz.**

An easy and inexpensive way to determine ovulation is to chart the **basal body temperature** (BBT) each morning immediately upon awakening. This is a time honored method of evaluating ovulation, but the problem is that it tells us that ovulation **has** occurred, but cannot predict it. The reason for the rise of temperature with ovulation has to do with the thermogenic effect of progesterone on the body's temperature regulating system— another example of a hormone having multiple actions in quite different areas of the body. This rise in temperature depends on the rate at which progesterone increases as well as the sensitivity of the thermostat. Therefore, there are a number of normal but different patterns seen on the temperature chart. Because the temperature regulating center is easily affected by activity, even getting out of bed before using the thermometer will probably interfere with the temperature pattern, so the reading must be taken immediately upon awakening. Use of a special thermometer is unnecessary, although basal body temperature thermometers with widely separated spaces and digital thermometers are easier to read, especially if you are bleary-eyed in the morning. Sometimes there is a dip in the reading just before ovulation, but this is variable and unimportant. Women who work at night will have no problem in keeping the chart if they arise at the same time each day. But if you work irregular shifts or travel through

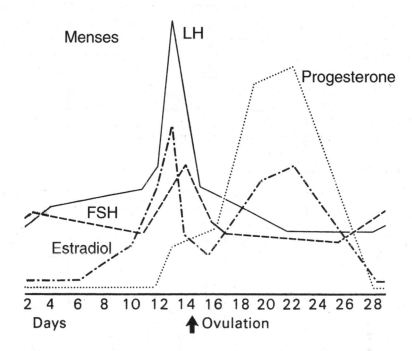

FIGURE 2.10   Interrelationships of hormone levels during the menstrual cycle.

different time zones frequently, the BBT may be unreliable and frustrating. Research has shown that the temperature may rise just before or a day or two after actual ovulation. Therefore, the BBT chart is more useful for documenting ovulatory function then precise timing of the event. Figures 2.11 and 2.12 demonstrate some common temperature chart patterns. Regardless of when in the cycle ovulation occurs, the luteal phase should last 12 to 14 days as evidenced by sustained temperature elevation, usually about one half degree or more above the baseline in Fahrenheit scales. Some women regularly have basal readings of less than 96 degrees, but this does not have any negative meaning.

Urinary kits designed to detect the presence of LH are extremely helpful in predicting and pinpointing ovulation. If you look at figure 2.10 again you'll see that this LH surge is a dramatic event and can be used with great reliance as a marker. Normally the LH surge begins about 2 a.m. and

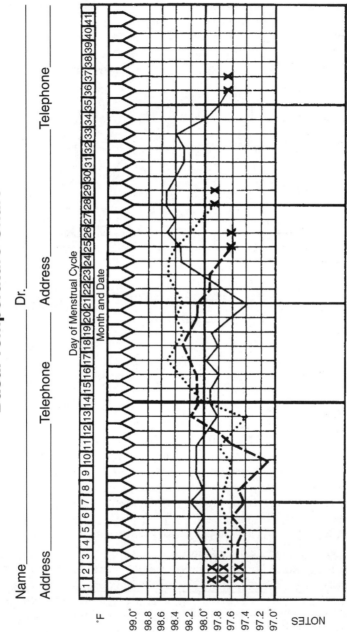

FIGURE 2.11   Basal body temperature (BBT) charts showing three normal patterns. Note that elapsed time between ovulation and the next menses averages 14 days regardless of when ovulation occurs in the cycle.

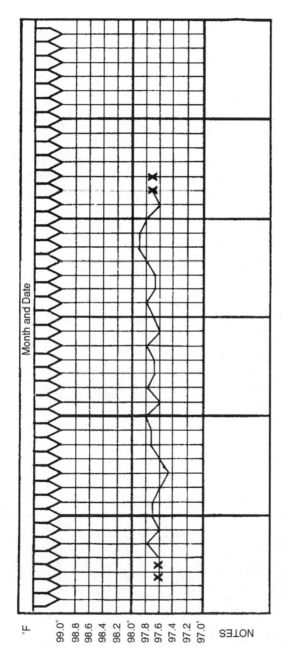

FIGURE 2.12   A BBT chart showing lack of elevation, and hence, indicative of anovulation.

may not make its appearance in the urine until substantially later in the day, dependent upon the state of hydration. Therefore, if you test early in the morning, and if you have not had any water before bedtime, the test may be falsely negative, and probably will still be positive the next morning, but you will have already ovulated. For this reason we tell our patients to test between 2 p.m. and 7 p.m. If the test is being used for sexual timing or for insemination scheduling, accuracy is important, especially if one remembers that the egg is fertilizable only for 18-24 hours after ovulation. These tests are generally very easy to use. Our patients tell us that the ones with the blue color end point are easier to read than those with a pink scale. These tests should be initiated a few days prior to expected ovulation since even though they are over-the-counter, the cost may be considerable. Prior to development of the urinary tests, serial blood tests for LH were performed, but because of the cost and the necessary trips to have blood drawn, this form of testing has given way to the urinary kits except during stimulated cycles.

Ultrasound has been used to detect ovulation. As the follicle matures, it grows in diameter about 2 mm daily, and is ready to be released at about 22 mm of diameter. This figure is quite variable, and applies to natural unstimulated cycles. Ultrasonic examinations when used to predict ovulation must be done in a serial fashion over the course of a few days, and therefore this method is logistically cumbersome and not cost-effective. Of interest, however, is the fact that the ultrasound has shown us that while mittelschmerz is almost always one-sided, it does not predict the side where ovulation is occurring.

3

Male Anatomy and Reproduction

The reproductive mechanisms in the male are less complex than in the female, especially considering the fact that there is no similar cyclical component. In fact, the production of sperm and their delivery seem simple compared with the many physiological events which must occur during the female cycle in order for reproduction to happen. In the male there is little separation of sexual and reproductive anatomy as is the case in the female, hence the diagnosis of male infertility and sexual dysfunction are often linked. Diagnosis of failures in male reproduction is difficult, and more often than not, the term **idiopathic male infertility** is used, which is a fancy term that means that the physicians cannot make a diagnosis to explain the cause of the problem. Our ability to diagnose and to treat male infertility has lagged behind the advances made in dealing with problems in the female. Research efforts and money spent on male infertility is but a fraction of that expended on the female side. This is unlikely to change in the near future now that in vitro fertilization with the direct insertion of sperm into the egg (ICSI) has proven to be so successful in bringing about pregnancy in the most severe forms of male infertility. In essence, we have a very successful method of treating a problem whose causes remain unknown.

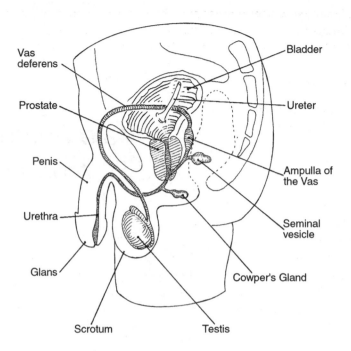

FIGURE 3.1   Male reproductive anatomy.

The Male Reproductive System

In contradistinction to the female, the male has most of his reproductive organs outside the abdomen (figure 3.1 illustrates the major parts of the male reproductive system). The **urethra** passes throughout the entire length of the penis. It is an internal canal which carries both sperm and urine from the body. The penis also contains a mass of spongy erectile tissue. When the arteries which supply this tissue dilate, and veins constrict, the penis expands to erection. The principal reproductive organs are the two testes, or testicles. These produce both sperm and hormones, the most important of which is **testosterone**. At puberty, testosterone causes changes in a boy's voice, facial hair, body build, and genital structure. If an otherwise healthy man loses one testicle through injury or surgery, there usually is no decrease in his fertility even though there may be a decrease in the total number of sperm present in the semen released at orgasm. The ability of the sperm to move properly, and the ratio of normally to abnormally formed sperm are far more important determinants of fertility.

Production and Transportation of Sperm

Sperm are produced within narrow tightly coiled tubes called **seminiferous tubules**. A normal male below the age of 40 usually produces about 125 million sperm daily (figure 3.2 is a schematic representation of a testicle and its ductal system). The walls of these many tubules contain cells known as stem cells. When these primitive cells divide, one of the two new cells remains in the tubule to repeat the process while the other new cell eventually becomes a mature **spermatazoan** (the technical name for sperm). It enters the passageway of the tubule while still quite immature and attaches to one of the many **Sertoli cells** (figure 3.3) which provide nourishment. With time the sperm moves through the tubule to the rete testis, which serves as a collection point or staging center for sperm entering from hundreds of tubules. The rete testis is linked to the **epididymis** by ducts.

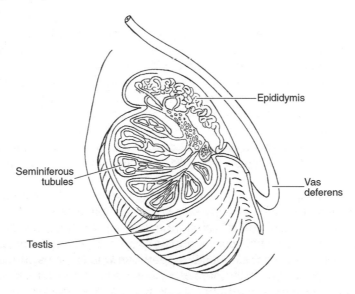

FIGURE 3.2 Cross section through a testis showing the coiled seminiferous tubules and the ductal system transporting sperm away from the testis.

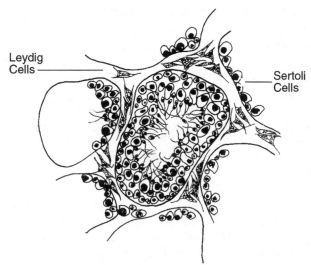

FIGURE 3.3 Sertoli cells, which "nurse" developing sperm, and Leydig cells, which secrete testosterone.

These sperm are still not yet mature enough to move properly on their own, but they are pushed through the ducts by contraction of the muscles in the walls similar to the peristaltic wave of the gastrointestinal tract. But because pregnancy has been induced with sperm taken directly from testis by needle aspiration or biopsy, we know that these sperm, although immature and incapable of intrinsic motion, have what it takes to bring about a normal fertilization if placed directly into an egg as is done with ICSI. It is within the epididymis that the sperm finally mature. The tightly coiled epididymis would measure about 20 feet if it were stretched out. Sperm spend almost two weeks in passage through the epididymis maturing further.

From the epididymis, the now mature sperm move on downstream to the **vas deferens**. This tube is fairly straight and approximately 14 inches in length. It rises out of the scrotum (the sac containing the testes) and connects with the seminal vesicle in the pelvis. The seminal vesicle, as the name implies, actually does not store sperm as was previously thought. Its main purpose, along with the prostate gland, is to supply an alkaline fluid (semen) in which the sperm are suspended. The process of sperm production and maturation takes about 72 days with at least 17 stages of sperm forms being recognized prior to storage in the vas. For this reason there is a built-in delay in seminal improvement as seem in the semen analysis following any form of direct treatment. Often this lag can last for three or more months especially following surgical treatment.

The vas is the structure which is cut and sealed during **vasectomy**, the male sterilization procedure. Unfortunately, it is also somewhat vulnerable to injury occurring during hernia repairs in the groin, especially when performed during childhood. Closure of either the epididymis or the vas results in **azoospermia,** or lack of sperm in the ejaculate. Some men are born with blockage in the vas, usually on both sides. Strangely enough, inheritance of a single gene for cystic fibrosis may cause congenital (meaning absent at birth) absence of the vas although it takes two copies of the gene for cystic fibrosis to cause the actual clinical disease state. DES, a synthetic estrogen used at one time for pregnancy support, has been implicated as a cause of congenital blockage of the seminal ducts in some men exposed to this drug while in utero. Blockages can also result from inflammation following infections of the genito-urinary tract. There is a simple test available to determine if the cause of azoospermia is a blockage or failure of sperm to be produced. Semen normally contains a simple sugar (fructose). By testing for the sugar in the semen a ductal obstruction can be diagnosed when fructose is absent; on the other hand, the absence of sperm in a semen specimen which contains fructose usually points to failure of sperm production. Normally, the amount of sperm in the ejaculate is about one tenth of the seminal volume.

The seminal vesicle and the prostate gland supply most of the seminal fluid, which is highly alkaline. This serves to neutralize somewhat the normal acidity of the vagina and thus enhances sperm motility, and also serves as a source of nutrition. Because the prostate gland is vulnerable to infections, it is a common culprit in mild infertility, with the motility of the sperm being affected, rather than the count.

Unlike a woman, who is born with a fixed number of eggs, a man produces billions of new sperm during his lifetime. Additionally, because this production continues well into old age, the man is potentially fertile deeper into life than the woman who undergoes menopause near the age of 50. Although men experience no cyclical hormonally related events such as ovulation, they do have a hormonally activated control cycle which involves FSH and LH (see figure 3.4). In men, FSH stimulates the tubules to produce sperm. The Sertoli cells, in addition to serving as nutritional sources for the developing sperm also produce a hormone known as inhibin which shuts down FSH production. When increased sperm production is required, inhibin production drops, which then allows FSH levels to rise, resulting in the formation of more sperm.

LH stimulates the **Leydig cells** (figure 3.4) in the testes to produce testosterone. When the level of testosterone rises, LH levels drop. This is reversed when testosterone levels are low.

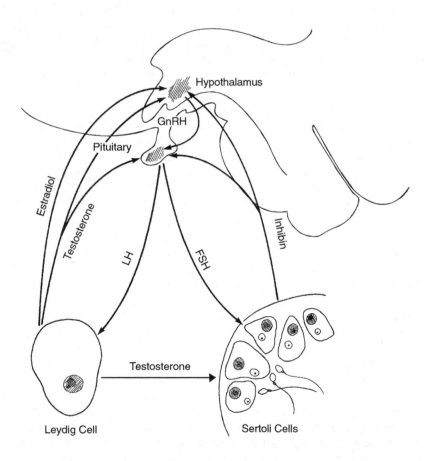

FIGURE 3.4 The male reproductive hormonal control system.

Sperm Delivery: Intercourse and Ejaculation

What effect does frequent coitus have on male infertility? The answer is that it increases the chances for conception — up to a point. A problem can arise if sexual activity is so frequent than a sufficient number of sperm cannot be replenished. Most young men can restore their sperm counts within 24 hours or less following ejaculation. In older men and in those with low counts signifying low production, the restocking process may take three or four days. Why are so many sperm needed to cause conception if only one sperm normally penetrates the egg? For every 14 million sperm ejaculated into the vagina only one to ten will reach the end of the fallopian tube! The sperm head contains enzymes which help to dissolve the cement which holds the **granulosa cells** together. These cells surround the egg within the follicle and adhere to it after ovulation. Thus, the sperm cells which do not actually penetrate the egg act as helpers for the one which finally produces the fertilization. It's a mistake to believe that long periods of sexual abstention can promote fertility by a sustained buildup of count. At some point the number of sperm made daily begins to equal the amount which die while being stored. More important is the fact that sperm motility starts to decrease somewhere between 8 and 10 days between ejaculations.

In order to deliver sperm into the vagina, the man must be able to both relax then contract involuntarily certain muscles that control erection and ejaculation. It is not surprising that certain conditions and neurological diseases can cause problems. The nerve damage eventually caused by diabetes mellitus, for example, can interfere with this process and leads to **retrograde ejaculation**, in which semen passes back into the bladder rather than out the urethra. This occurs because the diabetic process damages the nerves which control muscles that normally prevent a backflow into the bladder during ejaculation. This same malfunction can also occur as a consequence of surgery done near the junction of the bladder neck and urethra (usually performed to relieve obstruction of urinary flow). Drugs commonly cause problems with erection or ejaculation. Tranquilizers and antidepressants head the list. Agents used to treat high blood pressure also have a well deserved reputation for causing difficulty with either erection or ejaculation. On the other hand, drugs such as Viagra, used to treat impotence, are actually restorers of fertility in men who have reasonable sperm production but who were unable to deliver the sperm. The deleterious effect of some drugs also carries over to the area of anti-inflammatory drugs used to treat gastrointestinal disease such as regional enteritis or ulcers, with effects both on production and motility. The drug effect can be subtle as is the case with calcium channel blockers, used in the treatment of cardiovascular disease. In this example the drug interferes with the final step of capacitation necessary for sperm activation. Marijuana causes a decrease in testosterone production, which may lead not only to reduced sperm numbers, but additionally to a diminished sex drive.

Evidence has accumulated that smokers have a greater chance of decreased sperm concentration. The use of steroid preparations by athletes, particularly football players and weight lifters, has led to irreversible infertility in some. It is important for you to be frank with the doctor who takes a history concerning drug use since almost anything can be related to problems in production or delivery of sperm. It may be a good idea to write down all the drugs you're now taking and include as many others as you can recall from the recent past so that the physician gets the whole picture.

4

Normal Initiation of Pregnancy: Facts and Fallacies

How it Happens

The process of sperm migration through the female tracts is complex and large gaps remain in our understanding of the details. Fertilization, the actual entry of a single sperm into the egg, occurs in the ampullary portion of the tube, near the fimbriated end. Sperm have been recovered from the ampulla within a half-hour after deposit in the vagina. On their own, the sperm do not swim fast enough to reach the ampulla within that time frame. Therefore, by a process which is still mysterious, they are moved along by the assistance of the woman's transport system, probably uterine and tubal contractions. This is even more amazing considering that the cilia, the hair-like projections in the tubal lumen, beat in a waveform **toward** the uterus! The scenario reminds one of the salmon which fight furiously to get upstream in order to spawn. Sperm can live in the tube for as long as five days, although two or three is more common. This explains why conception often can occur when intercourse takes place well **before** ovulation; that is, usually the ovum enters the tube which already contains sperm lying in wait. On the otherhand, the egg maintains a fertilization potential up to 24 hours **after** ovulation. So the notion that extremely accurate and strict timing of intercourse around the time of ovulation is essential for fertilization to occur is a fallacy, provided that sperm are normal in number, and maintain normal motility for a reasonable amount of time. A regimented timetable for scheduled intercourse, under normal

35

circumstances, is counterproductive because it places a great deal of stress on both partners. In cycles where the egg is not fertilized, it will pass into the uterus, disintegrate and is absorbed by the body. This takes place in the fallopian tube in women who have tubal blockage either from infection and scar tissue formation or from sterilization.

When sperm encounter the ovum they surround it and release enzymes from the sperm head in order to break down the cement which holds together the granulosa cells still adherent to the egg. It is estimated that about 1,000 sperm are usually in the vicinity of the egg at this time. Keep in mind that somewhere around 150 million sperm enter the vagina during intercourse. Once a solitary sperm has actually penetrated the outer membrane of the egg a special mechanism within the egg is triggered which prevents other sperm from entering. Otherwise, we would have a condition known as polyspermic fertilization, in which an excess of genetic material would be present. Such an embryo would have too many chromosomes and would be spontaneously aborted.

Soon after fertilization, the embryo travels down the tube to the junction of the isthmus, where it spends three or four days developing. It divides first into two cells, then four, then eight, and so on. After four or five divisions the embryo enters the uterus but does not implant into the endometrium for about another 36 hours. By this time the cell mass has an inner fluid filled cavity and is known as a **blastocyst**. Even at this early stage differentiation already has begun, with some cells destined to become fetus and others beginning to form the placenta, commonly called the afterbirth, which is responsible after the seventh week of pregnancy for hormonal production and for exchange of nutrients and metabolites between mother and fetus. If, for any reason, the endometrium is not receptive, the early embryo will not implant. Once implantation occurs additional blood vessels develop within the endometrium at the site. As the process continues, some of the blood vessels in the wall of the uterus are entered, and bleeding may occur. This is "good bleeding" as opposed to that which is seen in a threatened miscarriage. Only blood tests and ultrasound examinations can tell the difference. About 20% of all pregnancies will have some early bleeding.

Additionally, women may experience groin pain early in pregnancy, especially with the first pregnancy. This is nothing more than the uterine ligaments beginning to stretch, and the pain is actually a good sign because it signifies uterine growth.

Attempting Pregnancy

How can you improve your chances for conception? Certainly exposure to sperm around the time of ovulation is a key factor. Since healthy sperm can survive in the fallopian tube for two days or more, intercourse at 36 to 48 hour intervals around the time of ovulation is usually sufficient to ensure an adequate number of sperm in the tube.

Aside from the basal body temperature (BBT) method, is there any way for a woman to tell when she is ovulating? Many women experience lower abdominal pain just before or just after ovulation. The popular term for this is **mittelschmerz,** which translated from the German literally means "middle pain". It may last from 12 to 36 hours. Some women can accurately predict ovulation because of changes which they notice in the vaginal secretions which actually reflect changes in cervical mucus quantity and quality. The urinary LH kits have been a real boon to ovulation timing. Ovulation will occur on the day following the first positive change in the kit. Intercourse on the evening of that day with a positive reading or the next morning will make it possible to have sperm in the fallopian tube as the egg enters. Even this hormonal shift does not prove positively that ovulation has taken place in the full physical sense of the word. The only actual proof of ovulation is pregnancy itself. For instance, the hormonal shift may occur, but the egg may never be physically extruded from the ovary. This phenomenon, called "intrafollicular ovulation" or "luteinized unruptured follicle syndrome", is seen most often in infertile women, but may occur from time to time in the normal population. The diagnosis must be made with serial ultrasonic examinations just before and after the presumed ovulation. Therefore, the logistical difficulty and the expense of the examinations preclude using this technique unless the index of suspicion is high.

Nicotine and Alcohol

Smoking has little effect on sperm production in the otherwise healthy male with a normal sperm count. But studies have shown that for those with marginal sperm production, smoking becomes an additional negative factor. The situation in the female is more clear. Women smokers are more likely to be infertile than their nonsmoking counterparts. Data from IVF programs show conclusively that the pregnancy rate in smokers is less than that for nonsmokers. Moreover, smokers have smaller babies than nonsmokers as a consequence, most likely, of reduced placental blood flow caused by spasm of the small blood vessels secondary to the nicotine effect. Women who continue to smoke have earlier menopause and lower estrogen levels while on hormonal replacement because the nicotine induces increased enzyme activity in the liver which breaks down the estrogen. Therefore, we can conclude that no part of the female reproductive system escapes the negative action of nicotine. Alcohol is another matter. While drinking during pregnancy is strongly discouraged because of the risk of the fetal alcohol syndrome, moderate social use of alcohol probably plays little role in aggravating infertility in either sex.

Body Build

As is the case with most other things in life, moderation is beneficial. Women who fall below a certain minimal weight for their height and who have reduced fat content frequently have an associated dysfunction in the hypothalamus which leads to anovulation or even amenorrhea (the complete absence of menstrual function). Some of these women fall into the category of "anorexia nervosa" which is a severe psychological disorder. Far more common, however, is a relationship of obesity to infertility. Massive obesity in the male may present as a problem in the mechanics of delivering sperm into the vagina. Artificial insemination may bypass the problem, although weight reduction is certainly a better first option. In cases where sperm production is marginal, the added heat in the scrotal area coupled with impairment of heat transfer may cause problems. It is not uncommon for rather large football linemen to be infertile during the season since they also wear plastic protectors and use hot whirlpools to a great extent, with the net result of exposing the testes to a great deal of additional heat. Fortunately, this effect tends to be transient, and wears off within a few months after the season ends.

Obesity in the female is more commonly associated with ovulatory disturbance than is an overly slender build. Studies have shown that as little as a 10 -15% loss of weight is helpful in restoring normal ovulation even though the individual remains rather corpulent. Ovulation induction in these patients initially may be unsuccessful even with large doses of medication, but they may become responsive following weight loss. The number of people who do well as defined by maintaining weight loss without some help is small. Over the years I have found that peer group programs such as Weight Watchers provide the best chance for sustained effect. Crash diets and supplements which fill the stomach have only a transient effect because eating habits and patterns have really not been altered.

Coital Position

Coital position usually is not a factor with respect to fertility except in couples with physical handicaps or in the case of extremely low seminal volume. The advice to lie in bed for 30 minutes following intercourse is worthless. It is perfectly normal for semen to leak out of the vagina following intercourse, and failure to do so raises the suspicion that seminal volume is low, or that there is retrograde ejaculation.

Ovarian Function

Contrary to popular belief, the ovaries do not necessarily alternate function; that is, ovulation occurs as a random event from side to side. There are women who seem to favor one side over the other, but only ultrasonic studies can document this. Of interest is the fact that when mittelschmerz occurs on one side, the ultrasound not infrequently documents ovulation on the other side. Women who have one ovary which functions normally will ovulate monthly. Rarely, a woman has lost an ovary on one side and a fallopian tube on the other. Conception can occur by a process known as **transmigration,** as shown in figure 4.1. The egg can be carried in the peritoneal fluid from one side to the other. At best, this is an inefficient method of transporting eggs, and frequently these patients will need IVF.

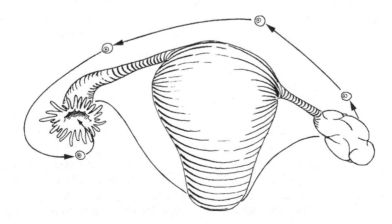

FIGURE 4.1 Illustration showing transmigration of ovum in a patient with one tube and one ovary on opposite sides. The ovum is carried passively by fluid normally present in the body cavity.

TWINNING

Twins can come about in two ways. For non-identical twins, two follicles rather than one ripen during a cycle. This is more likely to happen when ovulation inducing drugs are employed. Also, there is an age related surge in the late 30s and early 40s as a consequence of increased FSH levels. There is a tribe in Africa which has a high percentage of twin births; studies have shown that those women naturally have high FSH levels which cause multiple ovulation within a cycle. Identical twins occur when a single fertilized egg splits into two separate embryos. Identical twins by necessity are always of the same sex while non-identical twins may be either the same or discordant. Sophisticated blood tests can distinguish identical from fraternal twins.

UTERINE SIZE

It's not unusual for me to see a new patient who is apprehensive because her gynecologist told her that she has an "infantile uterus". Having a small uterus is absolutely normal for one who has never been pregnant, and the size of the uterus usually has little or nothing to do with fertility. An exception is the uterus of a patient exposed to DES. A large uterus may contain fibroid tumors **(myomas)** which can distort the cavity and cause infertility, miscarriage and/or premature delivery. A "tipped" uterus usually results from lax uterine ligaments, in which case there is no negative effect on fertility. If, however, a tipped uterus results from a disease process, endometriosis for example, that pathology itself is responsible for the compromised fertility.

Does the Pill Cause Infertility?

Many women are concerned about the long term effects of birth control pills on reproduction. There don't seem to be any negatives except that former pill users may take a few more months to conceive after stopping than women who previously used a diaphragm or condoms and who were presumably ovulating. Recent evidence has shown that birth control pills do not increase the size of fibroid tumors but actually may mildly retard their growth. What is often forgotten is that use of the pill confers substantial protection against development of ovarian cancer even years after the pill has been stopped.

The risk of breast cancer has always been a disturbing topic. Most studies show no link between the pill and breast cancer. There is some evidence that there is a risk when use begins early in life and is sustained over a long interval of time. A career woman who plans to contracept for a long duration may actually protect her fertility potential by use of the pill. By putting her ovaries in a state of metabolic hibernation she reduces her risk of endometriosis. Women were not bio-engineered for incessant ovulation. Only 100 years ago, when contraception was inefficient or nonexistent, women in the reproductive age group rarely experienced long intervals of uninterrupted ovulation; they were usually either breastfeeding or pregnant. Mechanical methods of contraception such as condoms, diaphragms and IUD's cannot afford this additional protective factor.

The pill is given frequently to women with mild ovarian hormonal disorders in order to regulate menstrual cyclicity or to induce periods for those who are amenorrheic. The appearance of regular menses while on the pill masks the underlying problem, but when the medication is stopped patients usually revert to the pre-pill pattern. So when I take a history of someone who complains about irregular periods after stopping the pill, they usually admit to irregular periods before using it. Women do not become more fertile than normal after pill use; there is, in fact, no "rebound" effect. However, if pregnancy occurs in the first cycle after discontinuation, there is a slight increase in the chance for twinning due to a pituitary "overshoot" of gonadotropins as the suppressive effects of the contraceptive pill are removed. These are, of course, fraternal twins. Use of the pill does not increase the risk for spontaneous abortion. It should not be taken during actual pregnancy because of the risk of causing fetal abnormalities.

Orgasm and Fertility

Female orgasm has no known effect on fertility. But if sexual intercourse brings little or no pleasure to either partner, or physical pain, the frequency of coitus falls off and so do the chances of getting pregnant. Women who view intercourse as a threatening event may be prone to tubal spasm which may interfere with sperm passage. This remains an unproved theory. When sexual dysfunction is psychological, a sexual counselor can be quite helpful. Sometimes artificial insemination must be used.

The Adoption Myth

There is a popular fallacy that adoption "relaxes" women who have trouble conceiving, and restores fertility. We all know of couples who adopted after a long duration of infertility who then conceived. For every five couples with that happy scenario there are 95 who remain infertile following adoption. After the first year without pregnancy, close to 10% will conceive in the next year or two, but the rate drops off to approximately two percent yearly for the next three years. Adoption certainly does not improve the status of diseased tubes or the effects of endometriosis. Statistically valid studies show that couples who adopt have no increase in fertility over those couples who do not adopt.

In this chapter we have just scratched the surface of some of the folklore connected with fertility. I have avoided some of the more far out anecdotes such as having intercourse with your boots on as an aid to having a male baby. These first four chapters are meant to give you a background in the terminology and a sphere of knowledge concerning the physiology of reproduction. We will now consider the actual fertility investigation upon which treatment is based.

5

The Fertility Investigation:
Who, What, Where and When

Ultimately you must decide when to initiate a consultation dealing with fertility. Moreover, you should not be rigidly locked into definitions. Instead, consider the ages of both partners, particularly the woman, the duration of time over which you have been trying to conceive, your degree of anxiety about all of this, and whether or not there is anything in your medical history which might be a factor in preventing or impairing conception. In the next few pages you'll learn what will happen during the first visit, which diagnostic tests might be performed and what the doctor hopes to learn from the results.

Seeking Treatment

Unfortunately, the place where you live may become a factor in the type of treatment you receive. If you are located near an urban center, you probably will have access to a number of specialists and facilities where the latest techniques may be applied. On the other hand, if you live in a rural area high tech treatment is harder to find. Some couples may travel a hundred miles or more for each of the office visits required in a step-by-step work-up. Today, more than ever, your health insurance may be a major factor in determining your selection of physicians and even the choice of therapies. Not all physicians are members of every insurance plan. The Health Maintenance Organization (HMO) plans in particular may be quite restrictive in the list of participating specialists. Additionally, certain diagnostic tests and therapies may not be included under your specific policy depending upon which program and riders your employer has chosen. Therefore, the physician may be faced with a dilemma of choosing between a covered therapy unlikely to succeed versus what is a more obvious first choice, but one which will entail a significant out-of-pocket cost.

The Experts

Who are the fertility docs? The obstetrician-gynecologist is usually the first to be consulted in matters of fertility. The practice of obstetrics carries with it inherent problems in office scheduling and does not mix well with the more orderly practice of fertility. This is not to say that an interested obstetrician cannot function in this area; however, most "fertility doctors" have eliminated obstetrics from their practice.

The American Board of Obstetrics & Gynecology has organized a Division of Reproductive Endocrinology and Infertility with its own approved training programs and examinations leading to certification. Many experts in the field have practiced fertility therapy for years and may not be formally certified, so lack of certification is not necessarily a sign of lack of expertise. A number of medical specialties focus on increasingly narrowing areas of fertility. For example, some urologists have become specialized in **andrology**, the study of sperm production and transport. Some internists specialize in endocrinology and focus on the role hormones play in reproduction, but they eventually have to refer couples to other physicians when diagnostic or therapeutic surgical procedures are necessary.

As with anything else in life, there can be too much of a good thing. The involvement of many specialists in the therapy of infertility is sometimes seen in large centers, but fragmentation of care is expensive, frequently emotionally frustrating and unsatisfactory to the patient. In most cases, a competent fertility specialist is able to oversee and conduct the diagnostic as well as the therapeutic aspects of care with limited referrals to other sites or physicians. Large fertility clinics can offer up-to-date services and techniques. This may translate to ancillary personnel such as sex therapists, psychologists, and specially trained nurse practitioners to deal with the "total problem" of infertility, which may include significant emotional distress. Sometimes the fertility expert will sense your anxiety and make a strong recommendation that you see a psychological counselor. By all means follow that suggestion since you'll find it enormously helpful. One of the drawbacks of a large clinic is that there may be lots of paperwork. Additionnally, intraoffice memos don't always wind up in the right place. In a university clinic there are young physicians in training who will participate in your care at various levels, although always (it is hoped) under supervision.

How do you go about getting help? The American Society for Reproductive Medicine (1209 Montgomery Hwy., Birmingham, Al, 35216-2809) can provide information and a list of physicians in your area who have indicated interest in this field. The ASRM WebSite (www.asrm.com) is particularly helpful as an informational source. RESOLVE, (RESOLVE, Inc., 1310 Somerville, Ma 02144-1731) is a lay group with many local chapters throughout the United States. This is both an educational and support organization. Local chapters are made up of critical consumers who can serve as a good referral source for physicians deemed competent to manage matters of fertility. RESOLVE also publishes national and local newsletters and has regularly scheduled meetings for its members. Family doctors and obstetrician/gynecologists are a good source for referrals. An increasing number of medical practices have WebSites—some good, and others not so good. Remember that these kiosks are non-regulated and that the content is not subject to any peer review process.

The Initial Interview

The initial consultation allows the health professional to assess the medical history of both partners with special emphasis on factors that might bear on the problem. If the consultant is a gynecologist, the female partner will usually have a complete physical examination, not just a pelvic evaluation. The male partner may also be examined. Physical findings that pertain to fertility status may be uncovered at this time. Simultaneously, the couple can essentially audition the doctor to see if he or she is someone with whom they feel comfortable and one who is willing to spend the time necessary to answer questions and to educate the couple. Printed material and in-office videos are of great value but do not replace a face-to-face session. Bring with you or have sent any previous medical records which might be helpful; I prefer to see actual pictures or x-ray films rather than printed reports which are always somewhat subjective.

Many fertility centers adhere to a fixed plan or work-up, a regimen procedure designed to touch all bases in a systematic approach. This certainly fits well into computer programs, and allows a group of physicians to effectively treat a high volume of patients, but this arrangement tends to become rather mechanized and impersonal. I still believe that each case requires its own approach to diagnosis and treatment, and that reliance on a computer program to map out the most appropriate strategy produces a diagnostic and therapy plan which may be inappropriate for that couple. Often just getting a good history will point to the problem. In our practice, we send each couple a questionnaire (figure 5.1) as the appointment is made for the initial visit. Each partner can fill out the form at home, not under pressure in an office. It is not unusual for us to get two different answers to the same question, particularly in the area of sexual function. At the time of the first visit we insist that both partners are interviewed together. In that way we get to know each couple and the general features of their case as well as how they interact when the problem is faced. We discourage the attitude that "it's her problem" or "he's the infertile one"; fertility is truly a partnership arrangement. The medical history is reviewed in depth and any medical records that are missing and which might be helpful are identified and a request made for copies. A basic plan of investigation is formulated with the tests being done over a relatively short period of time dependent upon the age of the female, the duration of infertility, previous therapies, and the degree of anxiety. It is important for the couple and physician to be on the same wave length so far as how vigorously diagnosis and therapy should be pursued. If, however, diagnosis has already been made elsewhere, and multiple factors have been excluded, it is unnecessary to start all over again. Once the diagnosis has been verified, all that remains is to discuss the various treatment options.

Evaluation of Male Fertility

The fertility investigation of the male hinges largely upon a single test—the semen analysis. The series of tests performed on the specimen tells most of what is needed to be known about sperm production and delivery.

FIGURE 5.1 Fertility history questionnaires that we use to obtain detailed information on each couple seeking treatment.

Fertility Questionnaire For Women

Date _____

Name _____

Address _____

Birth date _____

Husband's name _____

Telephone number at home _____ At work _____

Other name and number to be called in emergency _____

Insurance Information

Insurance company _____ Identifying numbers _____

Referring physician and address _____

Age at first menses _____ Date of last menses (first day) _____

Usual menstrual interval _____ Usual duration of bleeding _____

Cramps (please circle) Yes   No   Minimal   Moderate   Severe

Do cramps start before or after bleeding? _____

Are cramps always present?   Yes   No

Background Information

Please underline or circle all responses that apply and fill in blanks.

Chronic headaches, history of head trauma, seizure disorder, problems with sense of smell, visual disturbances, dizziness, loss of balance.

Rapid or marked changes in weight, increased thirst, changes in appetite, increased sweating, chronically warm or cold, history of painful swallowing, change of voice or hoarseness, insomnia, fatigue, tremors, craving for salt, loss of scalp hair, growth of hair on face or body in new places or in excess, change in size of clitoris, diagnosis of thyroid disease, diabetes, history of breast secretions or milky discharge from nipples.

History of acquired or congenital heart disease, scarlet fever, rheumatic fever, diagnosis or treatment of high blood pressure.

History of pulmonary (lung) disease such as tuberculosis, pneumonia, chronic bronchitis, emphysema, lung cysts or tumors.

History of gall bladder problems, hiatal hernia, ulcer, appendicitis, colitis, regional enteritis, pancreatitis, jaundice, hepatitis, liver problems.

History of anemia, need for transfusion, arthritis, kidney infections, nephritis, Bright's disease, urinary tract abnormalities, frequent urination, auto-immune diseases.

History of any other serious or chronic illness (describe) _____

Duration of marriage? _____ Duration of infertility? _____

Either partner previously married?   Yes   No

Children from prior marriage?   Yes   No

How long to conceive? _____ (male) _____ (female)

Outcome of pregnancies:

Delivery, miscarriage, abortion   Delivery, miscarriage, abortion

Year _____   Year _____

Complications: Yes No   Complications: Yes No

Fever: Yes No   Fever: Yes No

Previous methods of contraception: Pill Condoms Foam Diaphragm IUD Withdrawal Rhythm None

If pill, were menses regular before? Yes No

If pill, were menses regular after? Yes No

How long to resume menses when pills stopped? _____ weeks

If IUD, was device removed to conceive? for complications? (describe)

_____ other? (describe) _____

Usual frequency of sexual intercourse per week _____

Lubricants used: Yes No Specify _____

Does husband ejaculate during intercourse? Yes No

Does ejaculation occur outside vagina? Yes No

Does his semen leak out when you stand? Yes No

Do you douche before or after? Yes No

Is intercourse (coitus) painful to either partner? Yes No

Do you achieve orgasms? Never Rarely Usually Always

Has artificial insemination ever been suggested? Yes No Husband or Donor

History of Syphilis Gonorrhea Pelvic infection? Yes No

Do you work? Yes No

Type of work _____

Exposure to chemicals or x-ray in work or in hobbies?   Yes   No

Smoking habits: Yes   No   Pack/day

Alcohol: Yes   No   Drinks weekly

History of use of marijuana, opium or other addictive drugs: Yes   No

Medications used now or recently _____

Allergies _____

History of therapeutic x-ray treatment (not for diagnosis) or anti-cancer drugs or drugs for arthritis: Yes   No

Family History: Father   Alive   Dead   Cause _____   Age ___

Mother   Alive   Dead   Cause _____   Age ___

Sister(s)   Age(s) _____   Brother(s)   Age(s) _____

History of family infertility caused by endocrine (hormonal) disorder?   Yes   No

Previous hospital admission (any reason) Medical/Surgical

Where _____   When _____   Reason _____

1. _____

2. _____

3. _____

History of psychiatric treatment: Yes   No

Name of Doctor _____

Previous Infertility Studies

Drug treatment: Yes   No   Hospital Admission: Yes   No

Temperature charts?   Yes   No   Normal: Yes   No

Husband had semen analysis: Yes   No   Year ___   Normal: Yes   No

Post-coital test for sperm survival in cervix: Yes   No   Normal: Yes   No

X-ray of tubes and uterus: Yes No   Year _____ Normal: Yes No
Laparoscopy (telescope in abdomen): Yes No   Year _____ Normal: Yes No
D & C to examine uterine lining: Yes No   Year _____ Normal: Yes No
Hysteroscopy (telescope in uterus): Yes No   Year _____ Normal: Yes No
Immunologic testing for sperm allergy: Yes No   Normal: Yes No
Hormonal tests: Yes No   Results, if known _____
Chromosomal (genetic) studies   Tay-Sachs screening
Sickle cell screening   Thyroid tests
Skin test for tuberculosis   Year _____ Skull x-ray   Year _____
Diabetes test   Others _____

Previous Infertility Treatment

Any procedure on cervix such as biopsy, cauterization, cryosurgery (freezing): Yes No

Any procedure on uterus, vagina, tubes, ovaries, or operations for inflammatory or infectious pelvic diseases, operations for adhesions or endometriosis: Yes No

Stimulation of ovulation with oral or injectable agents such as estrogens, Clomid HCG, Humegon, Pergonal, others: Yes No

Treatment of endometriosis with drugs: Yes No

Treatment of tubes with medication via uterus: Yes No

Artificial insemination: Husband Donor Yes No

Use of fertility-promoting douches: Yes No

Fertility Questionnaire For Men

Date _____
Name _____
Address _____
_____

Height _____ Weight now _____ Greatest weight _____
Hair color _____ Eye color _____
Ethnic extraction _____
Birthdate _____
Telephone number at home _____ At work _____

Background Information

Please underline or circle all responses that apply and fill in blanks.

Rapid or marked changes in weight, increased thirst, changes in appetite, increased sweating, chronically warm or cold, painful swallowing, change of voice or hoarseness, insomnia, fatigue, tremors, salt craving, loss of hair other than on scalp, decreased beard growth, history of thyroid disease, diabetes, increase in breast size or sore nipples.

History of acquired or congenital heart disease, scarlet fever, rheumatic fever, diagnosis or treatment of high blood pressure.

History of pulmonary (lung) disease such as cystic fibrosis, tuberculosis, pneumonia, chronic bronchitis, emphysema, lung cysts or tumors.

History of liver or gall bladder disease, cirrhosis, jaundice, pancreatitis.

History of arthritis, auto-immune diseases, kidney infections or stones, gout, urinary tract abnormalities, other serious or chronic diseases.

Do you ever suspect that you have fathered a child outside this marriage?   Yes   No

How long ago? _____

Have you ever had reason to doubt your fertility outside this marriage?   Yes   No

Are you circumcised?   Yes   No

If no, does foreskin retract easily?   Yes   No

Have you ever been treated for gonorrhea, syphilis, prostatitis, or infection of testicles and/or seminal vesicles?   Yes   No

Has there been a recent change in libido or sexual drive?   Yes   No

Do you have difficulty in maintaining erection?   Yes   No

Do you ejaculate in vagina without difficulty?   Yes   No

Is urination or ejaculation painful?   Yes   No

Usual sexual frequency weekly (all outlets) _____

Has a doctor ever told you that you were infertile?   Yes   No

Has a semen analysis ever been performed?   Yes   No

When? _____ Where? _____ Results? _____

Has artificial insemination ever been suggested to achieve pregnancy with your sperm?   Yes   No   Yes   No

With donor sperm?   Yes   No   Yes   No

Any history of hernia repair at any age including shortly after birth?   Yes   No   When? _____

History of mumps?   Yes   No   Age _____

Any history of undescended testes?   Yes   No

Final outcome, if yes _____

History of injury to testes?   Yes   No

History or diagnosis of varicocele (varicose veins in scrotum)?   Yes   No

Treated _____

History of treatment in past to promote fertility?   Yes   No

Specify _____

History of genitourinary surgery?   Yes   No

Present means of employment _____

How long has this type of work been performed? _____ Years

Have you ever been employed in occupation with sustained high temperatures?   Yes   No

Have you ever been a professional driver, or do you drive long distances
as part of your employment?   Yes   No

Type of underwear worn: Boxer Shorts   Jockeys

Tobacco: Cigars   Cigarettes   Pipe   Amounts Daily _____

Alcohol - Drinks weekly_____

Drugs

History of use of marijuana, opium or other addictive drugs: Yes   No

Medication used now or recently _____

Allergies _____

History of therapeutic x-ray treatment (not for diagnosis) or anti-cancer drugs
or drugs for arthritis?   Yes   No

Family History: Father   Alive   Dead   Cause

                                      Mother   Alive   Dead   Cause

                                      Sister(s)   Age(s) _____

                       Brother(s)   Age(s) _____

Any history of family infertility or endocrine disease?   Yes   No

Specimen Collection

The semen specimen may be collected during an office visit or at home and delivered to the laboratory. In many cases, the health insurance contract dictates where the analysis is performed. In HMO situations this is often a capitated laboratory chosen as the lowest bidder. For the most part these laboratories live up to the standards set for the industry, but we have encountered some sites which consistently turn out reports which have little resemblance to reality. Most fertility practices choose to perform the analysis in their own laboratory which has close supervision and quality control, but as mentioned above, this is not always possible.

The patient masturbates into a sterile wide-mouth jar. The first few drops of semen usually contain the most vigorous sperm, and a wide-mouth jar helps prevent loss. Ideally, the specimen should be collected 2 to 4 days after the last ejaculation. If the specimen is taken sooner, the sperm count may not yet have been fully replenished. Waiting for longer than seven days will not increase the count, but may cause a decrease in sperm motility. If ejaculation can not occur within an office or laboratory setting, nothing is lost by producing the specimen at home, provided that it is delivered within two hours, and with the jar kept next to the body so that low temperature will not cause the sperm to lose motility. Most offices and laboratories have visual aids to provide stimulation for semen collection.

There are a few men who cannot produce a specimen by masturbation under any circumstances. Interrupting coitus in order to collect a specimen is not a particularly good method because semen leaks out before the first throbs of orgasm are recognized. Ordinary rubber condoms are unsatisfactory for collection because rubber adversely affects sperm motility. There are special plastic condoms made for specimen collection during intercourse which can be obtained readily from the physician or pharmacy. Although some religions forbid masturbation or the use of condoms, we have found that most members of the clergy accept this practice when it involves fertility enhancement.

After collection, the semen is tested in a laboratory to determine reproductive status. Before describing the tests, however, it is worth stressing that the analysis should be performed by technicians with experience and expertise in this area. A person who performs a semen analysis a few times monthly usually will not get consistently accurate results. Portions of the semen analysis can be performed with automated devices, which, generally speaking, give reliable and consistent results for sperm count and motility, but are less desirable for evaluation of sperm structure (morphology) than the human eye.

Semen Volume and pH

The first step in the analysis is to measure the volume of semen in the ejaculate. Each ejaculation normally contains between 2 and 5 mL, about a teaspoonful, of semen, depending on the duration of time from the last ejaculation. Less than 1 mL may be associated with infertility because few sperm will be able to reach the cervix since there is little fluid in which to swim, even if sperm **concentration** is normal. An analogy might be a small puddle of fluid (semen) in a large empty reservoir (the vagina). Under these conditions any swimming organisms would be restricted to an exceedingly small area. For reasons which remain unclear, semen volumes in excess of 7 mL are associated with some degree of sub-fertility regardless of the sperm count. Low semen volume may be the result of retrograde ejaculation, which can have many causes. Diabetes, for example, can damage the nerves controlling the bladder sphincter. This muscle normally blocks the entrance to the bladder during ejaculation, but failure results in semen passing into the bladder rather than out through the urethra. Certain medications that affect the nervous system, and particularly those used in treatment of high blood pressure may also cause retrograde ejaculation, or no ejaculation. Quite commonly the problem is encountered following urologic surgery, and cannot always be avoided, especially when the bladder and/or prostate gland are involved.

The pH of the semen should be measured. The normal pH is about 7.5 to 8.5, in the alkaline range. This counterbalances the normal acidity of the vagina, and helps to protect the sperm, which are acid sensitive, until they reach the safe harbor of the cervical mucus.

COUNTING THE SPERM

Sperm counts are performed by placing a portion of the specimen in a glass counting chamber and then using a microscope in the same way as performing a blood count. If the technician is skillful, repeated counts of the same specimen will not vary by more than 15%. But a repeat analysis on another occasion can normally be expected to show a variation of 40% or more, with greatest differences being noted in men with low counts. Therefore, several analyses may be necessary in order to determine the expected range in an individual. The automated devices use a recorder, a video camera attached to the microscope and a computer program. In most cases they are as accurate as the human observer except at the extremes of sperm concentration.

How many sperm does the man need to be normally fertile? Many specialists consider 20 million per mL as the acceptable lower threshold of normal fertility. But many normally fertile men have concentrations below this arbitrary figure. There's no argument that counts <10 million per mL are usually associated with significant subfertility. Although men are concerned about their sperm count, the truth is that a concentration of 90 million sperm has no greater fertility potential than a specimen of 20 million. The term used to describe specimens with concentrations < 20 million per mL is **oligospermia.** Forty years ago 60 million sperm per mL was considered the lower limits of normal. Twenty years ago, experts adjusted that figure down to 40 million, and we now accept 20 million. Since the methods of counting haven't changed until recently, why the lower sperm counts? One contributing factor may be the environmental stresses under which people live. In animal colonies, conditions of crowding and stress reduce sperm counts and overall fertility of the population, perhaps as a self-regulating defense mechanism. There is a seasonal variation in sperm concentration with a decrease in the summer months, but usually only to a minor extent.

A second factor may be the various poisons that are part of our contemporary life-style. A few years ago a report got media attention when the results showed that over the last few decades semen counts in the general population have declined. A number of good laboratories attempted to verify this finding. The results were mixed which can easily be explained by geographic differences in diet, use of drugs or pharmacologic agents, or exposure to some particular mix of toxins in the air or the water not present in all locales. A disturbing finding was that the laboratories which found a significant reduction in sperm count over a 40 year period also reported an increase in the incidence of testicular carcinoma, suggesting exposure to a common factor such as a known heavy metal toxin (arsenic, cadmium, mercury) and/or an organic compound such as dioxin and other similar defoliants. The database on industrial pollutants and their effects on us is expanding rapidly, and there's no reason to believe that sperm production should be immune from damage. Most of the efforts in this area have centered on the risk of cancer rather than the effects on fertility. We remember when aniline dye exposure was confirmed as a work-related hazard to formation of bladder cancer, followed by the association found to exist between asbestos exposure and a unique form of lung cancer.

Heavy alcohol consumption can dampen sex drive, and, by affecting the liver, can alter testosterone metabolism leading to seminal problems. There is almost universal agreement that smoking for the female constitutes a negative fertility factor, but the story is less clear for the male. Recent evidence has shown that male smokers have a higher percentage of broken strands of DNA, the genetic carrier which programs our cells, in their sperm compared with nonsmokers. Additionally data are beginning to accumulate which suggest that within IVF programs male smokers have lower pregnancy rates than their nonsmoking counterparts even when the results are corrected for smoking behavior in the female. No threshold number of cigarettes daily has been established as being completely without adverse effect. In actual practice, men who have normal sperm production will probably have few clinically detectable changes associated with smoking, but for men with impaired sperm production and/or function, smoking may aggravate the problem. Survey data show that there is a higher proportion of smokers in an infertile population than in a fertile control group. This does not necessarily document a cause and effect relationship but an association only, meaning that smokers may have some additional life-style exposure which is the actual toxic agent. Use of marijuana is associated with a reduction of testosterone production leading to diminished sex drive, sperm motility decline, and with heavy use, a drop in sperm production.

As a summary comment, the sperm concentration, unless it is down in the 10 million range or less, is the least important factor in a semen analysis, with count having little or no correlation with pregnancy rates for concentrations more than 20 million per mL. The semen analysis has as its greatest value the ability to identify the patient who has few or no sperm in the ejaculate, since in most cases there is no clue that this may be the case.

Sperm Motility

If sperm count is the least important component of the analysis, **motility** is the most. This term is a measure of the inherent ability of sperm to swim in seminal fluid and the female reproductive tract. What matters most is the total percentage of moving sperm rather than the total number of sperm. Specimens in which 40% of the sperm are active fall within normal limits. Below that threshold there is a drop-off of fertility regardless of count. This does not take into account either the vigor of the motility or the interval of time that it is sustained (see below). When the analysis is performed by a technician an estimate is made of the percentage of sperm swimming ,and on a 4-point scale the grade of motion is estimated, with an overall score of three or more as normal. Sperm are also graded on **progression** which is the ability to swim in a purposeful fashion. Sperm that swim in erratic circles do not contribute to fertility. Those sperm which do not move may not be dead, but immotile. In some cases reasonably normal motility can be observed for an hour or two after ejaculation with a dramatic decline over the next few hours. Therefore, in order to have a more accurate assessment, motility should be evaluated over a six hour interval as part of the initial screening analysis. At normal room temperatures, there should be no more than a 25% reduction of motility in six hours compared with the initial estimation. Remember that sperm need to survive in the female reproductive tracts for one to three days. Therefore, the common practice in commercial laboratories of examining the semen as soon as possible after collection and then discarding the specimen does not give the type of information which is needed.

Computer assisted semen analysis (CASA) has added a great deal to our knowledge base on sperm motion. An individual sperm can be isolated in the video frame and its motion followed and analyzed. The human eye cannot do this. Moreover, our eyes are drawn to that which moves; therefore compared with the computer, technicians usually over-estimate motility. Freshly ejaculated sperm have a tail (flagellum) beat of 7 or 8 times per second. In slow motion we see that normal sperm move in a particular wave form with the head held at a certain angle to the sperm body. The computer can measure the velocity of the sperm in a straight line and also measure what is called the curvilinear velocity and compare the ratio of the two. Over a 5 to 6 hour period after ejaculation sperm undergo a maturation process known as **capacitation** culminating in the **acrosome reaction** which exposes the enzyme system on the sperm head, giving sperm fertilization capability. During this interval of time the sperm dramatically change their motion characteristics. They become **hyperactivated,** with changes in tail beat frequency and amplitude, an increased angle between the head and body, increased velocity and curvilinear velocity, and changes in the wave form of motion. The computer can measure all of this but the human eye cannot. Failure to undergo these changes is correlated with an infertile specimen regardless of sperm count.

Morphology and Viability

Morphology refers to the appearance of the sperm. Figure 5.2 illustrates both normal and some common abnormal sperm forms. Among the parameters assessed are the ratio between the head and the body, comparison of the sperm head length to width, the appearance of the neck piece and characteristics of the tail. Two languages are spoken here. The World Health Organization (WHO) criteria are the standard and most widely used. When examined carefully, at least 40% of the sperm should have normal appearance. A newer system known as the Kruger score utilizes a much more rigid set of criteria with the result that anything over 14% is considered to be acceptable. The potential for confusion mounts when an individual has had semen analyses performed in different laboratories and results are compared. Therefore, it is important for the physician to know which system a particular laboratory employs. The computer programs are becoming more sophisticated in analyzing morphology, and are now beginning to be more reliably consistent, and will probably replace the technician, at least in laboratories performing a high volume of semen analyses.

A commonly asked question is whether sperm morphology has anything to do with birth defects in the offspring. This would be the case if it were true that abnormally shaped sperm more commonly had defects in the chromosomes and/or DNA content at the gene level. A few investigators have addressed this question, but the issue is far from settled.

Viability refers to the percentage of sperm in a specimen that are actually alive. Nonmotile but live sperm cannot be distinguished from dead sperm except with a special stain. Normally, at least 60% of the sperm should be live.

Viscosity, Clumping and Agglutination

Semen is normally quite viscous (thick) shortly after ejaculation, and may remain so for up to 30 minutes. It is believed that this viscosity enhances the ability of the sperm to remain in contact with the cervix by forming a "plug" at the cervical opening. The enzymes in the semen then thin this out until it becomes more liquid. Failure to liquefy may interfere with sperm migration through the cervix. If, under microscopic inspection, sperm seem to stick together in clumps, one becomes suspicious of a chronic infection in the male genito-urinary tract with the prostate gland usually involved. This is especially true if white blood cells are also seen microscopically. Usually the motility of the sperm is reduced under these circumstances, but long-term treatment with antibiotics may help. Somewhat different from clumping is **agglutination,** in which the sperm adhere to one another in a head-to-head or tail-to-tail fashion. This finding suggests that the immune system has perceived the sperm as being foreign and is producing antibodies against them.

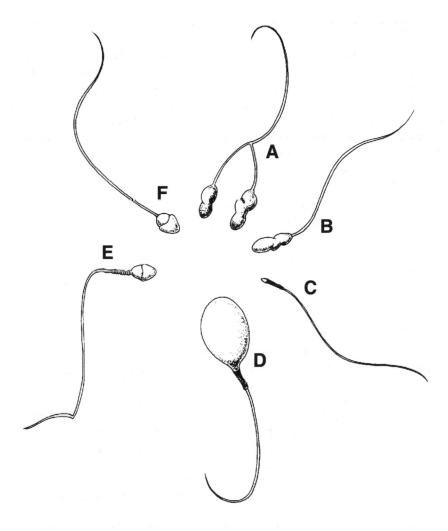

FIGURE 5.2   Various abnormal sperm forms commonly seen, including
(A) Double-headed variety, (B) Abnormal neck, (C) Microsperm,
(D) Macrosperm, (E) Tail abnormality, (F) Normal.

Fructose Test

Complete absence of sperm in the ejaculate may be caused either by failure of the testes to produce sperm or by a blockage in the ductal system which interferes with delivery. The fact that the epididymis produces a simple sugar, fructose, provides an easy and convenient method of differentiation between the two. If fructose is absent from the specimen the conclusion can safely be made that there is a blockage in the ductal system, but nothing can be inferred about production.

Medical History

If the semen picture is less than satisfactory the medical history may shed some light on the cause, although in about half the cases there seems to be no obvious answer.

Mumps. Mumps, in the male, can cause severe testicular pain, and if contracted after puberty may lead to permanent sterility.

Testicular torsion. No one who has ever had testicular torsion forgets it. This is an acutely painful condition as a consequence of the testicle twisting on the vas, blocking the flow of blood to and from the testicle. It is not common but can be promptly corrected by surgery, if the diagnosis is made early. If not, the testicle probably is permanently damaged.

Undescended Testis. Many infants have testes undescended into the scrotal sac at birth which then become normally placed within a week or two without any intervention. The temperature within the abdomen is significantly higher than within the scrotal sac, and therefore, even if the condition is surgically corrected in early childhood, the testis may not function normally when adult status is reached. Additionally, there is evidence that at least in some cases, the testis has not descended because it was abnormal to begin with.

Epididymitis. Infection of the epididymis, if not promptly treated with antibiotics can result in scar tissue buildup causing blockage.

Hernia Operations. Correction of inguinal hernia puts the vas at risk. It may be cut or clamped during the operation, particularly when the hernia is repaired during childhood before the vas is fully mature.

Prostatitis. The prostate gland may be infected with the result that sperm motility rather than production is decreased. This is usually reversible, but long-term antibiotic treatment may be necessary and recurrence is common.

Vasectomy Reversal. Reversal of sterilization may be successful with appearance of sperm in the ejaculate, but in about half of the cases sperm antibodies will have formed. These antibodies may impair sperm motility as well as ability to bind to the outer membrane of the egg and subsequent penetration. Insemination techniques may be of help, with IVF reserved as the ultimate solution.

Radiation and Chemotherapy. Treatments of malignant disease may be live-sparing, but may produce permanent sterility. Modifying factors include the age at which treatment occurred, the total dose, and type of agent used. Sperm production may be adversely affected for a period of years with subsequent recovery. Today, sperm banking prior to these treatments is being used with increased frequency in order to safeguard future fertility potential. In many cases the seminal quality is poor because of the systemic nature of the disease process prior to treatment; however, in vitro fertilization techniques, including direct insertion of sperm into the egg, can overcome this issue.

In Utero Exposure. Exposure in utero to drugs such as DES can lead to formation of cysts or blocks in the ductal system and some other anatomic alterations, but whether or not associated changes in sperm production follow exposure is not clear.

Drugs and Medications. As mentioned earlier, marijuana lowers testosterone levels with possible adverse effect on sperm motility more common than sperm production, and with an associated reduction in sex drive. Regular users of cocaine also have a reduction in sexual frequency. Many medications may interfere with sperm production, maturation, motility or delivery. Among these are anti-inflammatory drugs, certain antibiotics, some ulcer medications, and mood altering drugs. It is important that the fertility physician be apprised of any and all medications taken including those sold over-the-counter and at health food stores.

Hormonal Testing in the Male

Reproductive problems in the male caused by hormonal disturbance occur much less frequently than in the female. Decreased testosterone levels may be associated with a change in voice, rate and thickness of beard growth, sex drive, and general feeling of energy and well-being. Sometimes the patient's body build, hair distribution and muscular development suggest that hormonal testing is in order, but routinely, the yield of screening every male patient with seminal problems by using expensive hormonal tests is low. Thyroid disease in the male is much less commonly encountered than in the female. Usually the only hormonal tests needed to evaluate infertility in the male are serum levels of testosterone, FSH and less frequently, prolactin. Excessive prolactin production in the female may cause a milk discharge from the breast as is normally the case during breast feeding, but lactation in the male in the face of high prolactin levels is less commonly seen. Elevation of prolactin in the male reduces FSH and LH release causing both decreased sperm production and testosterone levels.

The Clinical Examination: What to Expect

The male is usually far more anxious than the female about to have a genital organ examination. Maybe this preview will be helpful. Physicians will look and palpate the penis, testicles, epididymis and prostate. We want to rule out conditions such as a varicose vein in the scrotum, scarring from previous epididymal infection, testicular atrophy, and prostatic infection. The examination for varicocele is performed with the patient in the standing position. With straining, as if constipated, any defect of the valves in the scrotal veins will be accentuated and either felt or seen as a distended blood vessel. The flow of blood from the scrotum through the veins should always be in the upward direction. Putting a Doppler flow microphone on the scrotum is even a more accurate method of diagnosing failure of the valvular system of the scrotal veins since it can detect the direction of flow. The clinical importance of this diagnosis will be discussed in the chapter on male infertility treatment. The physician will examine the urethral opening to be sure that it is at the end of the penis and not beneath the shaft.

Various illnesses can lead to atrophy of one or both testes. This degeneration may actually start during fetal life and be present at birth but remains unnoticed until the testes begin maturational development at puberty. Generally speaking sperm production is related to testicular size.

The size of each testis can be estimated or actually measured with volumetric cups. Normally, the right testicle is lower than the left for the simple reason that men walk better that way!

The epididymis is checked for areas of firmness which might indicate scarring from chronic infection. The prostate is felt through the rectum. This part of the examination is uncomfortable but certainly tolerable. A tender gland or one which is described as "spongy" or "boggy" usually indicates the presence of infection.

Evaluation of the Female

The evolution of specialty practice in medicine, particularly in the United States has conferred many benefits of diagnosis and therapy on patients, but the downside is that sometimes seemingly mundane issues may fall between the cracks. Such is the case regarding determination of the immune status and genetic risk factors of the patient about to conceive. As the pediatric programs for mass immunization have become increasingly more efficient, fewer children contract rubella (German measles) and/or rubeola (measles). While the natural disease produces antibodies which can last a lifetime, preventing a re-infection years later, this is not always true with antibodies induced by the vaccines. Therefore, every woman of reproductive age should be screened to see if her antibody titer is sufficiently high enough to protect against an exposure to the virus during pregnancy, since both of these viral illnesses have the potential to induce serious defects in the developing fetus. Essentially the same holds true for varicella (chicken pox). I continue to be amazed at the high percentage of patients who, at the initial interview, have no idea of their immune status, which should have been determined by the family doctor or obstetrician. When we find that a patient is not immune, vaccination is recommended, and the couple is told to contracept for three months to avoid a possible adverse effect of the vaccine on the developing fetus. At the same time it is true that at least for measles and German measles thousands of fetuses in utero have been exposed to vaccines without any apparent ill effect. Experience with the chicken pox vaccine is not as broad.

Women should also be aware of their blood type and Rh status. Women who are Rh negative may be sensitized during pregnancy with an Rh positive fetus, even if the pregnancy fails to progress past eight weeks. The actual effect is noted in the next pregnancy during which the mother produces antibodies directed against fetal blood cells which eventually will cause fetal demise or the necessity of intrauterine transfusion and early delivery. All of this can be prevented by a single injection at the time of delivery or miscarriage provided that the situation is appreciated. Toxoplasmosis is a disease caused by a cat parasite transmitted to the human by inhalation while changing a litter box. Normally, it causes a transient viral-like illness which is self limited, although it can infect the eye and produce chronic problems. During pregnancy, initial exposure and infection can lead to severe fetal central nervous system damage. Therefore, screening the patient for antibodies will tell us if she has been exposed and has already developed antibodies which will protect her in the future; if not, she is told to induce her husband to change the cat litter during her pregnancy.

We have entered the era of what I call "ethno-genetic" medicine. As an example, cystic fibrosis is the disease carried by about 1 in 25 of the Caucasian population. It is not sex linked and is a recessive gene with over 100 known abnormal copies (alleles). Standard screening tests survey about 70 of the most common possibilities and are over 90% accurate. The chances for a union between two carriers is 1/25 x 1/25 or 1/625. Classical genetic mathematics would tell us that from this union children would be born with a ratio of one completely normal: two carriers: one affected, for a clinical rate of about one in 2500 deliveries. The actual rate is somewhat less than that because of genetic screening and counseling done because of a previous delivery with an affected child or a positive family history. Considering the prevalence in the general population, the cost of screening, the extreme morbidity and shortening of life of victims and the cost of their long-term health care, the recommendations are that all Caucasian couples be screened. If the wife is screened and is negative for all of the abnormal alleles, the husband probably need not be screened; but testing him becomes mandatory if she has any abnormal results. Couples of Mediterranean descent are at risk for carrying genes causing thalassemia, which in its milder recessive form is expressed as a minor anemia but is much worse when both genes are abnormal. Patients of African heritage may carry genes for sickle cell anemia; this also can be screened with a simple blood test. Jews of Ashkenazi descent carry an increased risk for Tay Saks disease, Gaucher disease and Canavan type central nervous system spongy degeneration. There are package screening tests available for this triad.

Exactly what genetically carried disease states will be routinely screened prior to pregnancy will be the result of some interplay between government health regulatory agencies, the medical profession, and the health insurers, with the latter looking at this on a more strict cost analysis basis. The natural incidence in the population, either general, or by subgroup, the ease and cost of screening, and the cost of caring for the victims will determine the degree of cooperation that we might expect from that industry. Of course, a family history of genetically carried disease supersedes any discussion of routine testing. Giving the doctor a good family history will aid tremendously in helping to decide if you need any special genetic screening tests.

History and Physical Examination

The medical history which focuses on reproduction may give a hint as to the nature of the problem. Particularly important are details of previous pregnancies, miscarriages and deliveries. Any previous abdominal surgery or treatment for tubal infections has obvious importance. A menstrual history with respect to onset and regularity is also central. Reproductive performance in a previous union or marriage sheds additional light on the individual partner.

The physical examination is not limited to evaluation of the pelvic organs. Distribution of body fat, hair growth and muscle development is important, sometimes giving a clue as to hormonal disturbance. A nipple discharge may indicate elevated levels of prolactin, which can interfere with ovulation. Strenuous physical conditioning can reduce body fat to below the threshold necessary for normal release of FSH/LH with decreased estrogen production leading to first anovulation and then to total amenorrhea. Activities such as long distance running are more commonly associated with this result than aerobic exercise. What information can be obtained from the traditional pelvic examination? First, the vagina will be inspected for evidence of infection. Similarly the cervix will be checked for signs of inflammation and close attention will be paid to the opening to be sure that it is not scarred over or closed, at least in part, since this could interfere with sperm passage. As the examiner feels the tissues and moves the uterus, tubes, and ovaries, he or she can estimate the freedom of motion which might be reduced by scar tissue and/or adhesions following surgery, infection, or the inflammation associated with endometriosis. Is the uterus enlarged? Are the ovaries in their normal place, and are they of normal size and shape? Is the area between the back of the uterus and the rectum tender and nodular suggesting that there might be active endometriosis? These and many other questions go through the mind of the examiner during the physical examination.

Ovulation Detection

BASAL BODY TEMPERATURE CHART

A woman who regularly menstruates with a 25 to 34 day cycle probably ovulates in a normal fashion, but this is an assumption, and we can do better than that. The easiest way to detect whether ovulation has occurred is to use the BBT chart. Among its advantages are that it is non-invasive, painless, and has merely the cost of a thermometer to contend with. The downside is that it can be used only to document that ovulation has occurred but will not predict impending ovulation. Each day upon awakening, before leaving the bed, an oral temperature is taken and recorded as shown in chapter 2. Just before ovulation there may be a dip in the temperature as shown in figure 2.11. This is not a consistent characteristic in every cycle. As you have already read, the slope of the temperature rise is a function of progesterone production and the sensitivity of the body's thermostat to the hormone. If pregnancy does not occur, the corpus luteum ceases to produce progesterone, and the temperature falls back to pre-ovulatory basal levels as menses begins. The accuracy of the BBT chart can be thrown off by any number of things, including any illness which might cause a temperature elevation. Because irregular shift work interferes with biorhythms, some people may not be able to use the BBT.

URINARY LH TEST KITS

The urinary LH test kit is immune to the rhythm disturbance that might fool the BBT. These tests are extremely accurate and have great use in actually predicting ovulation. Timing of coitus may be important for couples who have infrequent sexual relations and in cases where regeneration of the sperm count is slow. Additionally, these kits allow for more accurate scheduling of diagnostic tests such as the postcoital examination, progesterone assays, and endometrial biopsy. Therapeutically, the kit is used to time insemination. Although the instructions enclosed may state that the first morning voided specimen should be used, this actually is not the best way to use these kits. Experimental work which we did years ago showed that the late afternoon or early evening specimen was more accurate in identifying the beginning of the LH surge than testing upon awakening. The first test should be done 3 or 4 days before anticipated ovulation, calculated by subtracting 14 from the usual cycle interval. Thus, a woman who normally has a 33 day cycle should ovulate around cycle day 19, counting the first day of menses as day 1, and she should begin testing on cycle day 15 to allow for normal cycle variation. Some of these kits are more easily read than others, and, in general, patients tell us that the ones with a blue end point are more easily interpreted than those which use a pink color system. The test may stay positive for two or three days signifying elevated LH levels during that interval of time, and in other patients a positive result will turn back to negative in less than 24 hours. Since identification of the initial surge is the issue, the only important thing to note is when the test becomes positive, after which continued sampling is unnecessary. Ovulation will usually occur within 24 hours from the first positive response. Therefore, intercourse on the night of the kit change, or insemination the next morning, will maximize chances of conception.

ULTRASONIC PELVIC EXAMINATION

Almost all fertility practices have in-office ultrasonic capability. The older methods of abdominal scanning, which require a full urinary bladder in order to visualize the pelvic organs have given way to a vaginal probe for pelvic organ inspection (which is independent of bladder status). When the examination is performed in a serial manner, starting just before expected ovulation, confirmation of actual physical ovulation can be made as the enlarging clear follicle suddenly changes its appearance to a smaller, less regularly shaped structure with increased ultrasonic echoes (figure 5.3a and figure 5.3b). While ultrasonic studies are really a necessity when gonadotropins are used for ovulation induction, use of the ultrasound to document ovulation in a normal, unstimulated cycle is neither time nor cost effective.

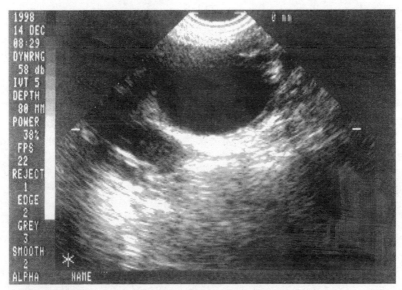

FIGURE 5.3a Ultrasonic appearance of mature ovarian follicle.

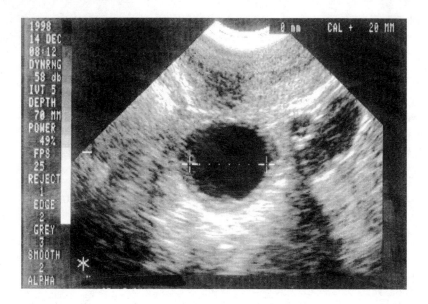

FIGURE 5.3b   Early corpus leuteum, showing on ultrasound increased internal echoes.

EVALUATION OF THE ENDOMETRIUM

The cyclical production of estrogen which increases during the follicular phase, and which then gives way to progesterone release from the ovary causes the uterine lining to change its microscopic appearance according to the hormonal mix which is stimulating it. An **endometrial biopsy** is the time-honored method of evaluating this relationship. It is a minor office procedure in which a small tissue sample is removed, usually with a fine bore suction device. When performed in the luteal phase, ovulation can be inferred, and the specimen can be used to see if its characteristics are normal for that particular stage of the cycle. Therefore, in order to be accurate, the biopsy must be " dated" from the time of ovulation. This is much more precise than using the onset of the last or next menses. Here is another good use for urinary ovulation detection kits. To the trained eye, the microscopic examination can place the lining within a day or two in a normal ovulatory cycle. Suppose we perform this test on the 24th day of the menstrual cycle in which the kit has turned positive on day 13, with ovulation occurring on the next day. That biopsy specimen should read out as a "post ovulation day 10". If, for example, the reading actually is that of a day 6 lining, the biopsy is said to be "out of phase". Another term used to describe this is "luteal phase deficiency". This result can come about because of insufficient hormone production, or the relative inability of the endometrium to respond.

On the surface, this would appear to be a valuable first line test in the infertility assessment. But if we dig a little deeper, we find that in about 30% of cases abnormal biopsies which are repeated in the next month are read as normal in the absence of any treatment. Variables also include the manner in which the biopsy was taken, the skill and consistency of the person reading it, and, of course, if the day of ovulation chosen as the landmark was correct. Moreover, it has been demonstrated that an abnormal biopsy is not an unusual event in perfectly fertile women. Considering all the above, and additionally the cost and discomfort of the test, the trend in recent years has been one of a marked reduction in the frequency with which endometrial biopsy is performed.

The endometrium can also be accessed with the office ultrasound. Both the thickness of the lining and its ultrasonic appearance can be followed in a serial fashion throughout the menstrual cycle. If an abnormality is seen, hormonal blood tests can help to differentiate whether this is basically an ovarian problem or a uterine response issue.

FSH AND LH MEASUREMENTS

The ratio between FSH and LH, along with other hormonal indices, is sometimes used as a diagnostic indicator of **polycystic ovarian syndrome (PCOS)**. When sampling is performed in the first few days of the menstrual cycle, assuming that the patient has a cycle, the LH level should be less than twice the FSH value. Ratios over 2.5:l support the diagnosis of PCOS.

The most important role for FSH determinations is in evaluation of ovarian reserve. With the scientific literature confirming and validating this screening test as one of great value, its use has blossomed in the last few years, and in my opinion it is important enough to demand a separate chapter, which follows this one.

Serum Progesterone Sampling

Because progesterone is produced in quantity by the ovary only after ovulation, and during pregnancy as well, its concentration in the bloodstream can be used as an indicator of ovulation. Since this involves a trip to the office or laboratory, a needle stick, and some cost, progesterone determinations are not used frequently for this purpose. In a cycle in which ovulation occurs, but pregnancy does not, progesterone levels usually peak

7 or 8 days after ovulation (see figure 2.10). In pregnant cycles, the levels continued to rise. Progesterone, like many other hormones, is released in spurts from the ovary, which causes a problem with random sampling. Studies have shown that there's considerable variation on an hourly basis in blood levels. Nevertheless, progesterone estimation in the luteal phase, especially in conjunction with ultrasonic inspection of the endometrium, has some value in assessment of corpus luteum function and endometrial response. The relationships between progesterone levels, endometrial biopsy results, and ultrasonic appearance are not always simple or easily interpreted. Some patients have satisfactory endometrial appearance in the face of rather low progesterone values and vice versa.

Evaluation of the Uterus and Tubes

Hysterosalpingography, HSG for short, refers to examination of the uterus and fallopian tubes with x-ray and a special dye. The test is performed in a radiology department early in the cycle, before ovulation. The timing is first to avoid fetal exposure during unsuspected early pregnancy; and second to reduce the potential of a thick uterine lining later in the cycle causing interference with dye flow and interpretation of the film. A speculum is inserted into the vagina and the cervix is cleansed. A catheter or a rigid device with a soft plastic tip is inserted into the cervix or just inside the lower segment of the uterine cavity. Radioopaque dye is then slowly instilled with a syringe so that the uterine cavity fills and dye enters the tubes with eventual spill into the pelvis. If the person performing the test avoids placing an instrument known as a tenaculum on the cervix, which causes pain and subsequent tubal spasm, the procedure should elicit no more than menstrual-like cramps. We routinely give our patients an agent such as Motrin just prior to the test; this seems to greatly reduce any associated discomfort. The truth is that the degree of patient pain is directly related to the skill and gentleness with which the instruments are placed. It is also important to realize that the dye is at room temperature and may be mildly irritating, so the dye should be passed slowly.

The HSG has some inherent drawbacks and inaccuracies. It is not very accurate in detecting adhesions around the ends of the tubes. If the test causes significant pain and cramping, a diagnosis of tubal obstruction at the junction in the uterus may be made in error. Any suggestion of abnormal results calls for laparoscopic examination of the tubes. Although primarily a test of tubal patency, the HSG gives considerable information about the uterine cavity so far as the possible presence of polyps, myomas, or adhesions is concerned. Hysteroscopy is necessary as a follow-up to further assess any cavity abnormality suggested by the HSG. While the films can be sent anywhere, and represent a permanent record, the fluroscopic views seen during the dye passage are very valuable. Therefore, ideally, the gynecologist or fertility doctor should be present for the study. The procedure itself may reactivate dormant infectious organisms in the tubes. Patients with a history of tubal infection probably should have prophylactic antibiotics given to avoid a re-infection that might be triggered by the test. If we unexpectedly find closed or damaged tubes, we put that patient on antibiotics afterwards for 5 to 7 days. Any current pelvic infection, or cervical/vaginal infection should be treated prior to this study, since lower tract organisms can be pushed into the tubes along with the dye. Women who routinely have antibiotic prophylaxsis for dental procedures because of atrial septal defects or prolapsed mitral valve should be covered as well.

The dyes used all contain iodine. Women allergic to shellfish or with a previous history of an allergic reaction to radioopaque dye have a few options. One is to use the dye with the least amount of iodine and to give them cortisone-like steroids for a few days before and on the day of the study. Another option is to skip the HSG altogether, and to go to laparoscopy as a first line test of tubal patency. Ultrasound also can be helpful in this situation. If a small catheter is put into the uterus and a salt solution with some bubbles is used, uterine cavity inspection and tubal evaluation can be performed. The images are more difficult to interpret than the x-ray pictures but usually are sufficient for diagnosis.

Postcoital Testing

It is important for the fertility doctor to ascertain if sperm survive once they come into contact with the cervical mucus. This is done with a painless procedure known as the **postcoital test,** in which a sample of mucus is collected after intercourse and examined under a microscope. Ideally, the mucus should be inspected 6 to 14 hours after coitus. Some patients will have normal results during the first hour or two of the interval with dramatic reduction of sperm motion afterwards. Because sperm should live in the cervical crypts for at least a day, examination later rather than sooner gives more meaningful information. The mucus can be taken from the cervix with any one of a number of suction devices which look like drinking straws. The pH is tested and should be neutral or slightly basic. If the pH is below six, sperm motility may suffer. The elasticity of the mucus is also measured by stretching it out until the strand breaks; it should stretch to at least six inches or more. The mucus should be clear and copious; under the microscope few, if any, white blood cells should be seen. Timing in the menstrual cycle is critical since some women have good mucus for only a day or two around the time of ovulation. We try to time all these examinations to occur on the morning after an LH kit positive response.

How are the results interpreted? Using a field magnification of 400 times, 10 or more nicely motile sperm in each of the sections viewed represents a normal result. Fewer than 5 per high powered field is a poor result. When very few sperm are seen, the problem may be that few sperm have actually entered the vagina, or that they have died rapidly and been removed by scavenger cells known as phagocytes. Large clumps of sperm stuck together or sperm with quivering motion suggest the presence of antibodies against sperm made by either the man or the woman. In some cases when repetitive postcoital tests continue to be poor, a crossover study may shed some light on the matter. Adding donor sperm on the microscopic slide to the mucus and placing the husband's sperm on a different slide with mucus of known good quality can help differentiate the source of the problem.

Second Level Tests

The foregoing has reviewed most of the initial or first line tests used in the evaluation of a subfertile couple. Many patients come to a fertility practice with many of these evaluations already performed. Most of the time they do not need to be repeated, but additional testing on a more sophisticated level may be necessary in order to fully delineate the extent of the problem. For instance, if someone comes to see me bearing x-ray films that indicate a tubal problem, assuming that the semen has been analyzed, and that ovulation has been documented, the next step probably will be laparoscopy to inspect and possibly repair the damage.

The Hamster Egg Penetration Assay

In this analysis, hamster eggs are harvested and the outer membranes are removed with enzymes. The sperm are prepared and incubated with the eggs. After a few hours the eggs are examined to see if they have been penetrated by the sperm (figure 5.4). This is a sophisticated test, difficult to

Figure 5.4
Hamster Egg Penetration Test

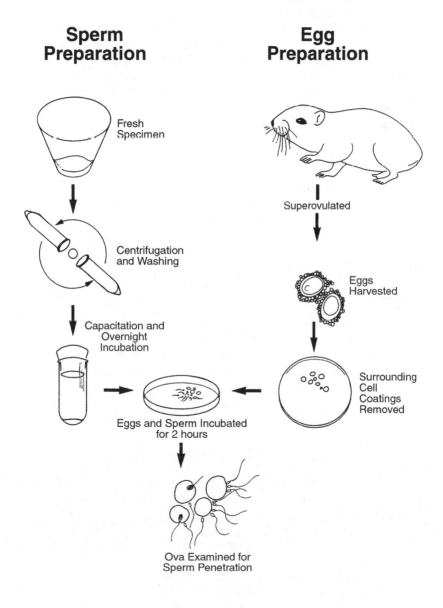

Sperm Preparation

Fresh Specimen

Centrifugation and Washing

Capacitation and Overnight Incubation

Egg Preparation

Superovulated

Eggs Harvested

Surrounding Cell Coatings Removed

Eggs and Sperm Incubated for 2 hours

Ova Examined for Sperm Penetration

perform, expensive, and non-standardized. Is it worth the trouble? Yes and no. The semen analysis may be absolutely normal, but the sperm may fail to penetrate the eggs. Does this mean that the individual is functionally sterile? Not necessarily. However, long-term follow up demonstrates that men whose sperm failed to penetrate any of the eggs are less fertile than those men with a normal result. The test seems to have its greatest value in the man who has had a varicocele repair because of poor semen quality. Men whose sperm continue to fail the test six months after surgery have a poor prognosis for pregnancy with coitus or insemination techniques, and usually require in vitro fertilization, sometimes with direct insertion of sperm into the egg in order to achieve success.

Testicular Biopsy

Even though the mere mention of this procedure is enough to make strong men cringe, the fact is that it is a minor process performed under local anesthesia in which a small piece of tissue is removed for microscopic inspection. Much valuable information can be gleaned from this study. Additionally, if there are no sperm in the ejaculate, and the test is being done to inspect for sperm production further upstream, a larger piece can be taken, and the sperm isolated and frozen for later use with intracytoplasmic sperm injection (ICSI) in conjunction with IVF. The appearance of the tubules with respect to scarring and the presence of sperm in various stages of development is a tremendous aid to diagnosis and subsequent counseling. Some men have what is known as the **"Sertoli cell only"** syndrome in which there are few or no sperm in the tubules. In actuality, about half of these men will have enough sperm to allow for microscopic harvesting and use in ICSI. Some of the biopsies show what is called **maturation arrest.** The picture here is one in which the sperm stop development prior to the stage where they become potentially able to fertilize. Even ICSI has limited success with sperm of this type.

Remember that when there's no sperm seen in the ejaculate, and when the fructose test is negative, indicating a block in the ductal system, the question of sperm production remains unanswered until a testicular biopsy is performed. Often, biopsy is done in the operating room with the surgeon prepared to correct the blockage if the biopsy shows normal sperm production. In any event, if sperm are present, the tissue should be processed so that the sperm can be recovered, and frozen for subsequent ICSI, since the operation to restore sperm flow may not be successful. Ultrasound is also used in the diagnosis of male infertility. The prostate and the ejaculatory ducts can be visualized and studied with this technique.

Pelvic Endoscopy

Endoscopy, literally "looking inside" allows the therapist to inspect the reproductive tract in its entirety. **Laparoscopy,** diagrammed in figure 5.5 is performed under local anesthesia with intravenous sedation or with general inhalational anesthesia. This is almost always an operating room procedure, although there is a move, mostly because of cost factors, to make this an office-based operation at sites which have the special equipment necessary to provide a reasonable level of safety. A telescope is inserted through the abdominal wall, usually at the navel. By merely moving the telescope and rotating it the surgeon can visualize all the pelvic reproductive organs, liver and gallbladder, the appendix, and virtually anything of interest within the abdominal cavity. Placing blue dye in the uterus with a syringe allows a surgeon to inspect tubal function as the dye exits the tubes. Do the tubes pass dye easily, without becoming distended? Is the vascular pattern of the tubal wall normal? Is there evidence of scar tissue? Does the fimbriated end of the tube appear normal, and does it make good contact with the ovary? Are there adhesions between the tube and the ovary? Is there evidence for endometriosis anywhere in the pelvis? These and a myriad of other questions go through the surgeon's mind at the time of the inspection. By inserting small ancillary operating instruments the procedure often

FIGURE 5.5   Diagram of laparoscopy.

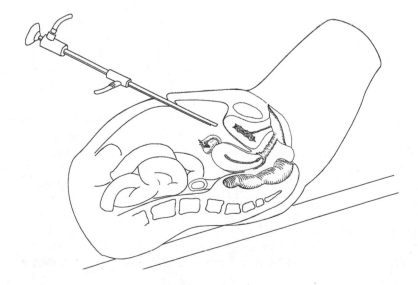

becomes therapeutic as well as diagnostic when any abnormality is found. Photo-documentation with stills or video allows for a permanent record of the findings and procedures with the possibility of additional consultation. The patient is usually discharged a few hours later. The surgical risks include those of anesthesia in general, damage to the intestines, major blood vessels, and bladder, and of course hemorrhage and infection as with any surgery. In fact, these complications occur infrequently.

Laparoscopy is recommended for infertility evaluation under the following circumstances:

1. Unexplained infertility in excess of one year
2. Infertility in women over the age of 35
3. When the hysterosalpingogram suggests tubal pathology
4. When pelvic ultrasound demonstrates an ovarian cyst which does not spontaneously resolve, or which shows characteristics of endometriosis or other ovarian lesions that warrant operative intervention
5. Failure to conceive after six months of satisfactory induction of ovulation or six months of well-timed donor insemination
6. Suspected endometriosis
7. Infertility with a previous history of pelvic surgery
8. Inspection concomitant with reversal of tubal sterilization
9. Infertility with a history of pelvic infection

Hysteroscopy, as shown in figure 5.6 is a procedure which allows direct inspection of the uterine cavity with a telescope. It frequently follows an abnormal HSG or ultrasound which has suggested the presence of adhesions, polyps, or myomas in the uterus. Abnormal uterine structural anatomy, such as a septum, can also be inspected. Diagnostic hysteroscopy is usually carried out with local cervical anesthesia and can be done in a well equipped office. For infertility investigations it is frequently done at the same time as laparoscopy in the operating room. Operative hysteroscopy, such as incising a uterine septum, cutting adhesions, and myomectomy is almost always done in the operating room. The hysteroscopic approach to tubal blockage at the uterine junction has, in many cases, replaced open microsurgery of the tube with results at least as good, if not better, and with substitution of a minor outpatient procedure for a major operation.

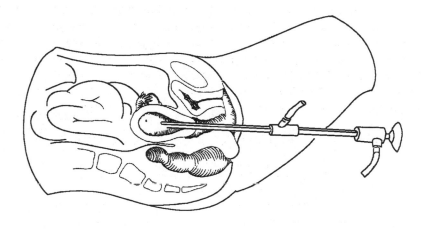

FIGURE 5.6   Diagram of hysteroscopy.

Falloposcopy, also call tuboscopy, allows one to visualize the interior of the fallopian tube by passing the instrument through a hysteroscope channel directly into the uterine end of the tube. Originally, the thought was that diseased tubes could be inspected and graded for severity as a preliminary to tubal repair. The success rate of IVF and its favorable "cost per baby" ratio to tubal surgery has diminished interest in this procedure which requires expensive and fragile instruments.

Additional Hormonal Testing

Thyroid disorders are rarely a cause of infertility, although there may be thyroid malfunction present coincidentally. Today, thyroid stimulating hormone (TSH) has become the most accurate sensitive screening test for thyroid deficiency (hypothyroidism). As the name implies, this hormone is responsible for governing the production of thyroid hormones within that gland. Over-active thyroid conditions are usually clinically very obvious with patients complaining of weight loss, increased appetite, sweating, rapid heart beat, tremor, and difficulty in sleeping whereas the under-active gland is much more subtle, with symptoms including lethargy or easy fatigue, weight gain, constipation, feeling of being cold all the time, and difficulty in concentrating. Thyroiditis is an autoimmune condition in which the gland first becomes over-active, and then from scar tissue formation, becomes permanently under-active. These patients require close supervision and management as they pass from one phase to the other.

PROLACTIN

Prolactin, the hormone normally increased in the postpartum period to promote milk production, can be elevated in the blood stream in the non pregnant state, either by over-activity of the cells in the pituitary responsible for its production, or by a tumor within that organ. Additionally, high TSH levels, present with hypothyroidism so mild that it is not clinically apparent and diagnosed only with blood tests, causes the prolactin secreting cells to work overtime. For that reason, prolactin determinations should always be accompanied by TSH testing to be sure that a prolactin elevation is not really a consequence of a sluggish thyroid. Many things affect prolactin levels within the bloodstream. Levels are at their lowest in the morning, but are elevated by eating, fear, pain, and breast stimulation. Therefore testing should be done with a fasting patient who has not had any breast stimulation that morning. Mood altering drugs, such as tranquilizers and antidepressants are common causes of prolactin elevation, once again documenting the importance of a thorough drug history at the initial interview; incidentally, tell the fertility doctor about any new or changed medications which may have come up after the first visit. When levels are very elevated, it is necessary to rule out a tumor in the pituitary; this is done with a CAT scan. The treatment for small tumors is the same as for over-active cell secretion—medication. The initial drug used for this, bromergocryptine, frequently causes nausea, nasal stuffiness, and a lowered blood pressure, sometimes causing posturally related dizziness, as with climbing steps. Cabergoline, a newer agent, needs to be taken twice weekly as opposed to daily, and has a much lower incidence of side effects.

Prolactin elevations interfere with FSH and LH release, so that first the patient has irregular menses with anovulation, but then she usually progresses to total absence of menses. Reversal of the prolactin elevation effect is rapid, usually within a few weeks. The reason for the amennorhea is that because the pituitary gonadotropins are shut down, the ovaries are unstimulated, and serum estrogen levels reach menopausal depths. For that reason, over and above fertility issues, prolonged amennorhea must be addressed, since osteoporosis can occur even in young women. Less than half of the women with prolactin elevations will have a true milk-like nipple discharge, so absence of this complaint does not rule out a prolactin elevation.

ESTROGEN LEVELS

Estrogen levels are seldom obtained as part of the initial investigation, since if the patient has any menstrual function, she has, by definition, sufficient estrogen to stimulate the uterine lining. Additionally, the normal range of estrogen concentration in the blood stream varies by tenfold throughout the menstrual cycle, so that isolated determinations are of little value. The story changes dramatically when gonadotropins are used for ovulation induction, since serial estrogen levels, obtained daily during the critical interval, along with ultrasonic ovarian evaluation, are used to determine the daily dose and the point at which an injection of hCG is given as the final trigger to bring about ovulation. Women with no menstrual function have insufficient estrogen levels to stimulate the endometrium, so quantification of this biologic effect has little value. Instead, a "progesterone challenge test" may be employed in which progesterone is given as a single injection, or by mouth over the course of 5-10 days, in an effort to provoke a menstrual episode. Failure to bleed documents that the endometrium has not been primed with enough estrogen to allow the progesterone to finish the process of maturing the lining before hormonal support is withdrawn.

THE ANDROGENS

Normally the testes produce a small amount of estrogens and the ovaries manufacture a bit of testosterone and similar androgens associated with male characteristics. Additionally, the adrenal gland in both sexes produces many of the same hormones. The level of any particular hormone in the blood stream reflects contributions from all of the production sites and must be considered from the perspective of the total mix. The appearance of the female patient who is "androgenized", with excessive hair growth on the face and chest, temporal recession of the hair line, oily skin and acne, and frequently, but not always, obesity, calls for a panel of androgens to be drawn as a screening test. The appearance of the patient is not always a good yardstick since many people of Mediterranean origins normally are more hirsute than Nordics, who may not show any of the characteristics mentioned above even when testosterone levels are quite elevated. High levels of androgens interfere with the cyclical interplay between the ovary, pituitary and hypothalamus, leading to irregular menses with long intervals (up to six months) and, in some, total loss of menstrual function. Many of these women are diagnosed as polycystic ovarian syndrome based on the hormonal pattern and the ultrasonic appearance of the ovary. We now know that insulin plays a pivotal role in this story, which will be continued in greater detail in the chapter on ovulation induction. By first suppressing and then stimulating the adrenal glands and ovaries with specific drugs, the source of the excess androgens can be identified and the proper therapy chosen. When the adrenal is involved, it often is a manifestation of a genetic propensity toward altered adrenal function, and is called an adult onset of mild congenital adrenal hyperplasia, most common in Ashkenazi Jews.

These hormonal aberrations almost always are on a cellular basis, but similar to prolactin excess, they may be caused by a tumor. Adrenal gland involvement may be from the gland itself or secondary to a tumor in the pituitary. CAT scans (an x-ray study) of the abdomen looking at the adrenal, which sits just over the kidney, and inspection of the pituitary with the same technique will pinpoint the site of the growth (the MRI is also helpful abdominally). Ovarian tumors which produce androgens in excess may be small and frequently are solid, rather than cystic, which means they might not show up on pelvic ultrasound. MRI (magnetic resonance imaging) is very helpful in delineation of these lesions, which are sometimes even missed at the time of laparoscopy. The androgen levels seen with tumors is sometimes so high that patients become masculinized, a step past androgenized, with beard growth, voice change, change in body habitus and muscular development. These tumors are usually, but not always, benign, and removal of the affected ovary alone under most conditions is sufficient.

Carbohydrate Metabolism Tests

It is not news that obese patients are more likely to eventually develop diabetes mellitus. Nor is it a secret that the patient with a typical polycystic ovarian syndrome picture is especially vulnerable. What is new, is the realization that insulin levels in these patients are frequently elevated as part of the initial presentation. The pancreas is already working overtime as a consequence of what has been called "peripheral resistance" to insulin's actions. If the insulin levels can be reduced, in many cases the androgen levels fall also, and normal ovulatory menstrual function may be spontaneously restored, or the patient who was previously refractive to ovulation induction with clomiphene citrate, now becomes responsive.

How do we test for this? Simple. A full 4 hour glucose tolerance test with insulin levels as well as glucose determination will be diagnostic. That involves going into an office or lab after an overnight fast, having a blood sample drawn, drinking something sweet, and having repeat blood sampling at 1, 2 and 4 hours later (bring a book to read). If insulin levels are found to be elevated, treatment with oral agents which sensitize the peripheral tissues to insulin are effective. This is another example of the domino effect of our hormonal systems, with insulin and its related growth factors directly controlling ovarian hormonal production.

Chromosomal Analysis

The chromosome is to the gene as the forest is to the tree. By that I mean that chromosomal rearrangements, deletions or absence are major findings—gross, even though the chromosomes are inspected under the microscope. Alterations on the level of the gene must be diagnosed with sophisticated methods of molecular biology, since minute changes or deletion In one of the basepairs of the DNA molecule can bring about profound changes in the individual; witness cystic fibrosis, phenylketonuria, sickle cell anemia and the glycogen storage diseases, to name but a few.

With the exceptions (so far) of the presence of one recessive gene for cystic fibrosis causing congenital absence of the vas deferens and partial deletion of a segment on the Y chromosome causing azoospermia or severe oligospermia, chromosomal analysis has little to offer the infertile couple. This is not the case, however, for the couple beset with repetitive miscarriage, in which chromosomal changes may be the causative factor. Most of these alterations involve **translocations,** a transfer of genetic material from one chromosome to another. Thus the total amount of genetic material within the cell nucleus may be normal, but the distribution is not. This leads to formation of **gametes** (sperm or eggs) which have an abnormal amount—too little or too much—-of chromosomal material, as a consequence of meiotic division when the total number of chromosomes are halved.

Chromosomal analysis, known as a **karyotype,** involves obtaining a tube of blood from which the cells are grown in the laboratory. When should this test be performed? We recommend it after three consecutive abortions, or after two in the case of women over 35. Because either partner may be carrying a translocated chromosomal fragment, both must be tested. In cases in which the ultrasound has diagnosed pregnancy failure, but the actual miscarriage has not yet occurred, the tissue is still viable, and direct genetic sampling of the fetal tissue allows for a chromosomal analysis of that fetus. The laboratory "hands on time" is major and the costs are accordingly high. Your insurance carrier, who might provide benefits for "infertility services" might not include "pregnancy wastage" in that package, so it behooves you to check on this. Results usually take 2 or 3 weeks as a function of the rate of growth of the cells.

There is no direct treatment for pregnancy loss as a result of these chromosomal rearrangements. A few in vitro fertilization programs offer "pre-implantational genetic analysis" in which each embryo can be sampled for abnormalities at the chromosomal or even gene level, prior to uterine placement. This is rarely insurance covered, and is available at only a few centers. Otherwise, the couple is left to what is similar to rolling the dice; eventually the right combination will come up, but many pregnancies may have to be initiated before success is achieved. Hormonal supplements have no role here. In almost every case, chromosomal deletions or additions are an all or none phenomenon, with the offspring being totally normal or a carrier of a translocation like one of the parents. The most notable exception to this rule is Down syndrome, with the person having 3, rather than 2, copies of chromosome 21. The sex chromosomes, X and Y, are also exceptions with a single X responsible for Turner's syndrome in women, with the person having short stature, ovaries without eggs, and sometimes associated cardiovascular changes. XXX females, sometimes called "super females" are anything but; they are almost always sterile. XXY males have **Klinefelter's** syndrome; they are usually tall with eunichoid proportions and build (like a pre-pubescent boy with long arms and legs relative to the trunk) and are almost always sterile.

Immunologic Testing

Considering that sperm contain protein foreign to the female, and that sperm enter not only the vagina, but eventually the uterus, tubes and abdominal cavity, all women should manufacture antibodies against sperm. The fact, however, is that this rarely occurs as a cause of infertility. Nothing in the routine semen analysis or postcoital testing is specific for antibodies. Clumping and agglutination of the sperm suggests the presence of sperm antibodies as is virtual absence of sperm in the postcoital test, when the male is known to have a normal analysis. Usually, women who have become sensitized to sperm, react to all sperm, but we have seen a few cases where they are "allergic" to their husband's sperm only. The reproductive tract system in the male is usually isolated from the blood stream, sort of like two pipes running in parallel, but with no connections. Sometimes, as a result of surgery, inflammation or trauma, sperm can leak into the circulation and present as a foreign substance to the cells charged with the responsibility of antibody production against various invaders. There are specific laboratory tests for detection of sperm antibodies in either partner. Treatment is discussed in the chapter on immunologic infertility.

Microbiologic Culture

Certain organisms have been associated with infertility, repeated pregnancy loss, or both. One of the most controversial of these is **ureaplasma urealyticum**, an organism having properties of both bacteria and viruses. It can be cultured from the cervix, when present, and is one of the "ping-pong" infections, passed back and forth between sexual partners, unless both are treated simultaneously. Symptoms may be absent or mild, a vaginal discharge or stinging with urination or urethral discharge in either partner. Treatment with tetracycline antibiotics is inexpensive and highly effective. About 30% of cervical cultures will be positive for this organism, which, obviously, is widespread in the general population. The literature that deals with whether or not its presence is reproductively deleterious is about equally divided pro and con. Since it's easy to treat, most of us will treat husband and wife concomitantly to eliminate this organism.

There's no question that a culture positive for **chlamydia trachomatis** in either partner calls for treatment of both. This organism is responsible for more cases of tubal damage than with gonorrhea, but is often less clinically apparent at the time of the initial infection. A thick mucoid cervical discharge can be noted, albeit as a non specific sign of chlamydial infection. This too, is a ping-pong infection, with no immunity conferred after the initial exposure. Treatment with tetracycline derivatives to both partners simultaneously is highly effective, but positive pre-treatment cultures need to be repeated. Exposure to the organism results in long term antibody levels detectable in the bloodstream, years afterwards. This allows us to screen the woman with a chlamydial antibody titer to determine if she might have sustained tubal damage as a result of a clinically silent infection well in the past. Even if the tubes appear to be normal by HSG inspection or with laparoscopic examination, the cilia which line the tube may be permanently lost and this patient needs IVF, since no surgery can restore these cells. The trouble with this neat story is that chlamydial organisms can be responsible for illness elsewhere in the body, with chlamydial pneumonia, caused by a slightly different subspecies, as one example. The antibody test may not be specific enough to differentiate between the two, in which case clinical judgment usually is brought to bear. Since pelvic chlamydia can live in the tubes for years, long after cervical cultures become negative, and because treatment is easy, safe, and usually effective, a positive antibody titer almost always calls for treatment of both partners, even if the cervical culture is negative at that time, in order to be as sure as possible that no live critters are hiding anywhere.

This has probably been a long and arduous chapter for you to complete; I've tried to make it informative without being overly technical. Much of what we do in therapy is based on these diagnostic studies. In order to understand what your therapeutic options are, you must first have some knowledge of the physiology involved—what's broken or not working, and how can it be fixed or by-passed.

6

Normal and Subnormal Human Fertility: The Necessary Statistics

Don't cringe or panic! This chapter may even be enjoyable as well as informative. We'll start out with a report by Zinaman and co-workers which appeared in Fertility and Sterility (65:503, 1996), the official journal of the American Society for Reproductive Medicine. I've chosen this paper to discuss because the protocol of the study was well constructed, the findings are of interest, and some of the problems in study patient selection are obvious. The objective was to examine fertility and pregnancy wastage rates in a group of presumed fertile couples. The plan was to follow 200 couples who had just stopped contracepting in order to conceive over a 12 month interval of time with sensitive pregnancy tests being performed in the last half of the menstrual cycle for the first three months. The population base consisted of men from 20 to 51 years of age with a mean of 32.3 years, a standard deviation (SD) of 4.8, and with women from 23 to 37 years with a mean of 30.6 and a SD of 3.3. What can we conclude from these data? First, the men tended to be older than the women, and the range of ages was greater. The **mean** represents the average age obtained by adding up all the ages and dividing by the number of subjects. This is different from the **median,** which is the age at which half the subjects are older or younger. If the median is more than the mean, the sample is not distributed equally around the mean, and for this example would contain an excess of older men. **Standard deviation** is a term which expresses the extent of variation around the mean. For instance, we might examine a population with a mean age of 30, but with a range of age between one and 90, compared with a group with the same mean age but with a range between 24 and 36. Obviously, the second group is more homogeneous; the SD expresses this with a specific quantifiable measurement. The volunteers for this study were recruited by radio announcements, newspaper advertisement, and direct physician referral. The female population was 91.5% white, non-Hispanic; 2.0% were Hispanic; and 4.0% were African-American. College or graduate school education was reported by 80.9% of the women. Family income was well above average. Current smoking was reported by 6.5% of the women, and 77.5% reported alcohol consumption in the 30 days previous to enrollment. Thus, you can see that this study group may have reflected the population around the center which was performing the investigation, but was not truly representative of the general population in North America considering ethnic proportions, education, income, and alcohol (more) and smoking (less) use. The subjects were volunteers who learned about the study from the media or from a physician, thereby creating bias or at least another variable in the selection process. Additionally, the initial telephone screening process, while limiting the female age group to 21-37, also required them to have regular menstrual cycles between 25-33 days. At any time in the general population, about 15% of women in this age group not on oral contraceptives pills will have menstrual cycles which fall outside these limits, further reflecting the fact that the study group does not represent the so-called "normal population" chosen completely at random.

Although this was a study designed to examine the fertility rate in a group of presumed fertile couples not undergoing treatment, the investigators counseled the subjects on coital timing and frequency. This constitutes a form of treatment. The majority of women (52.5%) were **nulliparous,** which means that they had never before delivered. Of this group 72% became pregnant at least once within the one-year study period compared with 88% of previously delivered women. Are these results different? A statistical term used to express whether differences between groups are truly real or a finding which occurs at random that does not reflect reality is the p value. The p for the results above was 0.008, which means that this difference would be seen by chance in eight of 1,000 trials. The usually accepted maximal p for statistical significance is $p=0.05$. Therefore, the observed difference was a real one. A pregnancy was recorded according to the pregnancy test results, which during the first three months, was performed daily in the last half of the menstrual cycle in order to pick up those "occult" or "biochemical" pregnancies completely unsuspected by the patient who usually had her menses on time.

Figure 6.1 shows the cycle - specific pregnancy rates over the study

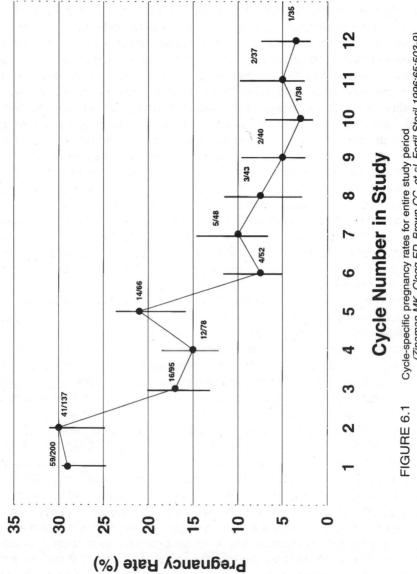

FIGURE 6.1   Cycle-specific pregnancy rates for entire study period
(Zinaman MK, Clegg ED, Brown CC, et al. Fertil Steril 1996;65:503-9)

interval. The numbers in the figure reflect pregnancies as the numerator and the number of subjects as the denominator. So for the first month we see there were 59 pregnancies in 200 couples. Of the 141 couples remaining, four dropped out of the study, leaving 137, of which an additional 41 conceived in the second month, and so on. Data presented in this fashion are known as a "life table analysis," an actuarial method of tracking the rate of an event over defined time segments. The name given to fertility per menstrual cycle is **fecundity.** As you can see, fecundity was greatest in the first two months, with a rapid decline for the next three months, and a low conception rate for the remainder of study. This is, indeed, the usual finding in studies of this type. The most fertile people conceive quickly, but there is a spectrum thereafter, just as there is for performance in anything else. We arbitrarily define infertility as lack of conception within a year, but some people will conceive without any treatment in the next year or two; we'll address that shortly. In the study mentioned here, 18% of the couples had failed to conceive by the 12th cycle. This is greater than the figure obtained by the National Center for Health Statistics of 8%, and greater than the usual figure of 12% in similar studies. The difference may represent under- reporting in one study, and different population bases.

The fecundity data can be used to create what is called a **"cumulative pregnancy rate"**. Using the data from figure 6.1, the curve in figure 6.2 was constructed. Note the degree of success in the first two months which then declines and flattens out between months five and six. If this were a pregnancy rate curve for a monthly treatment, we would rightfully conclude that if it had not worked by six months or so for an individual, we should move on to a different therapy. These kinds of cumulative pregnancy rate curves can be established for almost any therapy. It is important for both the doctor and patient to understand how they can be used to determine the treatment plan. The same method can be applied to a one shot therapy such as surgery for tubal damage. Here, the question is asked "how long should we give this to work before going on to IVF as a tubal bypass?". The answer is that most of the surgical treatment curves flatten by 18 months postoperatively.

Getting back to our example study, the total miscarriage rate was 32%, 29%, and 33%, respectively, in cycles one through three in which sensitive pregnancy tests were performed. Of the 19 lost pregnancies in cycle 1, seven (37%) were without subject awareness; the numbers for cycles 2 and 3 were 7/12 and 1/5, respectively, for a total of 42% of all of the miscarriages. This is not cycle dependent and is constant throughout most studies. In summary about 30% of all pregnancies will fail, according to the definition of a positive

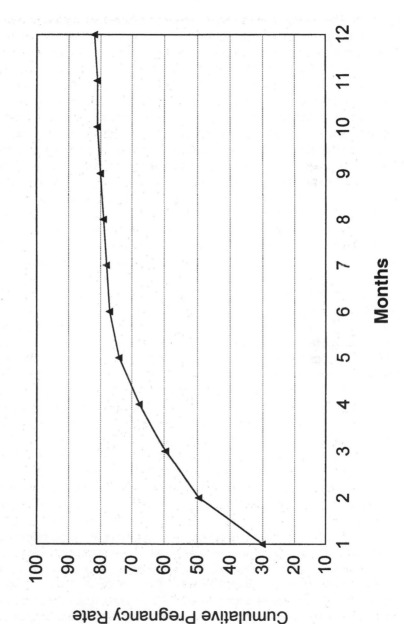

Figure 6.2
Cumulative pregnancy rate

pregnancy test only, with about 40% of those being completely unknown to the patient unless documented with early pregnancy tests done before the onset of the expected period.

Let's look more closely at pregnancy rates according to diagnostic classifications in subfertile populations who are untreated. Logically, this is of importance because for any treatment being evaluated, some of the people for whom the therapy is said to be successful would have conceived without intervention. Good studies recognize this, and include in the protocol provision for random assignment of patients to an active treatment arm and an untreated, control, group. Similarly, drug studies employ a randomly assigned group which is given a placebo agent with no activity. This is best done in what is known as a "double blind" fashion in which neither the investigators evaluating the effect nor the patient knows which group he/she is in until the study is over and the results have been tabulated.

You may never have heard of Walcheren. At the time of the study it was an island in the southwest of the Netherlands. One hospital and one gynecologist serviced the reproductive needs of this rather homogeneous population. Between 1985 and 1994, 726 couples were seen in consultation because they had failed to conceive with at least one year of unprotected intercourse. A standard diagnostic work-up was employed including semen analysis, BBT chart, progesterone determinations, postcoital testing and HSG/laparoscopy (Snick et al, Hum Repro 12:1582, 1997.) What do the results tell us?

First, the mean duration of infertility was 20.7 (SD 13.9) months and the mean female age was 29.1 (SD 4.5) years. Therefore, we conclude that there was great variation in the duration of infertility, with a minimum of 12 months, but the female age variation was small. As a commentary, the age of the female population in this study is about five years younger than what would be seen in this country, probably reflecting in part our tendency to delay childbearing coupled with easier access to a socialized health care system in the Netherlands. From the original group, 342 were untreated and were observed for mean of 17.3 (SD 22.5, median 8.0, range 1-107) months after registration. Armed with your new knowledge of statistics, you'll probably comment that at least half of the patients were followed for substantially less than the arithmetic average, and that the variation of follow-up was great. Nevertheless the study gives us meaningful information. The untreated women had 239 conceptions with 201 live births. The abortion rate is less than in the first study, but this investigation did not employ early pregnancy tests. The mean time to conception for those with a live birth was 8.1 (SD 10.0, median 4.0, range 1-73) months. Note that of those who conceived, half did so by four months, far less time than the average. While the paper states that they were untreated, I'm sure that during the work-up some attention was paid to counseling regarding coital frequency and timing, which is frequently therapeutic when there are problems with cervical mucus and/or seminal quality.

Statistically, the principle of cumulative rates can be used to "normalize" the data so that we can project the pregnancy rate if all the patients not receiving treatment had been followed for 36 months. When that exercise is done, we come up with a live birth rate of 46%. If an ovulatory defect were found and not treated, the birth rate was reduced by 60%, and for an untreated tubal problem, the reduction was 90%. Unexplained infertility had the best prognosis. The results also support previous work pointing out that sperm count, alone, does not have a good correlation with pregnancy rates. That reminds me to point out that this study focused on birth rates; be careful when you read literature as to what the end point is — pregnancy or delivery. The other important finding in this study was that live birth rates were inversely proportional to the duration of infertility; in other words, the longer a couple was infertile, the less likely they were to conceive.

A similar study appeared in Fertility and Sterility in 1995 (64:22) with John Collins as the lead author. Results from 873 untreated Canadian couples observed for 21.0 (SD 23.0, median 12.9, range 1 to 89.2) months were included with observations made on an additional 1325 patients prior to any active treatment. The untreated couples had 340 conceptions but 263 live births, a seemingly high abortion rate. The time to conception in successful pregnancies was 10.4 (SD 12.1, median 6.0, range 1 to 73.9) months. Live birth rate was highest for couples with secondary infertility, females < 30, and infertility < 36 months. Projected live birth rates after 36 months of observation only were 33% for unexplained infertility, 23% for ovulatory problems, and 29% for low sperm count. Women with milder stages of endometriosis had a 20% success rate, but the more severe grades had only a 5% live birth rate.

These studies have been presented first, to give you experience in critical appraisal of what you might read, but second, to furnish you with some data whereby you can set the tempo for your treatment, once a diagnosis has been made (or not made). As is always the case, these decisions will be influenced by duration of infertility, female age, the severity or extent of the problem, your degree of anxiety, and (unfortunately) your insurance coverage for fertility services.

The next example to be considered here asks a basic question — how often do fertile couples have abnormal fertility tests? Doctor Guzick and his associates (Hum Repro 9:2306, 1994) addressed this issue in 32 couples in which the female was about to have a laparoscopic sterilization. At least one commonly performed fertility test result was abnormal in 22 couples. Ten of these were related to semen analysis and/or post coital testing, again documenting that results of the semen analysis, especially the count, may not accurately reflect the fecundity within that couple, unless the numbers are very low. Remember, normally fertile couples may have abnormal fertility test results such as low sperm count, occasional anovulation, and hormonal patterns or levels that may fall outside the normal range. An abnormal finding or test result in the infertile couple may, or may not, be causally related to the problem.

The last statistical tool which we'll introduce has to do with assessment of risk factors. Suppose we have some preliminary information which suggests that women who consume at least three Milky Way bars weekly have an increased risk of having twins. We construct a careful study with sufficient numbers of control, non-users of the product matched to the test group for age, reproductive performance , smoking and drinking habits, and anything else we can think of. We observe the groups over a reasonable interval of time, and then compile the data. And yes! There is a statistically significant difference in the twinning rate. But we would like to know in simple terms what is the magnitude of the increased risk of having twins if our women eat three Milky Way bars weekly. The terms **relative risk (RR)** and **Odds ratio(OR)** are used daily by gamblers, often subconsciously, and can be applied here. So we do the calculations and determine that the risk compared with the control group is 3.7 times. But we also know that depending on the sample size and particularly on the frequency with which the observed event occurs, there will be variation of the results if the trial is repeated, with the degree of variation proportionately more marked for events which occur infrequently. For example, if something occurs 3 times per thousand in one trial, and we repeated the study 100 times, we might find a range from 0 to 13 per thousand. This method of quantifying the expected spread is one of setting **confidence limits (CL),** usually encompassing the expected results 95% of the time, and rejecting as a quirk the total 5% extremes, both high and low. Just one more point. A result of RR=3.7, CL= 1.6 to 9.8, means the difference is statistically significant with a computed odds ratio of 3.7 times, but that the actual ratio could lie anywhere between the lower and upper limits. Obviously, the tighter the spread, the more the ratio reflects the true figure. If, however, the lower limit dips to below I, as in RR=3.7, CL= 0.8 to 5.6, we cannot say, with statistical correctness, that the two groups being compared have a true difference. Consider flipping a coin ten times in a row, with 100 such trials. Intuitively, we would expect a mean and median to be close to five for either heads or tails, but we also know that a 6:4 and 7:3 ratio would not be rare, and even more infrequently, we might see ten consecutive heads. The rules of statistics help us to avoid making the mistake of concluding that there is a difference when none exists, and also of saying that there is no difference when one actually exists.

Medical statisticians are concerned about the effect of duration of infertility in analysis of various therapies. They have paid less attention to "duration of remaining fertility potential." That is to say that a two year history of infertility in a 38 year-old woman calls for more immediate and aggressive treatment than a four year history in one who is 29.

I've tried to make you conversant with a few basic concepts of medical statistics so that you can better understand the strengths and weaknesses of some of the material which follows. Today, it is possible to download enormous amounts of material from the Internet, some of it original and some of dubious veracity. If you choose to use those sources be critical in your appraisal of how the data were obtained and whether the conclusions are valid.

7

Ovarian Reserve Testing

Demographic data from official United States surveys point out the need for testing ovarian reserve in a population which increasingly is delaying reproduction. In 1925, the childless rate for women > 35 was 11%; by 1991 it was 21%, and it is now in the neighborhood of 25%. More impressive is the fact that in 1994 one-third of all first births were in women > 35. The ability to conceive, especially when measured as a monthly event (fecundity), decreases with age while miscarriage increases. Therefore, the issue is not simply one of the decline in the egg reservoir that eventually leads to menopause, but additionally a diminution in egg quality. We know that the uterus, per se, does not become the limiting feature, because egg recipients in their 40s and 50s have miscarriage rates which reflect the age of the younger egg donor. Is there a subset of the population that we could study in an effort to ascertain reproductive potential over a lifetime? Some of the orthodox Amish sects which neither smoke, drink nor contracept and who marry early have been surveyed with this question in mind. There is a median of about eight births per couple with 3 to 4 miscarriages, but the median age at the last delivery tends to be between 38 and 39. Because these groups intermarry frequently and the genetic pool is relatively small, the recessive gene problem is magnified, and the spontaneous abortion rate may be slightly increased as a result.

Another interesting way of looking at female fecundity as a function of age is to examine the results of artificial donor insemination in a large group. This was done in France, a country in which all donor sperm comes from a central source, with standardization of the specimens and with accurate data retrieval . Fecundity per cycle rates were 11.0 for women < 25; 10.5 for those 26-30; 9.1 in the 31-35 group and 6.5 for those > 35 (Schwartz and Mayaux, N Engl J Med 306: 404, 1982). The sample size consisted of 2193 women whose husbands' were azoospermic. The effect of age was slight but significant beyond 30, and became marked after 35 years. The probability of success with treatment up to 12 cycles was 73% and 74% respectively, for the two groups under 31. This dropped to 61% in the 31-35 group and decreased further to 54% for those beyond 35. So for some women the effect of age was only one of taking longer to become pregnant, although for others, it was failure.

I have included an abbreviated author's citation, first to credit a major contribution to our knowledge fund, and second, to allow those who have access to a medical library or online medical databases to read the original. I will continue to summarize the literature but in special and specific cases furnish you with the reference of what is considered to be a good review, or a landmark report.

A number of studies have found no difference in estrogen levels in blood at the time of ovulation when young women and older women were compared, although it is a well-established fact that the follicular phase is shortened in the later reproductive years. Progesterone determinations in the luteal phase show no difference according to age. The only hormonal indicator of impending or incipient ovarian failure is FSH in the first few days of the cycle independent of age. Screening for FSH levels on the third day of the menstrual cycle is an excellent means by which to identify patients with decreased ovarian reserve, with results applicable both to egg quality and quantity. A major advance was achieved in 1987 when Navot described the clomiphene citrate challenge test (C3T), which has been popularized by Scott and other authors. This test is similar to the cardiac stress test, in which a tracing is taken before and after exercise. In this circumstance, the organ being stressed is the ovary, the stimulus is clomiphene citrate (Clomid or Serophene), and we use hormonal blood test results instead of a cardiogram tracing.

As commonly employed, FSH and estradiol are measured on the third day of the cycle. The reason for the estrogen determination is that in cases of impaired ovarian function, the granulosa cells surrounding the follicles produce less inhibin B than is normal, which allows the FSH levels to rise with greater stimulation of estrogen production than should be present early in the cycle. The bottom-line of all this is that paradoxically, high estrogen levels early in the cycle may be a sign of poor reproductive potential, especially when concentration in the blood exceeds 65 pg/mL (picograms per milliliter), independent of FSH level. The FSH levels should be in the normal range, which is usually 3 to 9.6 milli-international units (mIU) per milliliter. This will be dependent on the laboratory, so a list of laboratory standards is necessary for proper interpretation. The test is currently done against a standard derived from human pituitary extract rather than the older urinary standards which gave results that were roughly double those currently expected. This day 3 determination is the baseline reading. The patient then receives 100 mg of clomiphene citrate, as two 50 mg tablets taken together from cycle day 5 through 9. The blood test taken on day 3 is then repeated on day 10. The dose of the clomiphene citrate is independent of weight, and the days are independent of the menstrual cycle history. Our own research has shown that day 3 results do not differ statistically from days 2 or 4, so that there is a leeway of one day, plus or minus, if day 3 proves to be extremely inconvenient for blood sampling. The day 10 sample seems to be a fixed point in time, however. The estrogen level on day 10 should be at least double that seen on day 3. But the amount of rise has nothing to do with any fertility quotient. The only reason for measuring estrogen on day 10 is to be sure the patient has a hypothalamus which is sensitive to the clomiphene citrate which will, in turn, stimulate the pituitary and the ovaries. If the patient is not sensitive to the agent, the test is invalid. The FSH concentration, on the other hand, should remain in the normal range. Women with one ovary may have somewhat higher levels without a significant reduction in fertility potential. Women recovering from chemotherapy affecting the ovaries may take two or three years to stabilize, so that early testing may give a bleaker picture than actually is the case. Because clomiphene citrate is an ovarian stimulant (used clinically for over 30 years) some women will become pregnant in the test cycle as a therapeutic benefit.

Our current philosophy is to screen all infertile women seeking care with us who are at age 35 or over regardless of any known fertility problems. Additionally, patients with unexplained infertility at any age, those with irregular ovulation, patients who have a poor response to ovulation induction, and those with repeated miscarriage are also tested in this manner.

Let's discuss an excellent review article which takes a life table analysis approach to an infertile population according to age and results of ovarian reserve testing with both Scott and Navot among the authors (Hum Repro

10: 1706, 1995). About 1200 women from an infertile population were screened by C3T. Patients with tubal disease, adhesions or male factor were eliminated from the study, leaving 588 available for follow-up, with 505 having normal tests and 83 showing reduced ovarian reserve. For the whole group, the mean age was 34.1, SD 0.2 years, certainly a homogeneous group with respect to age and about what is seen in usual clinical practice. The mean duration of infertility was 3.2, SD 0.3 years, so this was legitimately an infertile population. The mean follow-up interval was 15.2 (SD 0.3, range 1 to 43) months. Table 7.1 shows the distribution of clinical diagnoses in the study patients according to the results of ovarian screening. Note the high percentage of abnormal results in patients who had been labeled as "unexplained infertility". Treatments included ovulation induction and insemination. Figure 7.1 shows the cumulative pregnancy rate, irrespective of age, according to normal or abnormal C3T results. Please note that these are pregnancy rates and not delivery rates.

Distribution of clinical diagnoses in women with normal and abnormal clomiphene citrate challenge tests

Category of Infertility	Normal Ovarian Reserve		Diminished Ovarian Reserve	
	n	%	n	%
Ovulatory disorder	22	44	30	36.1
Luteal phase defect	58	11.5	5	6
Cervical factor	47	9.3	4	4.8
Unexplained	178	35.2	44	53
Total	505	100	83	100

TABLE 7.1   Scott RT, Opsahl MS, Leonardi MR et al.

Human Reprod 1995;10:1706-1710

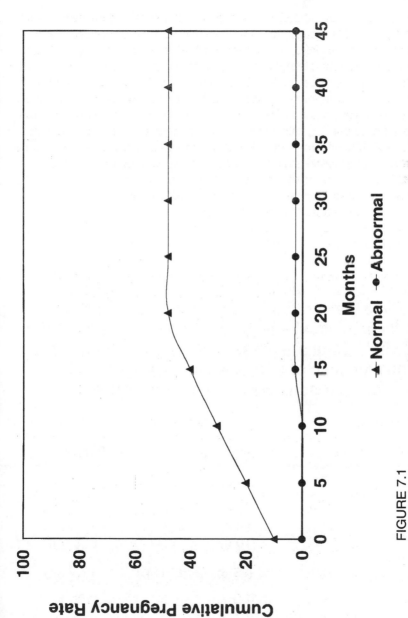

FIGURE 7.1

Cumulative pregnancy rates in women with normal ovarian reserve screening (normal, n = 505) were significantly higher than in women with evidence of diminished ovarian reserve (abnormal, n = 83) (P < 0.001) (Scot RT, Opsahl MS, Leonardi MR et al. Human Reprod 1995;10:1706-1710)

Table 7.2 is quite illuminating, with the data presented by age vs. results. We see that while it is always better to have a normal reserve test, a normal result in a forty-year old does not mean that she has the reproductive potential of a younger woman. In fact, there was a steady age-related decline in pregnancy rates among those with normal test results. Also note the relatively high percentage of abnormal results in the 34-36 and 37-39 year old groups – the most common categories we treat. If we momentarily eliminate the data dealing with diminished ovarian reserve in the 31-33 year old group because of small numbers, we see that the test is amazingly accurate in its prognostic ability to identify those who will not conceive. It has no real use as a positive, rather than a negative, predictor. Since women with elevated FSH levels have high miscarriage rates (in the 50% zone) the test becomes that much more accurate with respect to the bottom-line.

Table 7.2
Incidence of normal and abnormal clomiphene citrate challenge tests and the associated pregnancy rates within the individual age groups and for the population as a whole. Data are presented in contingency table format for ease of interpretation but all statistical comparisons were done via life table

Age Group (years)	Normal ovarian reserve n (%)	Pregnant (%)	Diminished ovarian reserve n (%)	Pregnant (%)
< 30	92 (94.8)	61 (66.3)	5 (5.2)	0 (0.0)
31-33	150 (93.2)	85 (56.7)	11 (6.8)	2 (18.2)
34-36	48 (87.1)	63 (42.6)	22 (12.9)	1 (4.5)
37-39	85 (80.1)	33 (38.8)	21 (19.9)	1 (4.8)
> 40	30 (55.6)	3 (10.0)	24 (44.4)	0 (0.0)
Total	505 (85.9)	245 (48.5)	83 (14.1)	4 (4.8)

Scott RT, et al. Human Reprod 1995;10:1706-1710

We recently evaluated the results of C3T testing in 210 patients prior to IVF who were 35 and over, or with a history of poor response to ovulation induction . FSH values in this high risk group were abnormal in 23 on day 3 as defined by 10 mIU or over, and were abnormal in 35 on day 10, with 27 of this latter group abnormal on day 10 only. This underscores the need for the whole test rather than a day 3 only screen. No patient in this group with an FSH of 13 or greater had a liveborn. Based on this result which mirrors the general literature on the subject, we will not perform IVF on patients who have FSH values in excess of 13, although we will treat patients in the office with values to 17 after a long discussion about the situation and the need for a reduced expectation of success with any approach other than an egg donor. Different physicians are more or less rigid on this subject than we, and you need to discuss this with your therapist. When I tell a patient with an FSH of 17 or more that she will not get to a viable delivery without an egg donor, that is said with only a 2% error, which is a highly accurate predictive statement. There is no absolute cutoff value that I know of beyond which there is no delivery. Every year we have a handful of patients who achieve what is really a miracle pregnancy. Dr Scott's team recently evaluated the outcome of pregnancies in 1034 patients with abnormal ovarian reserve test results. The crude pregnancy rate (any positive hCG test) was 2.7%; the abortion rate was 71.4% (20/28) with a net delivery rate of 0.7%. Pregnancies were achieved in natural cycles, clomiphene citrate or gonadotropin stimulated cycles, and with IVF. Before continuing expensive and complicated treatments, you should have some awareness of what your success rate might be. A single elevated FSH determination is like an indelible tattoo; even if retested, the reproductive potential in a month with normal results is no better. When results start to drift into the high normal range, they should be repeated at six month intervals. The C3T is especially helpful when we unexpectedly identify a patient in the twilight zone of FSH 10-13. We then can inject some urgency into the treatment protocol and become more aggressive in management than we otherwise might have been. Identification of women whose reproductive potential is virtually nil saves a great deal of wasted financial and emotional effort and points the way to serious consideration of an egg donor or adoption before the couple has exhausted their resources.

8

Emotional Aspects of Infertility

Andrea Mechanick Braverman, Ph.D.

"I grew up playing with dolls and knew for certain that I wanted to be a Mom more than anything else in the world. Each month I don't get pregnant, I feel like a small piece is taken from my heart and may never return. I could get through anything if someone would just tell me that I would get pregnant eventually. Not knowing if I'll get pregnant one day is what keeps me constantly worried"

Ellen, age 32

Infertility steals spontaneity, self-esteem, intimacy and dreams. Unsure about the future, many infertile men and women are left in limbo because they are afraid both of planning for a pregnancy and the possibility that they will never conceive. Infertility catches people unaware. Children are rarely raised with awareness that they may be infertile one day. To the contrary, health classes focus on reproduction and contraception and seldom is the word infertility ever introduced to health class. Did you know much about infertility until you wanted to have a baby?

We grow up with the assumption that we are fertile. Our parents were able to conceive and deliver; often our siblings, cousins, and friends have been able to get pregnant without a problem. Most couples consider when, and not if, they will conceive. Attempts to time pregnancies are made with consideration of career choices, vacation plans, or seasons. Due to the focus on planning pregnancies around the couples' lifestyle, some may have a hard time acknowledging that there may be an infertility problem.

Conversely, other couples have had exposure to infertility through family or friends' experiences and have a heightened awareness about the possibility of infertility. Combined with experience, some couples may be sensitized to infertility due to their age or medical history. Nonetheless, the majority of men and women have not entertained the notion that they may not be parents even if they choose to be.

Reactions to Infertility

We come to confront our infertility in a variety of ways. Like many other difficult events in life, we can go in and out of stages of denial, acceptance, anger and resolution.

After nearly a year of attempting to get pregnant on their own, Sue and Bill went to see their doctor. Sue remarked, "I just couldn't believe it. I knew I could get pregnant. I figured it was my job, but I still didn't get pregnant after the hectic rush was past."

Denial is a common reaction to infertility. As discussed previously, most people do not attribute infertility to their lack of pregnancy. Work, diet, sleep habits, and other variables are often blamed before people consider a medical problem. Denial protects us from trying to absorb difficult information. Bad news can be let in slowly and stopped when the person feels overwhelmed.

Contacting a doctor means acknowledging that there may be a medical problem. This can be threatening to either the male or female partner. Fertility, virility, and masculinity/femininity can all be confused easily. As each person feels vulnerable when diagnosed with a fertility problem, s/he conjures up what that diagnosis means to her or him. Upon occasion, some individuals are so overwhelmed by the prospect of being diagnosed with an infertility problem, that they will avoid the feelings by refusing to seek medical assistance.

It is not easy to hear that you have an infertility problem. Reactions range from disbelief to fear to anger. There is no one "correct" or "better" response to being diagnosed with a problem.

"When the doctor told me I had no sperm, I felt like someone had pulled that amazing tablecloth trick where they remove the tablecloth and leave everything else still standing on the table. Outside, my life looked as before - normal. Inside, I felt empty. It was a bad dream that wouldn't end."

Aaron, age 29

Being diagnosed as infertile demands that we re-evaluate how we view ourselves. As they go through this process, many people feel that they have been set apart from their friends and family. This sense of separation and, for some, isolation, can be devastating.

Since the infertility problem can sometimes be identified with an individual, the infertile partner can often feel responsible or guilty. Knowing intellectually that you do not have control over your body is very different from accepting it emotionally. Since we want the best for our partners, knowing that your infertility is causing emotional distress for your partner can be difficult at best. An added difficulty for men may be the knowledge that their partners must endure the major burden of diagnostics and treatment.

Sometimes, the past can play a role. For some men or women who have had a pregnancy before and terminated the pregnancy, infertility can feel like a punishment. Sometimes it reawakens a sense of sadness or feelings of an opportunity lost.

"The doctor reassured me that the abortion I had when I was 18 years old didn't do any damage. But I can't help wondering if maybe there's something there that he can't see."

Emily, age 25

It is important to confront these thoughts and feelings. Like any wound, only exposure to sunlight and air will help the healing process. You cannot "will" yourself to stop thinking or feeling. However, you can put a stop to the negative messages you give yourself, e.g. "it's all my fault" or "it's my punishment", etc.

Reactions by Friends and Family

Friends and family want to be supportive and say the right thing. However, few people know what to say to you when you have fertility problems. First, friends and family are skittish because fertility does involve sexuality, a subject which is usually private. Second, they may be uncomfortable discussing anything personal. Third, they may be simply afraid of intruding into your privacy.

Family and friends want the best for you. Consequently, they will try to provide support and sometimes stumble in the process. Encouragement such as "I just know you'll get pregnant - you'd make such great parents" or "Just relax - don't try so hard" is intended to be helpful. These "helpful hints" usually have the opposite effect because these comments often have an underlying message, which is absorbed by the infertile person and is completely missed by the person giving the advice. The message is one of blame. It is your fault that you are not pregnant because you are 1) too stressed; 2) trying too hard; 3) working too hard, or; 4) too something else. Although the medical literature is mixed on the relationship between stress and pregnancy outcome, no one supports the age-old advice of "just relax and you'll get pregnant" as the cure for infertility. Relaxation will certainly help quality of life, but it is simplistic to blame infertility on stress alone. If you are interested in reading more about the relaxation response and stress management, there are some excellent resources available; these are listed either through RESOLVE (mentioned later) or at the end of this chapter. The bottom line in the debate with stress and infertility is that you did not cause your infertility by being stressed nor are you preventing yourself from getting pregnant.

Friends and family do not want to see us sad or hurt. Therefore, the advice ladled out is targeted to reduce the sadness and hurt. If a cycle is unsuccessful, the emotional impact of that cycle is often minimized by well-meaning family or friends.

"Two days after my negative pregnancy test, I was still very quiet at work. A close friend and colleague asked me what was wrong. When I told her, she responded by telling me I should be over it by now and maybe I should see a counselor. After all, she said, it's not like you lost a baby."

Roslyn, age 29

Since there was no pregnancy, others may not see the reason for sadness. For the infertile man or woman, the cycle may feel like a pregnancy loss. Each month, there is a child imagined and each cycle represents hope. A cycle that does not result in a pregnancy may tap into feelings of hopelessness or increase a sense of isolation.

Anger

Anger is a constant companion for some people and an occasional unwelcome visitor for others as they experience infertility. It is easy to feel angry and there are many potential targets. Global questions such as "why me" can elicit feelings of anger toward your body, pregnant women, medicine, God, friends, and family. Anger is physically and emotionally draining to experience and anger can add to the feelings of being overwhelmed and exhausted.

Most infertile men and women do not feel angry all the time. However, the occasions where anger does intrude are disruptive and discouraging. The goal is not to eliminate anger; the goal is to manage the anger. If you tend to get angry easily, you need to develop strategies to cope with it. If anger does not present a problem, it does not mean that you won't find other areas that do.

Anger can be dealt with in many ways so that it does not build or prove to be destructive. Many people find "venting", i.e. talking about what bothers them, to be a very effective tool for managing anger. Others find more help through exercising and releasing energy or frustration. Like most things in life, the most effective tool is the one that works for you. Experiment with different coping strategies. One day try exercising and another day try talking. You might even want to try keeping a journal of what gets you angry so that you can identify triggers or be creative with other coping strategies.

Coping Styles

Coping strategies are also helpful when dealing with other strong emotions like depression or anxiety. Identifying triggers and experimenting with coping strategies can alleviate some of the intensity of these feelings. The purpose of developing strategies is to reduce the load placed on your shoulders by these feelings. For example, if you are feeling very anxious all day long, the relief of feeling anxious for only some of the day is welcome. Ideally, it would be nice to get rid of the anxiety altogether, but this is usually an impossible goal.

There is often a discrepancy between what we feel and what we think we should feel. This may translate into the belief that coping with infertility means never feeling sad or angry.

"I see pregnant women everywhere. The other day I realized all the women in my office were either pregnant or had just delivered in the last year.... It has gotten to the point where I don't like going to the mall because I'll either see big bellies or strollers. Then I feel mean and hateful. I didn't used to be like this."

Debbie, age 36

Feelings are never right or wrong. What we do with our feelings can be. If someone were to say to you, "I'm so angry I could kill you", would they be wrong? However, if they actually harmed you, then there would be agreement that the behavior was wrong.

Feelings about infertility are neither right nor wrong; we do not always agree about the "rightness" or "wrongness" of how we handle the feelings. Avoiding baby showers may be considered the "right" way to handle upset feelings about infertility. Others may consider avoidance "wrong". This conflict can occur within a couple where one partner feels that their behavior is a reasonable response to the infertility while the other does not. Or there may be a family situation where non-attendance at a family shower, christening or briss would be considered selfish, mean or evidence of poor coping styles. The infertile individual may view non-attendance as 1) an essential coping technique for him or herself, or; 2) as a favor to the family to not appear and be weepy or upset. Two different people can view the same behavior very differently and, in this case, both are convinced they are right because of their own point of view.

There are no prescriptions about handling different pregnancy related situations. Remember that you can always make a different choice at a later date. If baby showers are too difficult in the middle of a cycle, send a gift and a note and choose to attend a shower where it will not be harmful to you. Catalogues can provide an alternative to the baby department in the store. If not attending a family christening would be very hurtful to a beloved family member, make a strategy to work with the situation: 1) try talking to the family members; 2) work on your treatment plan and options prior to the christening to ward off feelings of hopelessness; 3) sit in the back of the church where tears may not attract attention, or; 4) have key support persons surround you during the christening.

It is not necessary for your partner to have feelings identical to yours to make going through infertility easier. It can be helpful that both of you have different feelings. Some men and women mistake the differences between them for lack of feelings or caring. Usually, differences reflect coping styles and not underlying feelings.

"I feel so useless when my wife cries. I should be able to fix things, or at least help her. But whatever I say seems to make the situation worse. She knows I love her, but she thinks I don't care as much as she does. I care. I just don't think crying about it helps."

Christopher, age 39

Some experts suggest that there are gender differences in coping styles with infertility, but the core feelings of wanting a child and the resulting sadness are similar regardless of gender.

If talking about the infertility experience truly helps you, but not talking about it truly helps your partner, how do you reach a compromise? For some, compromise involves having a fifteen minute rule in the evenings in which you discuss the infertility for fifteen minutes (or whatever length of time you set) and infertility is not discussed for the rest of the evening. Others have utilized turn taking, where discussion takes place on certain nights and other nights are rest nights from talking. Obviously, any plan needs to be flexible enough to account for new information or major events.

Intimacy

As mentioned before, infertility can be tremendously isolating. This isolation can extend to the relationship between the couple and their feelings of intimacy. Both partners can be worn down from the demands of treatment, both physical and emotional. Patience can run dry depending on how each partner is feeling during the cycle.

"We used to talk on the phone during the work day to catch up on the day. I really enjoyed hearing about his day and the problems at work. Now, I'm so exhausted by the fertility stuff that I don't have the energy to really listen... I want an evening back where we aren't tired, where we don't have ISSUES to discuss."

Amy, age 35

Communication can become focused on infertility and everyday events are shelved in favor of dealing with the latest news or crisis. Couples can feel "out of touch" with one another as a result.

As treatment continues, many couples will report a return of intimacy. If communication is good between the partners, infertility can be the uniting force against a world that is not in emotional synch with them. It is not uncommon to hear couples state that infertility has brought them closer together. However, many couples find that communication gets increasingly difficult as energy is drained and emotions run high.

Partners must be able to communicate with each other even though they may not completely understand the other's reactions or feelings. Couples need to be united in their goals, whether this means agreeing on a treatment course or supporting each other's coping style. Sometimes, having other support sources, e.g. friends, family members, support groups or books, allows couples to preserve their intimacy because they are relieving the burden that infertility places on the relationship.

Sexual intimacy can also be greatly affected by infertility. Once couples get into treatment, they become acutely aware of ovulation time and the need to have sexual intercourse. For some treatments, the doctor's office will instruct the couple when to have intercourse according to the results of an ovulation predictor kit. Spontaneity rarely begins with a call from the doctor's office.

"It is hard to feel romantic and warm when there is a cast of thousands in the bedroom. I feel like they make an announcement on the loudspeaker at the doctor's office to alert all staff to the fact my wife and I are going to make love that night. Sex is scheduled like doing the laundry and making dinner. I'm not sure I remember what spontaneous is anymore."

David, age 33

Sex can become a task for the couple. Embedded in the task is a great deal of pressure to attempt pregnancy in that cycle. Men will report resentment at feeling like they are the "sperm suppliers" and their partners are not interested in them or their feelings. In addition, there is tremendous pressure to perform. If the man fails to be aroused, he may feel that he has failed his wife in helping her to get pregnant or he may feel that he is less masculine by not being able to be aroused on command.

To retain sexual intimacy, it is helpful to recognize the pressures and limitations infertility places on the relationship. Despite what many people who have not gone through infertility suggest, it is not always fun to have to have sex. Acknowledge the predicament together; then look at ways to find some humor about the situation.

Try to accommodate the stress and find methods of reintroducing intimacy. The process may involve planning sexual relations earlier in the evening than right before bed or it could involve taking turns in initiating foreplay. As everyone knows, the most sensitive sexual organ is the brain. It may be helpful to start any sexual intimacy with telling your partner how much you love him or her; this ensures that communication is part of the sexual relationship. Romance can also be added as part of the timed intercourse as well as for the other parts of the cycle. Some couples find it nice to add non-intercourse sexual encounters between their prescribed sexual activities. This type of encounter involves sexual touching without the goal of intercourse. Having time for backrubs, showers together, or foreplay during the month can add a sense of intimacy and fun to the relationship.

Work and Play: To tell or not to tell?

There is no simple answer with regard to whether or not to share your infertility with friends, family or others at work. The decision to share is a deeply personal one and has many considerations. First, it is important to know whether disclosure would feel like a violation of your privacy or a relief. Obviously, these feelings would give strong guidance about whether to disclose your infertility. Second, consider the person(s) to whom you are disclosing. Are they people who have shown sensitivity and support in the past? Last, it is important to identify the goal of sharing or not sharing.

For many, the goal of not sharing is to protect privacy and/or to avoid managing others' feelings, reactions and questions. For others, the goal of sharing is to reduce the sense of being alone or the burden of keeping the feelings engendered by the infertility locked up inside. For most people the decision to share or not share falls somewhere in the middle. Many select key support people with whom they share their infertility but remain private with others. The need to tell or not tell also will fluctuate as you go through treatment and it is important to revisit the issue from time to time as cycles progress and treatment changes.

Work is complicated with regard to disclosing because disclosure may have very real consequences. Unfortunately, some work environments may have a prejudice against promotion or work assignments to an employee who is trying to get pregnant, e.g. being put on the "Mommy track". Yet, for women whose treatment requires regular visits to the doctor or early morning monitoring through blood tests and ultrasound, not disclosing to their employer presents other problems.

Due to the time demands, some women have chosen to inform only key supervisors with the understanding that the information will go no further. Other women have elected to share with a wider circle of co-workers because there is less stress in having everyone aware of the situation. Yet others have kept their privacy and were able to negotiate flexible schedules for their treatment times.

Should you choose to disclose to friends, family or co-workers, it is important to remember that you can still set boundaries. In other words, you may share your information and instruct the people with whom you share about how you want that information handled. You can ask that the information not be shared with anyone else; you can request that they ask questions or not ask questions about your treatment. There is latitude to share the infertility but keep private the times you are actually in cycle. Most people whom you will tell will be grateful for guidelines about how they can help you, e.g. whether they should ask about the infertility or wait for you to tell them more.

RESOLVE

An excellent resource for infertile men and women is RESOLVE, a non-profit group dedicated to the support, education and advocacy surrounding infertility. Based near Boston, the national organization also has local chapters. Many of the local chapters offer information sessions, conferences, support groups, and telephone support networks. For information or membership, you can write or call (617) 623-0744. Or contact RESOLVE through their Website: www.resolve.org.

Resources
1 Choosing Assisted Reproduction:
   Social, Emotional and Ethical Considerations.
   Susan Cooper and Ellen Glazer. Perspectives Press, 1998.
2 How to Be a Successful Fertility Patient.
   Peggy Robin. Quill, 1993.
3 What to Expect when you're Experiencing Infertility: How to Cope with the Emotional Crisis and Survive.
   Debby Peoples and Harriet Ferguson. W.W. Norton & Company, 1998.

Donor Insemination
   Helping the Stork: The Choices and Challenges of Donor Insemination.
   Carol Frost Vercollone, Heidi Moss, and Robert Moss. MacMillan, 1997.

Gestational Carrier
   A Matter of Trust: The Guide to Gestational Surrogacy.
   Gail Dutton. Clouds Publishing, 1997.

Pregnancy Loss
   Surviving Pregnancy Loss: A Complete Sourcebook for Women and their Families.
   Rochelle Friedman and Bonnie Gradstein. Citadel Press, 1996.

Adopting After Infertility
   Adopting After Infertility.
   Patricia Irwin Johnston. Perspectives Press, 1996.

Childfree Living
   Sweet Grapes: How to Stop Being Infertile and Start Living Again.
   Jean Carter and Michael Carter. Perspectives Press, 1998.

9

Treatment of Ovulatory Problems

Do Fertility Drugs Cause Cancer?

Let's deal with the unpleasant stuff first. Much of what follows is essentially a distillation of an excellent review of the question concerning a possible link between use of fertility enhancing drugs and ovarian cancer written by Richard Paulson (J Assist Repro Gen,13: 751, 1996). Ovarian cancer is the fifth leading cause of cancer related death in women with an average age of 54 at the time of diagnosis. A genetic pre-disposition has long been recognized, and certain dietary patterns have been implicated in increasing the risk. Use of "dusting powder" containing talc applied to the vulva is blamed for some ovarian cancers, since particles presumed to be talc granules can be found microscopically in the tumors, having gotten there by being carried up passively through the reproductive tract. These small particles then act as irritants inducing cancer in some physical-chemical fashion. The known reproductive links to ovarian epithelial cancer (which accounts for 80% of ovarian cancers) include continuous ovulation and lack of pregnancy and delivery. Known protective factors are use of birth control pills (with the decrease in ovarian cancer proportionate to the total duration of pill use), and breast feeding, both of which reduce the number of total ovulations over a reproductive life time. Therefore, one might suppose that infertility associated with anovulation might actually be protective, or at least neutral. The truth, however, is the opposite.

The first study which strongly suggested a link between use of fertility drugs and ovarian cancer was published by Whittmore et al (Am J Epidemiol, 136: 1184,1992). An odds ratio, statistically adjusted to OR = 27.0 (CL= 2.3-315.6) was given for infertile women with drugs used vs. women not infertile. Infertile women who did not use drugs had an adjusted OR=1.6 (CL= 0.74-3.3). We know from our previous statistical discussions that the variation in the first calculation is tremendous, and that the second risk factor is statistically not significant because the low-end of the confidence limits falls below 1. This study had large numbers of subjects, but out of 34 cancers occurring in infertile women, only 12 had ever used fertility drugs. Thus, the conclusions were based on a small number of actual cases. It also should be noted that when a pregnancy was achieved in the previously infertile group the relative risk became 0.6 (less than the controls) and continued to drop with succeeding pregnancies. The history of use of these agents was on a recall basis rather than from medical records, thus introducing a significant potential for error. The main criticism, however, had to do with the fact that the data for this study were originally collected between 1956 and 1986. Given the fact that the mean age for ovarian cancer diagnosis is 54, these women would have been taking drugs about 20 years or more previously. Clomiphene citrate was not approved for use in the United States until 1967, and the first human menopausal gonadotropic agent approved for use was Pergonal in 1969. Therefore, the likelihood of any of these patients using these drugs is small.

Upon the heels of the first disturbing report there appeared another epidemiologic study attempting to link use of clomiphene citrate with ovarian cancer (Rossing, et al. N Engl J Med, 331: 771, 1994). The group of women studied had been evaluated for infertility in the Seattle area between 1974 and 1985. In 3,837 patients,11 tumors were found, of which only four were invasive epithelial; five were borderline tumors and two were granulosa cell tumors. Compared with matched controls, the adjusted OR was 2.3, CL 0.5-11.4, for any clomiphene citrate use (obviously not significant). Further analysis, using as a criterion 12 or more monthly cycles with the drug, gave an adjusted OR=11.1 (CL = 1.5-82.3). No increased risk was found for the association with clomiphene citrate used for less than 12 cycles. Epidemiologists who conduct these kinds of studies concentrate on associations which may or may not be cause and effect related. The suggestion that there was a threshold at 12 months is biologically not plausible. Again, conclusions were based on a small number of frank invasive cancers. The clomiphene citrate link was not found in a study done in Israel. Three other studies done in Europe, where these agents have been used for a longer duration, failed to show any linkage. A more recent study from Italy (Parazzini et al Hum Repro, 12: 2159, 1997) with 971 women below the age of 75 with documented invasive epithelial ovarian cancer vs. 2758 controls showed no difference for ovarian cancer risk between infertile women taking fertility drugs and controls . A Danish study published in 1997 (Mosgaard et al, Fertil and Steril, 67:1005,1997) concluded that infertility without medical treatment produced a roughly twofold risk for ovarian cancer vs. controls. Treatment with fertility drugs did not increase this risk whether the patients got pregnant or not.

Confused? So are we. A dispassionate review of the literature on the subject would have to conclude that a case for an increased risk of ovarian epithelial cancer as a consequence of taking fertility drugs has not been made. Dealing with the infertile population subset that already has an increased risk makes for statistical land mines. Moreover, variables such as prior use of birth control pills known to ameliorate the risk introduce additional confounding variables. There's no question that this issue bears close scrutiny, but let me point out that there is no argument over the conclusion that infertile women who take these drugs and deliver become low-risk rather than high risk individuals.

Causes of Ovulation Disorders and Some Cures

Ovulation is the key to conception. In most fertility practices, ovulatory disturbance accounts for 30% to 40 % of patient flow. For ovulation to occur, a cascade of hormonal products must be produced in proper sequence in the right amount and at the right time. It's no great wonder that even a mild disturbance in this sensitive system is enough to cause big trouble. Thyroid malfunction can certainly interfere with ovulation, but mild defects have little or no connection. Signs and symptoms of thyroid over or under activity are usually so dramatic that diagnosis already has been made before the patient is seen by a fertility doctor. Hypothyroidism is easily managed with oral synthetic hormonal supplements. Hyperthyroid states can usually be managed with medication, but may eventually require surgery or a radioactive approach. The adrenal gland can also malfunction, making too much or not enough of its vast hormonal mix. As discussed previously, the adrenal glands can be screened with serial stimulation and suppression tests. Tumors can be differentiated with CAT scans and with MRI. Most of the time when the adrenal glands are the reproductive culprit the problem is one of simple over production of testosterone and related androgens. The solution is equally straightforward, and consists of orally administered small doses of Prednisone or similar cortisone-like drugs. This serves to suppress the overall activity of the adrenals with reduction specifically of the androgens.

In some women, estrogen levels do not increase enough in the follicular phase to cause LH release as the natural trigger for ovulation. A very simple, low-tech method of dealing with this is to give estrogen in small gradually increasing amounts to stimulate a normal train of events. Figure 9.1 illustrates this concept, using conjugated equine estrogens, (Premarin) 0.3 mg in each tablet. This is a very old form of therapy which pre-dates use of clomiphene citrate. It has none of the disadvantages associated with that drug, which will be discussed shortly. On the other hand, it works in a relatively small proportion of patients. Note that this is, indeed, a low dose estrogen protocol, since use of higher doses will be counterproductive, causing suppression rather than stimulation of ovarian function as seen with doses comparable to those used in oral contraceptive pills. As old as this protocol is, conjugated estrogens have never been approved for this use, as they are for menopausal hormonal replacement. Many of the hormonal treatments mentioned are not Food and Drug Administration (FDA) approved for that specific indication, although the drug itself has been registered and approved for other uses. This is not unusual, since surveys reveal that 30% of all prescriptions are for drugs used in circumstances other than that for which they were originally approved. Additionally, doses that were used for the registration consideration in pre-approval drug trials are exceeded in everyday practice.

Very often hCG (human chorionic gonadotropin) is given in conjunction with the low dose estrogen protocol when ultrasound examination demonstrates a follicle of mature appearance. The hCG acts as a surrogate for LH, causing ovulation to occur about 36-40 hours after a single injection of 5,000 or 10,000 units (Pregnyl or Profasi). This use for hCG is also not FDA or HPB approved, although it has been used for 40 years and is the hormone which naturally rises during early pregnancy.

A number of different disturbances in the area of the pituitary and hypothalamus can cause major ovulatory disturbance. Pituitary tumors of various cell types can be responsible, but in addition to the amenorrhea which usually occurs, other symptoms such as severe chronic headaches and loss of visual fields points to a CAT scan for definitive diagnosis. Most of the time these tumors can be removed by a neurosurgeon and menstrual function restored with or without medication. When the hypothalamus for some inexplicable reason decides to go into a resting state, the pituitary stops releasing FSH, the ovaries go into metabolic hibernation, and the patient becomes amennorheic and estrogen deficient. Neither the estrogen approach nor clomiphene citrate will usually work in this circumstance; use of the injected gonadotropins is almost always necessary. When

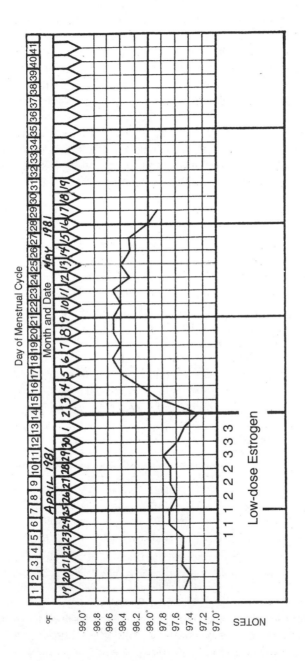

FIGURE 9.1 BBT recording of an ovulatory cycle with use of serially increasing oral doses of estrogens.

amennorhea and estrogen deficiency result from an excess of prolactin from a very small tumor in the pituitary or from excessive cell activity, medication can solve the problem with prompt restoration of menses and cessation of **galactorrhea** (milk discharge from the breasts) if it is present. Because pregnancy is, itself, a stimulus for prolactin secretion even before delivery, these very small tumors may grow and cause pressure on the optic nerves which pass close to the gland. When a tumor has been demonstrated, following the patient through the pregnancy with examination of the fullness of the optical fields by an ophthalmologist is necessary. Remember that sometimes clinically inapparent hypothyroidism with TSH elevation as the only abnormal test result may be responsible for prolactin elevation. Bromocryptine was the first drug really useful in control of prolactin excess. Taken once or twice daily, it is also associated with some annoying side effects such as nasal stuffiness, headache, gastrointestinal upset, and sometimes low blood pressure related to sudden changes in body position. Much of these can be avoided if a tablet is inserted daily into the vagina instead of the oral route. Absorption is better, and the dose necessary to restore normal prolactin levels is less. Now that we have cabergoline as a twice weekly oral medication with few side effects, women who tolerate bromocryptine poorly have an excellent alternative.

Heroin is one of the agents which can be extracted from opium, grown from poppies in many parts of the world. Morphine is a derivative of this family of biologicals. But we all manufacture similar compounds which are active in our central nervous system, called collectively **opiods.** The cells acted upon by these molecules have, quite naturally, opiod receptors on their surface. A group of pharmacologic agents known as opiod receptor blockers, as the name implies, can occupy these receptor sites and thereby inhibit any opiod effect whether from naturally produced compounds or from exogenously administered drugs that might be given as part of a normal surgical anesthetic protocol or associated with illegal drug use. These blocking drugs are almost always used intravenously as narcotic antagonists, but some, such as naltrexone, are active orally. What has this to do with ovulation? Well it seems that some women who are anovulatory and fail to respond to clomiphene citrate, have high levels of naturally produced opiods floating around in their brain, because when given this drug, many will start to ovulate with or without use of clomiphene citrate. This, of course, is preferable to the usual next step of switching to the external gonadotropins such as Follistim (Puregon) or Gonal-F, which are expensive, need to be given by injection, and which are more often associated with hyperstimulation and multiple birth. This form of therapy for resistant anovulation has some following in Europe, but definitely is not blessed by the FDA. Because the market is small, and the trials necessary for approval expensive, naltrexone, although approved and marketed in the United States for other indications, probably will never be submitted for this purpose. It seems to be most helpful in cases of hypothalamic shutdown of gonadotropin releasing hormone (GnRH) associated with amenorrhea. Success in restoring ovulation is usually reached within a month, so that a long, drawn-out trial of therapy is not necessary. Anovulation may return promptly when the drug treatment is stopped. This seems to be quite safe, and I have used this treatment with some success, but it is definitely not main stream therapy.

Polycystic Ovarian Syndrome

Before discussing the two main stalwarts of ovulation induction, clomiphene citrate and the gonadotropins, we need to spend a little time on the **polycystic ovarian syndrome** (PCOS), which in one form or another is responsible for a major proportion of ovulatory problems. First, it has been recognized for years that there seems to be a familial pattern, with inheritance best explained as an autosomal dominant, meaning that it can be transmitted by either parent as a single copy of the gene, and does not need to be present in both copies of the gene in order to be clinically important as is the case with most recessive gene disorders. Premature balding of one's father has been associated with an increased incidence of PCOS. The gene controls some of the steps in production of the androgens, which usually can be demonstrated to be elevated in PCOS patients. But this one gene explanation is probably over-simplified because of new findings implicating carbohydrate and insulin metabolism as important factors.

What is PCOS and how is it diagnosed? A group from the Middlesex Hospital in London (Hum Repro, 10:2107,1995), screened all patients referred to the reproductive endocrine clinics with a pelvic ultrasound and hormonal profile. The typical appearance of the PCOS ovary is one of an enlarged organ with multiple small cysts or follicles around the periphery of the outer shell (cortex) of the ovary. A population of 1741 women who met ultrasonic criteria and who did not have another endocrine disorder responsible for increased androgens formed the final study group. The mean LH level for the entire group was elevated, but 60% fell into the normal range; the same picture held true for the ratio of LH to FSH, which was >2:1 for the group, but which was not invariably elevated. An elevated testosterone concentration was recorded in 29%. Body mass index measurements defined 38% as obese. **Oligomenorrhea** (infrequent menses) was present in 47%, 30% had normally occurring cycles, 19% had amenorrhea (no menses), 3% had frequent bleeding episodes in the abnormal interval range, and 1% had heavy menses. **Hirsutism,** excessive hair growth on the trunk, arms and face, was noted as mild in 21%, moderate in 41%, and severe in 5% of the group. Acne was present in 35%. Of the 465 who had attempted pregnancy, 49% had primary infertility, 26% were secondarily infertile, and 25% were of proven fertility. Taking all the data into account, the ovarian ultrasound appearance was the single most diagnostic piece of information. Even this has its problems with respect to reproductive prediction, since 25% of the patients in the study with ultrasonic findings compatible with PCOS had proven to be fertile. Previous studies of groups of "normal" women with regular menses and without hirsutism have found a prevalence of about 20% of PCOS according to ultrasonic studies. Just as there is a significant overlap of hormonal values between normal patients and those with PCOS, there also seems to be lack of a clear-cut ultrasonic definition.

The biochemical markers traditionally employed are a LH/FSH ratio > 2:1 or 2.5:1, depending on the author, and high levels of testosterone and androstenedione. Besides blood levels reflecting menstrual cycle timing, concentrations of these hormones will change significantly as spurts are released from the ovary (shown in previous studies where samples were taken every 20 or 30 minutes). Not all patients are obese, but in those who are, diabetes is present in 10%.

The typical clinical presentation of a PCOS patient is one with infertility (if she is attempting pregnancy), menstrual disturbance as documented above, and perhaps a family history of similar symptoms and signs in a sister. She will tend to be obese, have oily skin, and possibly acne, especially if she is of Mediterranean heritage. Hirsutism, expressed as increased hair on the chin, and along the jaw line just in front of the ear may be disturbing to the patient. Increased hair on the forearm is nonspecific. Inspection of the scalp and the hairline will usually reveal some temporal thinning, as a male-type balding pattern, and **alopecia,** as a decrease of hair density in the midline of the scalp. When the patient disrobes, increased midline abdominal hair is frequently apparent, sometimes with loss of the typical female pubic hair pattern of an inverted triangle. Increased hair around the breast nipples is a nonspecific finding. Patients with increased insulin levels may show a curious velvet-like elevated, pigmented skin change around the neck and upper torso called **acanthosis nigricans.** The story of PCOS, insulin, and insulin-like growth factors and binding proteins is still evolving, and I will simplify and shorten what are thought to be the important aspects of the tale. Patients with PCOS often exhibit what is known as "peripheral insulin resistance". In order to maintain normal blood glucose levels, the pancreas works overtime and releases large amounts of insulin. Insulin is known to sensitize those cells in the ovary responsible for androgen production to LH. Although there is a surge of LH at ovulation, it is released from the pituitary throughout the cycle, causing the sensitized ovary to manufacture an excess of androgens. A number of drugs which can be taken orally have the ability to reduce the resistance to insulin, and can actually reverse this entire process with restoration of normal hormonal profile, and even ovulatory menstrual cycles. PCOS patients, who previously did not ovulate with clomiphene citrate, even at high doses, frequently become responsive. While there is now a sizable literature on use of these drugs primarily for improvement of reproductive performance, this is not an FDA-approved indication, and therefore you may meet with some resistance when mentioning it as a possible therapeutic approach. Weight loss, alone, has been associated with normalization of many of the biochemical markers associated with PCOS syndrome. A sustained, effective weight loss program producing a significant amount of loss, in the neighborhood of 15% for those under 200 pounds, will result in a spontaneous pregnancy rate of about 20%. It has been our experience that few patients can sustain such a program on their own; crash diets and dietary bulk additives are notorious for ultimate failure because basic abnormal eating habits remain unaltered. The best results are attained with programs like Weight Watchers, based on sensible dieting, education and peer pressure.

Ovulation induction protocols for PCOS patients are similar to those employed for anovulation in general with the exception that there seems to be a wider spectrum of response. Some PCOS patients are extremely resistant to the actions of clomiphene citrate but tend to hyperrespond to the gonadotropins, which must be given very carefully to avoid severe hyperstimulation. This will be discussed shortly, but first, to complete the approach to induction of ovulation in the PCOS patient, we need to look at the rebirth of a surgical procedure which seems to have benefit in re-establishment of ovulation for these patients.

Ovarian Wedge Resection

In 1935, doctors Stein and Leventhal reported seven obese, hirsute women with menstrual disturbance treated by surgically removing a wedge of ovarian tissue at the time of laparotomy in the same fashion as one would cut and remove a serving of pie. Indeed, PCOS for many years was known as the Stein-Leventhal syndrome. While many investigators reported results with surgery that were reasonably good with restoration of normal menses, pregnancy rates over the years were somewhat disappointing, and were assumed to be less than expected, given the ovulation rates, because of adhesions which formed between the tubes and ovaries. The beneficial effect on restoration of normal menstrual function was sometimes transient, but could just as often last for years.

As laparoscopic surgery became established as a viable alternative to laparotomy for many procedures, attention was once again directed toward a surgical solution to the PCOS problem. To date, the literature dealing with laparoscopic surgery for PCOS syndrome over the last decade is clear enough to draw some general conclusions. First, the procedure is quite different in concept from the classical wedge resection. The laparoscopic techniques all involve making small punctures in the outer portion of the ovary, preferably into the superficial cysts which define PCOS. Electrosurgical and laser energy systems have been used with equal results; just mechanically passing a needle into the cyst wall to allow the fluid to drain may be just as good. Of great interest is the fact that hormonal levels in the bloodstream which previously were abnormal, revert to normal within a few days after surgery, with FSH rising, LH falling, and androgens declining as well. The exact mechanism to explain this is still a mystery.

Pregnancy rates with reasonable duration of postoperative follow-up are usually reported in a range of 35% to 55%, rising to over 60% for patients who additionally receive medical therapy for ovulation induction. In most series, patients having this surgical treatment have been selected because they failed to respond to clomiphene citrate and the gonadotropins. Occasionally, patients were offered a choice, and although this was not a true randomized process, the pregnancy rates for medical vs. surgical therapy were about the same. The discrepancy between pregnancy rates and ovulation rates was small even though it has been demonstrated that some mild adhesions may form as a consequence of the procedure. The beneficial effect on ovulation may last for months or even years after surgery. Compared with use of gonadotropins, surgery offers considerable benefits including avoidance of the increased risk of multiple gestation, no need for intensive monitoring, no risk of hyperstimulation and the probability of a long-lasting effect. The downside includes the risk of the surgery itself (quite low) and probable formation of some adhesions between tubes and ovaries (which doesn't seem to make any difference). Another possible benefit of the surgery has to do with lowering the LH levels, which not only spur androgen production, but which also are thought to increase the miscarriage rate. There is increasing evidence that PCOS patients with high LH levels who conceive have higher miscarriage rates than the general infertile population, and that these rates can be reduced by pre-treating with agents like GnRH analogs (such as Lupron) or by laparoscopic surgery.

The present paradigm for treatment of infertility in PCOS patients who are anovulatory calls first for a trial with clomiphene citrate, followed by gonadotropins, if need be, with surgery or IVF as a last resort. But the surgical approach is becoming more popular, and on a cost per baby level is as attractive as gonadotropins with the added advantage of long-term reduction of the other clinically troublesome effects of PCOS.

Clomiphene Citrate

The best recent review of clomiphene citrate (CC) is that of Dickey and Holtkamp (Hum Repro Update, 2:483, 1996). The first author is one with long clinical experience with the drug; the second helped to develop it while working in the pharmaceutical industry. This section will start with a summary of that review. After clinical trials, and FDA approval, the drug was introduced in the United States in 1967. Clomiphene citrate is actually a mixture of two very similar forms of the same molecule having both estrogenic and anti estrogenic actions in various parts of the body. It is marketed in the United States under the trade names of Serophene and Clomid. In places where it is made by generic manufacturers (the patent has long ago run out), there may be some concern over batch-to-batch variation because of the manufacturing process yielding slightly different proportions of the two molecules.

This drug, which is not a steroid according to its structure, revolutionized treatment of anovulation because of the high percentage of patients with a positive response. It soon became apparent, however, that the ovulation rate was roughly twice that of the conception rate. What are the reasons for the great discrepancy? The first obvious answer is the presence of other factors in the couple which adversely affect fertility, such as a seminal or tubal problem. Less obvious, but true, is the fact that serial ultrasound studies indicate that as many as 25% of CC cycles with hormonal, endometrial biopsy, and BBT changes suggestive of ovulation are unassociated with actual physical extrusion of the egg from its follicle. Subsequent studies have indicted CC as exerting anti estrogenic effects on cervical mucus and the endometrium which are counterproductive to initiation of pregnancy.

The usual starting dose of CC is a 50 mg pill, given for five days, commencing on the fourth or fifth day of the menstrual cycle. Half of the dose has been eliminated from the body in five days after the last dose, but excretion continues for six weeks. Because its action is mainly at the hypothalamic level, and because certain compounds in the bloodstream enter the brain with difficulty, it is important that the total daily dose be taken at one time. Because the estrogen receptors in the hypothalamus become occupied by CC without an estrogen response, gonadotropin releasing hormone (GnRH) is increased, with the result that FSH levels are increased and ovarian stimulation occurs. Patients with a hypothalamus unable to respond in this fashion are CC resistant. While the initial dose is usually 50 mg, there is a weight-related dose response curve. Although FDA approved to 100 mg daily, doses of up to 250 mg have been employed. Some doctors have found that over 150 mg daily, extending the treatment from five to up to ten days is more helpful than dose increase. Ovulation usually occurs 5-9 days after the last dose but may be as early as three or as late as 11. Figure 9.2 depicts a common BBT chart response to ovulation induction with 100 mg daily of CC given for five days. If ultrasound is employed as a monitor of follicular development, it is important to realize that follicular maturity is not reached at the usual diameter in unstimulated cycles of about 20 mm but at 24 mm - 26 mm, which is key if hCG is to be used as a surrogate for the LH surge. Because of its anti estrogenic action on cervical mucus and the endometrium, the lowest dose that provokes ovulation should be used. A satisfactory postcoital test obtained prior to CC use needs to be repeated once therapy is begun.

The literature is divided on the question of whether adding estrogen will counteract the adverse effect of CC on cervical mucus. Because estrogen levels are higher, sometimes by five-fold, at ovulation in CC cycles compared with spontaneous ovulation, adding more estrogen intuitively seems fruitless, especially considering that estrogen receptors in the cervix are occupied by CC for weeks. Both endometrial biopsy and ultrasonic assessment of endometrial thickness suggest that the anti-estrogen effect of CC is common. To make matters more confusing, CC has been used to treat luteal phase deficiency, but can also cause it.

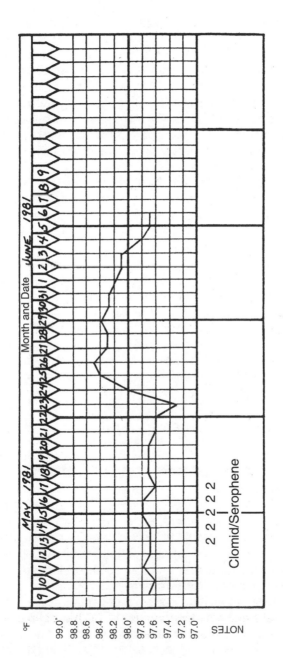

FIGURE 9.2 BBT recording of typical clomiphene citrate-induced ovulatory cycle.

In well chosen patients, apparent ovulation rates are over 80%, but pregnancy rates are in the 10% - 20% range monthly with a cumulative pregnancy rate of less than 50% at six months, which is the usual maximal duration of treatment currently recommended. Patients with elevated androgens, especially if the adrenal glands are involved, will have an improvement in pregnancy yield if small doses of steroids such as Prednisone are added daily. Because CC will usually induce multi-follicular development in both ovaries, there is an increase in multiple gestation which is not dose dependent. In most large series the twinning rate is between 6%-10% with triplets or higher order as 1%.

Ovarian enlargement as a concomitant to stimulation is expected but rarely reaches a size significant to be a clinical problem. Hot flashes occur in about 10% of the patients and actually can be interpreted as a good sign reflecting increased FSH release. Pelvic discomfort and breast tenderness have been reported usually as mild and transient side effects. Mood swings, particularly depression in patients with a history of depressive disorders, are common, but also self limiting. Because the curvature of the eye may slightly change, contact lenses may become tight, causing ocular symptoms and headaches. About 2% of patients report seeing halos or streaks of light, disturbing enough to stop therapy. The congenital abnormality rate in the offspring for major defects is no different than for the general population. There is some argument as to whether there might be a slight increase in cleft palate and anal stenosis, but if there is an increase, it seems to be on the border of statistical significance.

Ovulation Induction with Gonadotropins

Shortly after introduction of CC, human menopausal gonadotropins (hMG) became available for clinical use. Over the last thirty years many millions of gallons of urine obtained from menopausal women have been processed in order to extract FSH, present in high quantity as a consequence of the normal pituitary response to ovarian aging. Even after numerous purification steps, the final product always contains LH as an unnecessary and potentially deleterious contaminant. Additionally, even with strict quality control, there seems to be some evidence of significant batch-to-batch variation in potency. For many years Pergonal was the only preparation available in the United States. It continues to be marketed in ampoules containing 75 IU (USA and Canada) or 150 IU (USA only) of powdered drug which must be reconstituted in solution prior to injection. Serono, the manufacturer, is having increasing difficulty in maintaining the source of the preparation, and will probably phase out production as the recombinant pure FSH agent attains widespread use. Fertinex (Fertinorm in Canada) and Metrodin were improvements on the original product so far as purification and reduction of LH and inactive protein contaminants were concerned, but were still urinary based. Organon's hMG is known in the United States as Humegon, and is packaged in the same strengths as the Serono product. Ferring, a German-based large pharmaceutical company has been approved to market a similar product in the United States (not as yet in Canada) under the name of Repronex.

The shortcomings of the urinary-based preparations were appreciated for years, but the solution had to await perfection of recombinant genetic techniques. Once the DNA sequence which controls production of FSH was determined, it became possible to genetically engineer hamster cells in tissue culture to produce pure human FSH with no variation in potency and with no LH or other protein contaminant. Besides eliminating variation, these new forms of gonadotropin therapy can be self-injected just under the skin whereas the older forms were intramuscularly delivered. At the moment there's no orally active gonadotropin available, but research is intense in that area. Organon's drug is marketed in the United States under the name of "Follistim" and in Canada "Puregon" while the Serono product goes under the name of "Gonal-F" in both countries. The two are not completely identical, but no practical differences in terms of patient response have been identified. There is possibly one category of anovulatory patients who might need some trace amounts of LH in the preparation in order for optimal results to accrue. This is the patient with deep hypothalamic shutdown to the point of having virtually no endogenous LH in the bloodstream. While high-levels of LH may be deleterious to the developing egg, low levels become necessary for continued maturation prior to actual ovulation. Thus, some patients may do better with Humegon or Pergonal than the more pure drug. Pure LH has been developed as well, and could be given, when necessary, in precise doses.

Ovulation induction with gonadotropins, either hMG, or pure FSH, often written as r-FSH to denote the recombinant origin, is indicated in a variety of clinical situations. Certainly the first would be the patient with severe hypothalamic amennorhea with low FSH and estrogen levels, who usually will be refractive to CC stimulation. Examples include women with extremely low body mass from eating disorders or overconditioning, long distance runners, and those with various pituitary disorders. The next group includes those with normal or low FSH levels and some estrogen production who have not ovulated with CC or who have not conceived after six ovulatory CC cycles. This group includes the PCOS patient and garden variety anovulatory woman. The third situation relates to patients with incipient ovarian failure as a consequence of age, ovarian response to chemotherapy, or loss of ovarian substance from surgery. In this circumstance FSH levels are elevated, and the expectation of a satisfactory response must be lowered.

Ovulation induction, in normally ovulating women, is also used as an adjunct to fertility therapy with many names used to describe this process. Among the most popular is "controlled ovarian hyperstimulation" (COH). The largest number of patients in this category are those being stimulated within an IVF cycle in order to produce multiple eggs for retrieval. Additionally, COH is used in the treatment of unexplained infertility, endometriosis associated infertility, and a few other minor indications.

The protocol for ovulation induction varies according to the particular clinical situation. If the patient has PCOS, the dose schedule employed, at least for the first cycle, is apt to be on the low side because of the increased risk of a more than brisk response. Patients will usually have a similar ovarian response to stimulation from one cycle to the next, so that it is quite unusual for a patient to go from being a poor or slow responder to the opposite. Most patients will be started on two 75 IU ampoules daily, mixed together and given as a single injection either intra-muscularly or subcutaneously, depending on the specific drug used. Alternatively, a single 150 IU ampoule or vial may be used. More than sufficient diluent is supplied; FSH is very soluble, and the total volume needed to bring it into solution is quite small. Patients who already have demonstrated the need for large amounts of FSH may be started on as much as 450 IU daily, sometimes given in two equal doses. This seems to be the upper limit of dose over which increases have no effect. If the patient is in an IVF cycle, the philosophy of stimulation becomes different than in an office situation. In the former, the goal is to get as many eggs as is safely possible. In IVF there is some control over the multiple pregnancy rate according to the number of embryos placed into the uterus, but this does not hold true for office cycles with multi-follicular development and maturation. Generally speaking, the goal in an office cycle is to achieve maturation of 1-4 follicles with a corresponding estradiol concentration.

The first dose is usually given on menstrual cycle day 2-5, irrespective of whether the period was spontaneous or induced. Sometimes a baseline pelvic ultrasound will be obtained during the first few days of the cycle, particularly if the previous cycle was stimulated, in order to see if there are any residual ovarian cysts left over, whose presence, if unknown, might interfere with subsequent ultrasonic interpretation. Nothing much happens with respect to ultrasonic ovarian appearance or to serum estrogen levels for the first five days of stimulation. This is essentially the priming dose which sets the stage for what follows. We usually start to monitor estradiol levels after five days of stimulation. When rising values indicate increasing follicular maturation, ultrasound is added. We are interested in the number of maturing follicles, their rate of growth, and the relationship to the estradiol values. Figure 9.3 is an example of a typical office-based ovulation induction cycle with Follistim (Puregon), followed on a computer printout. The patient had been refractive to CC, and the decision was made to switch to Follistim (Puregon), starting with 2 ampoules of 75 IU each daily. On the fourth day of the cycle, the endometrial thickness (EM) on ultrasound was 6mm and there was a 16 mm cystic structure in the right ovary left over from the preceding CC cycle. Follistim (Puregon) (coded as "L") was given on days 4 through 7 and the patient was assessed on day 8 at which time the estradiol (E2) was 180 pg, developing follicles were present, and the EM was 9 (the left over structure from the previous cycle had either become smaller or had vanished). Two more days at the same dose were given. On the 10th day, the estradiol had risen to 343 pg, and 5 potential developing follicles were visualized on the ultrasound with greatest diameters ranging from 10 through 15 mm. The same dose was employed for days 10 and 11, and by day 12 the estradiol was 545 pg, the two "lead" follicles had reached satisfactory size and the EM had increased to 12 mm (anything over 9 mm at this point is quite acceptable).

Figure 9.3 Office stimulation flow sheet

Pt. Name:	Account No.:	Age: 35 — Doctor: BG
Husband:		DOB: 00/00/00
Phone: 000-000-0000		Cycle #: 3
Cycle Type: 2	Started: 07/12/98 LMP 07/12/98	Donor Egg:
Suppressive: n	Started: 00/00/00 Stopped: 00/00/00	Embryo Freezing:
Planned Tx:		Cycle Type History: 032

The Diagnosis for this Evaluation consists of the following factors:

Med Protoc: L
Ordered: Luteal Prog & Coitus   Meds:

			Meds				Hormone Levels					Left Ovary		Right Ovary	
Date	Day	#	Dose F OralE Typ Ser LH FSH HCG Time PRO Typ	E2	LH	PRO FSH	Beta	EM	P	1 2 3 4 5 I ≤		1 2 3 4 5 I	
7/15/98	4	7	2L					6	3		F	16	1
7/19/98	8	9	2L	180				9	2	11 10	2 F	9	1
7/21/98	10	11	2L	343	3			9	2	15 13 11	3 F	10 10	2
7/23/98	12		10.0 6:00P	545	5			12	2	18 17 14	3 F	13 12	2
7/30/98	19			>40									
8/10/98	30			29			35						

The hCG was given and the patient was instructed to have coitus the next night (insemination was not suggested for this particular couple because we didn't believe it would add much in their case to the pregnancy rate). One week later the serum progesterone was monitored and was >40 ng, with anything over 20 ng quite satisfactory (note there was no progesterone supplementation used). Ten days later, about three days after the expected menses which did not appear, the β hCG titer indicating pregnancy was positive at 35 mIU. The patient used 16 ampoules, two daily, over the course of an eight day stimulation and produced, apparently, two mature follicles. She had four sets of blood tests during the cycle and an equal number of ultrasound examinations including the baseline—a fairly typical and quite satisfactory response.

As with a natural cycle, FSH is responsible for follicular development, but LH, or in this case hCG as a substitute, is required for ovulation. When the lead follicles have reached a critical size of 17-18 mm in diameter, hCG, usually 10,000 IU of Pregnyl (Organon) or Profasi (Serono) is given with the expectation that ovulation will start in about 38 hours. Therefore, if we're going to perform insemination, the hCG is given at midnight, and the semen specimen is delivered at 8 a.m., two mornings hence, processed and used for insemination at about noon. Note that the follicles do not develop in concert. We know from retrieval in IVF cycles that some are more mature than others. Ovulation of this "cohort" of eggs occurs not simultaneously, but over the course of a few hours. Some of the follicles which appear to be healthy by ultrasonic criteria, actually contain eggs which have ceased to continue development, and add nothing to fertility; these eggs are called "atretic". The hCG is withheld if results indicate that more than the maximum number of follicles desired have matured, increasing the risk of both hyperstimulation and high order multiple pregnancy. Some physicians use hormonal support routinely in the luteal phase of gonadotropic stimulated cycles in the form of progesterone vaginally, orally, or by injection with small booster shots of a hCG as a less popular alternative. Commonly, luteal phase progesterone levels are monitored about seven days after ovulation, and ovarian size is assessed by physical examination or ultrasonography.

The usual process of follicular development and maturation starts late in the cycle with a cluster of eggs being recruited for activation in the next cycle. From this cluster, or cohort, one follicle emerges as the dominant one, destined to become the source of the single egg released at ovulation. Occasionally, two follicles share the honors giving rise to non-identical twins. When gonadotropins are injected early in the cycle, the process of **atresia** in which all of the follicles except one cease development is abrogated, giving rise to multi-follicular ovulation. The hypothalamus and pituitary are programmed to release LH to cause ovulation at a point dependent upon estrogen levels and their rate of rise. This governing system cannot differentiate an estrogen level which is derived primarily from a single, almost mature egg, from an estrogen level resulting from six still immature eggs. This results in a tendency for LH to be released prematurely, causing adverse effects on the eggs or even ovulation of immature eggs. One way to get around this is to use the GnRH agonists which inhibit pituitary release of LH; we'll discuss that a little later.

The obvious goals of gonadotropin therapy are somewhat incompatible with each other. Up to a point, increasing the dose will increase the percentage of patients who ovulate and also will increase the number of eggs ovulated per patient with a corresponding increase in pregnancy rate. The downside of this is expressed as an increase in severe hyperstimulation syndrome which can be life-threatening, and an increase in multiple gestation with the latter carrying risks of increased miscarriage and extreme prematurity, to say nothing of the social, emotional, and financial aspects for the next eighteen years. Even with close monitoring of the patient, the therapeutic tightrope does not allow much leeway for error. A poor cycle which has to be canceled for lack of response still costs a great deal of money for drugs and studies. Canceling a cycle because of the risk at the other extreme is even harder to do, and many times patients and physicians are at odds under these circumstances.

The expected results are greatly dependent on the indication for therapy, the age of the female patient, and the presence of multiple adverse fertility factors. Generally, about 90% of patients will ovulate with gonadotropic therapy. Cycle fecundity rates are usually reported as falling between 15%-25% for the first three or four cycles after which there's a drop-off. For that reason, continued therapy past four cycles is discouraged. Patients with pure hypothalamic amennorhea have the highest pregnancy yield and usually require the least amount of drug. As with CC, there is a weight-related dose curve. The pregnancy rate for patients who previously have failed with CC is, not surprisingly, less. A study of women not conceiving with CC who later were treated with gonadotropins was done in Spain (Balasch et al, J Assist Repro Gen,13: 551, 1996). These women were treated with a low dose approach with safety being the prime concern. A total of 234 patients received a total of 534 cycles of treatment with hCG withheld in 65 cycles because of poor response and in 28 cycles because of over- response. Of the remaining 441 cycles, 95% were ovulatory, and according to ultrasound, only one dominant follicle developed in 47.3%.

Pregnancy was established by 39.7% of the patients with a cycle fecundity of 17.4% and a cumulative conception rate of 33.5% by the end of the second cycle. Twins were seen in 15% of pregnancies and the miscarriage rate was a low 10.8%. More than 80% of all pregnancies were achieved in the first three cycles of treatment. Small booster doses of hCG were used, but no cases of severe hyperstimulation were seen. I bring this study to your attention because it documents that even in what is considered to be a difficult group of patients, good results can be achieved in the absence of severe side effects with careful attention to detail.

Clomiphene citrate sometimes is used in conjunction with the gonadotropins for two different reasons. The first has to do with a cost-saving approach with the total dose of gonadotropins about half what would normally be used alone. Although employed enthusiastically by some practitioners, this is not a popular protocol, even considering the fact that a full cycle of Follistim (Puregon) or Gonal-F will cost close to US $1,000 for the drug alone. The use of the r-FSH preparations may well increase in the future due to a reduced availablity of the urinary products.

Side effects of gonadotropin therapy are mainly those which follow an over- enthusiastic ovarian response, which cannot always be avoided even with close supervision. Expect to have some degree of ovarian enlargement and pelvic fullness or discomfort; if you don't, the response was probably insufficient. Mild forms of hyperstimulation are limited to ovarian enlargement and slight discomfort. When the ovaries become really massive and porous, there is a shift of fluid from the cardiovascular system to the abdominal cavity and sometimes to the thorax. The blood volume becomes concentrated, kidney function decreases, and serum electrolytes are thrown out of balance. Under these circumstances, the patients can become hypercoagulable with the risk of forming clots or emboli in major blood vessels, lungs, or brain. This is certainly a serious complication, and the patient must be hospitalized for fluid management, and possibly prophylactic anti-coagulation. Fortunately, this degree of hyperstimulation occurs in less than three percent of cycles. The other complication has to do with the multiple pregnancy rate, with results widely varied according to whether a conservative or aggressive philosophy is followed with respect to stimulation and the number of potentially fertilizable eggs present at ovulation. The multiple pregnancy rates for gonadotropin used in the office as opposed to IVF cycles, run somewhere between 12% and 20%. The spontaneous abortion rate figures range from 12% through 29%, being largely dependent on the mean age of the population sampled.

Gonadotropin Releasing Hormone and Ovulation Induction

Naturally occurring GnRH is released in spurts from the hypothalamus and acts on the pituitary to cause release of stored FSH and LH. Because of the hyperstimulation potential and multiple gestation rate encountered with use of the gonadotropins, the concept of inducing ovulation with pulsatile bursts at 90-110 minute intervals of GnRH delivered intravenously or subcutaneously via a small pump has the appeal of offering a more physiologic, softer approach which employs the pituitary as an intermediary rather than bypassing it. This, however, turns out to be a technique which after at least 15 years of experience, has never become popular. True, most of the cycles produce one ripe egg, and the incidence of both hyperstimulation and multiple birth are dramatically reduced (but not to zero). Mitigating against wide-spread use is a low per cycle pregnancy rate and the need to wear a portable pump for about 25 continuous days, with venous phlebitis a risk of that route, and subcutaneous irritation with the other. You probably will have little or no success in finding a physician still using this method of ovulation induction.

The Role of GnRH Agonists in Ovulation Induction

If GnRH is given continuously, the pituitary first becomes stimulated to release FSH and LH, but this effect is transient, and soon the gland becomes suppressed in a process known as "down regulation". It was recognized that this would be very helpful in avoiding inappropriate release of LH during cycles of COH with gonadotropins. The problem is that the natural or native hormone is metabolized so quickly by the body that the concept was impractical. When the synthetic forms of GnRH were developed, built into the molecular structure were changes designed to retard the rate of metabolic breakdown and to increase potency. We now have available agents such as Lupron, which can be taken on a daily basis as a subcutaneous small injection like insulin (not the long acting monthly depot form used for treatment of endometriosis) and Synarel, a similar agent, delivered as a nasal spray. The usual course followed is to start the analog on the 21st day of the cycle; menses will occur on schedule or with a slight delay, and estrogen testing will document that the suppressive action has begun, usually by 10-12 days after initiation of analog treatment. At this point, stimulation with gonadotropins is begun, but the pituitary contribution to the total FSH level in the blood is nil, and LH release from the pituitary is minute. Probably 90% of all IVF cycles use this approach to safeguard against inappropriate LH release causing the cycle to be canceled prior to egg retrieval or having eggs of poor quality. On the otherhand, probably less than 10% of office COH cycles are run in conjunction with down regulation. Additional cost may be one factor— there is the cost of the analog which is considerable, and because patients who are down regulated require greater doses of gonadotropins, that cost also must be factored in. Until there is a multi-centric study documenting that routine down regulation for office COH reduces the cost per baby according to cycles initiated rather than completed (thus addressing the canceled cycle issue), it is unlikely that this will become a routine addition to the basic protocol. The claims that down regulation with the analogs produces a cluster or cohort of eggs which are more uniform in developmental stage and of better overall quality has not been universally accepted. The chief reason for analog suppression in gonadotropin stimulated cycles is to avoid inappropriate LH release.

The analogs have yet another role to play in ovulation induction. Because the initial response is that of stimulation, they can be given early in the cycle in conjunction with gonadotropins as a stimulus rather than started late in the preceding cycle and waiting for onset of suppression. This is known as the "flare", or short analog protocol. It has some value in poor responders, especially those with elevated FSH values. It is not widely used, and consensus is that routinely the long analog protocol is better than the short, perhaps in part, because LH levels are elevated with the short regimen. Waiting in the wings are true GnRH antagonists, used in Europe and currently in clinical trials in the United States. These agents have no stimulatory action, and cause immediate suppression of endogenous FSH and LH release.

10

The Cervix and Uterus in Reproduction

The cervix is the staging area for sperm about to ascend to the upper reproductive tract. Its crypts act as reservoirs for sperm; its normally alkaline mucus secretions protect sperm from the acid environment of the vagina. Changes in the cervix of a congenital nature, or those occurring after disease or surgery, may be responsible for infertility.

Disorders of the Cervix

The Diethylstilbestrol (DES) Syndrome

The reproductive effects of DES are now seen infrequently because its use as a hormonal supplement in pregnancy complicated by diabetes and in pregnancy threatened by abortion came to a halt close to 40 years ago. This is a potent synthetic agent which acts as an estrogen in the body although its chemical structure is quite different from the normally occurring estrogens. When exposed in utero during development of the reproductive system, changes can occur in the fetus which are present at birth (and therefore congenital) but which are not apparent on the usual newborn physical examination. Among these changes are clusters of glandular cells in the vagina called 'vaginal adenosis' which years later lead to a form of cancer in some patients. The DES affected cervix can assume a variety of different appearances, and because of the adenosis potential, it is often subjected to many biopsy and laser procedures with the result that a narrowing of the cervical canal is produced— cervical stenosis. Cervical mucus production which was often compromised to begin with as a consequence of the anatomic changes present at birth, is often made worse by the surgical procedures which tend to remove those cells that were responsible for mucus production, thereby creating a major impediment to sperm migration. We will cover the uterine aspects of this syndrome shortly. It is important to realize that almost any abnormality present at birth which is attributed to a drug exposure during pregnancy can occur spontaneously. That is true for the DES syndrome. Insemination with sperm being deposited directly into the uterine cavity can successfully bypass the cervical problem. The DES cervix has an obstetrical importance as well, since it may become unable to contain the growing pregnancy, and in some cases it dilates long before fetal maturity. This particular problem may be addressed directly by putting a stitch around the cervix as reinforcement; this is known as a cervical **cerclage.**

The Inflamed/Infected Cervix

Sometimes, when the cervix is inspected visually during a vaginal examination, it can appear as quite red and inflamed. Often this is nothing more than a cervical **eversion,** which is an innocent out-rolling of the endocervical canal lining in much the same fashion as the appearance when bluejeans are rolled up at the cuff. Too often this is treated as a disease process, and the cervix becomes abused with unnecessary procedures. Eversion and hyperplasia is commonly associated with long-term use of birth control pills and will regress after they are no longer taken without any adverse effect on fertility. True inflammation as a consequence of infection can produce a very hostile environment for sperm.

Cervicitis can result from a variety of organisms— bacterial, viral, fungi and as with chlamydia, an organism different from any of the above. Normally a variety of microorganisms reside in the vagina and cervix as usual inhabitants. Antibiotic treatment for any reason, such as with a sore throat or ear infection, can upset the balance which normally exists in the vagina causing an overgrowth of organisms resistant to that agent. Lactobacillus is the major inhabitant of the vagina, but it is quite sensitive to almost all of the antibiotics used today. Some women are on long-term or chronic antibiotic therapy which poses a therapeutic dilemma. One way of dealing with this situation is to use vaginal tablets containing lactobacillus to restore normal balance. Sometimes cervical cultures are helpful to identify bacteria which may be the source of the problem. A general culture will not identify chlamydia or gonococcus; a special specific culture medium readily available is necessary. By creating inflammation, acute and/or chronic herpes of the cervix can be a problem. Fortunately, frequent recurrences (not re-infections) can be controlled with orally administered anti viral medications taken daily for many months. As we've said earlier, ureaplasma is an organism which may or may not be a reproductive pathogen. Fortunately it, as well as chlamydia, is sensitive to tetracycline drugs, but both partners must be treated simultaneously, and the positive culture must be repeated after therapy to be sure that a cure, indicated by negative culture, has been achieved. Chlamydia, of course, has tubal connotations which far outweigh any negative cervical effects. An acute chlamydial infection is frequently associated with a thick, yellow cervical discharge. Yeast infections of the vagina and cervix are common, and usually can be treated with vaginal preparations or with a single dose of oral medication. The patient with recurrent infections should be screened for diabetes.

Most treatments for vaginal-cervical infections use orally administered agents and/or local vaginal medications such as creams, suppositories, or gels. Sometimes this is not sufficient, even when used repeatedly, as may be the case with chronic tonsillitis— but the cure is not to remove the cervix. The least invasive approach is to destroy the first few layers of surface cells using cold rather than heat. This process is known as **cryocautery,** which destroys cells by freezing and thawing without producing any scar tissue, and which doesn't cause widespread loss of the mucus producing cells. Use of a hot instrument, a true cautery, is to be discouraged. The initial hope that laser energy applied to the cervix could leave a border of unaffected tissue has not stood the test of time. An electrosurgical approach to diseased cervical tissue, the 'large loop excision procedure' (LEEP) seems to be associated with less negative reproductive effects on the cervix. When an abnormal pap smear demands a biopsy procedure to rule out cancer of the cervix, small bits of tissue can be taken under microscopic guidance **(culposcopy),** but sometimes a true **cervical cone biopsy** is necessary. In that case the procedure can be done taking the minimal amount of tissue necessary to make a diagnosis.

Cervical Mucus

Some women, even at ovulation, consistently produce cervical mucus which is inadequate in amount or quality. This can sometimes be improved with small doses of estrogen prior to ovulation. The risk is that at some point the dose of estrogen will be sufficient to inhibit ovulation as is the case with birth control pills. Cervical mucus which is acidic rather than alkaline does not offer safe passage for sperm. Cervical mucus pH can be tested with a strip of sensitive paper. An old remedy was to use an alkalinizing douche just before coitus. This doesn't work, because water and mucus don't mix. In some cases the pH of some of the secretions of the body can be modified by using six bicarbonate of soda or Alka-seltzer tablets taken orally as two tablets three times daily, for a few days preceding ovulation. This is occasionally successful, and should be given a try before initiating intra-uterine insemination (IUI) for poor postcoital test results in the presence of persistently acidic cervical mucus. Cough medicines which liquefy pulmonary secretions have been advocated as a therapeutic approach to cervical mucus problems. There has never been published a valid study which would suggest that this has any merit. The problem with cervical mucus deterioration as a consequence of clomiphene citrate use is not readily solved by adding estrogen just before ovulation, since estrogen levels are already many times normal. If there is an adverse effect, IUI may be considered, but the same changes seen in the cervical mucus may exist in the mucus present in the uterus and tubes as well. Usually this finding dictates an early switch to gonadotropin therapy for ovulation induction.

Cervical Stenosis

Cervical stenosis, with constriction of the cervical canal at the vaginal opening, throughout its length, or at the entrance to the uterine cavity can be caused by infection, but more often by surgery done as a biopsy procedure, to remove early cervical cancer while preserving fertility potential, and to treat chronic infection. Whatever the inciting cause, cervical stenosis can be very difficult to treat. While it is true that if blood and menstrual debris can exit the cervix, sperm should be able to ascend, the clinical picture is not that simple. Although the cervix can be dilated in the office or operating room, scar tissue tends to reform during the healing process with the net result one of little or no improvement. Placing a surgical drainage device in the canal during the healing interval keeps the raw tissues apart, and helps to ensure a good therapeutic result. This is an uncommon cause of infertility, but in the absence of any other factors, results following surgery can be dramatic with pregnancy achieved within a few months. Additionally, the severe cramping that some women have as a consequence of outlet obstruction to menstrual flow is relieved.

The Uterus

Infection and its Aftermath

Infection of the uterine lining **(endometritis)**, may occur in conjunction with pregnancy or from an infection acquired sexually or during insertion of an intrauterine device. Diagnosis is usually made based on symptoms of pain, utero-cervical discharge often rather ugly and odiferous, and sometimes fever. An endometrial biopsy gives a tissue diagnosis, and cultures of the endometrial cavity can be taken in order to pick the most appropriate antibiotic regimen. The uterus is amazingly resistant to permanent damage from these infections. Sometimes they become chronic, and diagnosis becomes difficult because blind endometrial biopsy may miss the involved areas. Hysteroscopy allows inspection of the entire uterine lining so that directed biopsy can be taken. Treatment is usually three weeks of tetracycline or a penicillin derivative.

The one type of infection which is most likely to cause permanent scar tissue formation within the uterine cavity is that associated with pregnancy. The quintessential example is the patient who has retained placental fragments which go unrecognized for a week or longer after delivery. Removing the now necrotic and infected tissue can be very difficult, and is usually performed with a sharp curette, because the tissue is so adherent to the wall of the uterus that suction instruments are ineffective. Whether the patient is breast feeding or not, estrogen levels are quite low in the first month following delivery. The **Asherman** syndrome of endometrial scarring with possible total obliteration of the uterine cavity is most likely to occur when the clinical situation is one of retained products of conception associated with infection and low estrogen levels. This also occurs following incomplete abortion, whether spontaneous or induced. Scar tissue interferes with implantation sites and with blood supply causing infertility and/or repeated miscarriage. In its most severe form, the cavity is totally obliterated, and the patient is completely amennorheic in spite of BBT charts and hormonal tests which indicate normal ovulatory function.

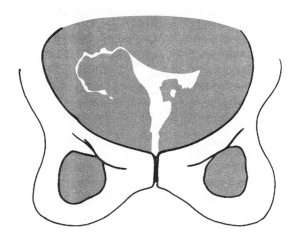

FIGURE 10.1 X-ray appearance of intrauterine adhesions causing a "filling defect" within the uterus. The defect appears as a dark irregular area surrounded by a white dye.

The diagnosis and evaluation of the extent of the problem usually is made with HSG or hysteroscopy. Figure 10.1 shows a mild case with an irregular defect in the uterus caused by the x-ray dye running around the scar tissue.

Treatment consists first of antibiotic therapy to deal with any residual infection. Then, hysteroscopy is employed with ancillary instruments to cut the adhesions from the uterine wall. In severe cases, this cannot be done as a single operating procedure, and multiple surgeries may be required. The bare patches which remain beneath the scar tissue must be stimulated with estrogen to regenerate something that approximates normal endometrium. Additionally, the problem which must be addressed at the time of surgery is to prevent contact of the rough, raw opposing surfaces which would lead to almost instant reformation of adhesions. Somewhat paradoxically, the solution is to insert an inert (no copper and non-hormonal) intrauterine device. The IUD acts as a barrier to surface contact and is left in for about six weeks during which high dose estrogen followed by progesterone is given. The IUD is then removed, and the cavity is inspected with a hysteroscope. Sometimes the scar tissue has extended into the tubes at the uterine junction. The pre-operative HSG will give this information on tubal patency, so that hysteroscopic surgery can be extended into the tubes, and results can be assessed during surgery with laparoscopy utilized simultaneously to document passage of dye from the ends of the tubes.

About 70% of women treated for intrauterine adhesions will eventually deliver, but this figure falls to 40% for those who start with total amennorhea. Endometrial scarring has no known long-term deleterious effect outside of reproduction; it does not cause cancer. But even after surgery has been successful, and pregnancy has been achieved, a long-term effect can be seen. Failure of the placenta to separate from the uterus after delivery is more common in patients previously treated for this condition. Blood should be readily available at the time of delivery, and the facility should be one in which an immediate postpartum hysterectomy (removal of the uterus) can be performed, if needed.

The DES Syndrome

Not all women exposed to DES in utero suffer any changes in reproductive anatomy or function. Women at risk who have a normal appearing cervix rarely have any uterine or tubal manifestations of DES effect. When the cervix is malformed, however, the uterus may also be affected. Typically, the HSG shows a small uterine cavity, which is classically in the shape of a "T" (figure 10.2) rather than the normal pear-shaped configuration. The hysteroscopic appearance of the cavity is also greatly altered, with the endometrium frequently exhibiting furrows or folds. The ultrasound may demonstrate a thin lining during the part of the

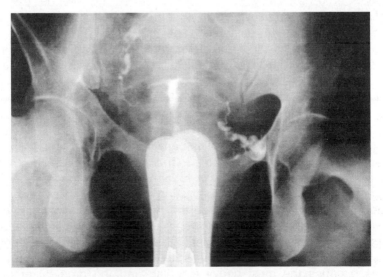

FIGURE 10.2 A hysterosalpingogram of a typical DES exposed uterus.

menstrual cycle when it should be thick and lush. Even when stimulated with large doses of estrogen, given over a long interval, the lining often fails to respond, probably based on the inadequate vascular anatomy beneath it or alteration of the receptors necessary to bind the estrogen so that it can have an effect. In either case, this does not auger well for pregnancy, and some of these patients will need to consider a gestational carrier as a solution. In less severe cases, the DES uterus can support a pregnancy initially, but then becomes irritable as the pregnancy progresses necessitating bed rest or use of drugs to induce uterine relaxation in order to prevent premature delivery. This is in addition to concern over the cervix's ability to remain closed until the onset of labor. Because use of DES had geographical hot spots, especially the east coast, I have had some considerable experience in treating its reproductive sequelae. The point that I wish to make is that the x-ray appearance of the DES uterus in no way predicts its reproductive potential; only the actual prior pregnancy performance can do that.

Fibroids: A Reproductive Nuisance

Within a gynecology practice fibroids **(myomas)** usually become clinically important when their individual size or multiplicity cause heavy and/or prolonged menses, discomfort from size alone, or bowel or bladder symptoms from pressure secondary to increasing uterine size. Pain sometimes is an accompanying symptom brought about by distortion of the uterus or partial outlet obstruction of menstrual flow. Malignancy is uncommon, and is somewhat age dependent. Reproductively, the effects of fibroids can occur with less dramatic symptoms than those mentioned above, and at smaller size.

Myomas are age dependent, with 25% of women over 35 years of age having at least one, but not necessarily clinically important, fibroid. Because of the tendency for pregnancy later in life, myomas constitute an increasing part of our reproductive practice. They are more common in ethnic blacks and less common in Asians than in Caucasians. Fibroids run in some families, and when inherited, tend to appear at an earlier age. While estrogens stimulate growth of pre-existing myomas, birth control pills do not, and they actually may decrease the rate of growth. Growth is erratic, occurring in spurts, sometimes after years of no size increase. As shown in figure 10.3, myomas can arise anywhere in the uterus. Size is less important than location. Lesions within the cavity are known as submucosal myomas, and these cause the most heavy bleeding and the greatest amount of reproductive impairment. Myomas which are just below the outer layer

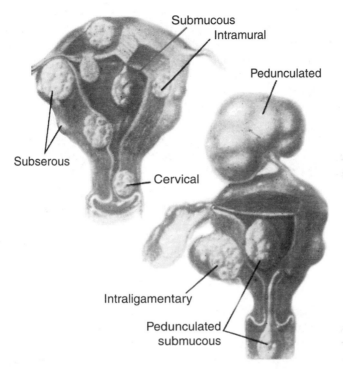

FIGURE 10.3 Myoma sites

of the uterus are called subserosal myomas. The myomas can grow to great size with just a stalk connecting them to the uterus. Myomas completely within the uterine wall are described as mural fibroids. The presence of myomas is not necessarily associated with infertility, unless the total bulk of the lesions is great and/or the uterine cavity becomes distorted as in figure 10.4. Submucosal myomas may have an IUD-like action, as well as interfering with sperm migration. The endometrium over a mural fibroid may be quite thin with distortion of the normal vascular pattern. Because pregnancy is a great stimulus to uterine growth, myomas can become huge, and cause the uterus to become irritable leading to premature labor and/or placental separation (abruption). They can also interfere mechanically with fetal growth. Large myomas may block the birth canal and necessitate cesarean section for delivery. Following delivery, fibroids may interfere with the ability of the uterus to contract, causing heavy bleeding sometimes quite difficult to control.

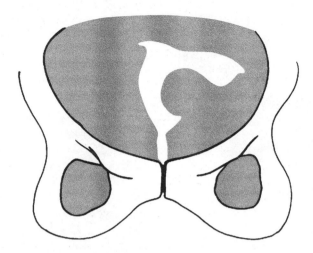

FIGURE 10.4   X-ray picture of uterine distortion caused by myoma.

The decision to remove myomas when they become symptomatic enough to bother the patient or cause anemia from blood loss is not difficult, but the decision to operate solely for reproductive purposes in the absence of symptoms or **menorrhagia** must be made based on prior reproductive performance (if any), the age of the patient, and the size and location of the lesions. Usually in a young patient it is suggested that she try a pregnancy to see if she can deliver without surgery, unless it is believed that fibroids are causing infertility, or unless the size and location of the lesions clearly dictates operative intervention. Removal of myomas is called myomectomy. When the uterine cavity is entered either purposefully or inadvertently during surgery, the usual recommendation is that future delivery be performed by cesarean section prior to onset of labor. Therefore, the decision to operate may actually entail two, rather than one, procedures. The risks of surgery, must also be considered. Anesthesia is a very small item in this category. Heavy bleeding intra-operatively can occur and may necessitate transfusion, and rarely, hysterectomy. Infection is uncommon. The reproductive risks of myomectomy also extend to formation of adhesions which by themselves can cause subsequent difficulty in conceiving. Also remember that some women are essentially programmed for fibroid formation; about 20% of women having myomectomy will have significant new myomas within five years following surgery. Myomectomy performed for reproductive purposes is sometimes a stop-gap measure before an eventual hysterectomy.

The operative technique for myomectomy performed at laparotomy is schematically outlined in figure 10.5. I use an injection of Pitressin, an agent causing uterine and blood vessel contraction, in the line of the intended incision. The myomas usually can be bluntly separated from surrounding tissue once the proper plane has been reached, similar to extracting a walnut from its shell. The uterus is then carefully reconstructed in layers. Submucus myomas are removed with a hysteroscopic approach through the cervix using an instrument called a resectoscope, which is also used during prostatic surgery. The laparoscopic approach to myomectomy is valid, but there continues to be argument over whether this should be applied to women who wish to reproduce following surgery. The reason is that it may not be possible to structurally repair the wall of the uterus as well with this approach as with open laparotomy. Case reports in the literature of uterine rupture before and during labor following myomectomy performed laparoscopically are cause for concern.

There's a role for the GnRH analogs as pre-operative therapy. Because of the suppressive action, low estrogen levels, similar to those seen during menopause, can be maintained for months with injections given monthly or as a single three-month duration dose. First, cessation of heavy menses allows the patient to restore normal hemoglobin levels such that she enters the operating room not anemic. The main reason for use is that because myomas are so estrogen sensitive, shrinkage occurs as a drug effect just as is the case during menopause. The maximum shrinkage usually occurs by the third month of therapy, and averages about 40% of myoma volume with large degrees of variation. Additionally, but of equal importance, this treatment reduces blood flow to the myoma which makes surgery that much easier.

The decision for myomectomy sometimes can be a very difficult one. A fertility specialist accustomed to myomectomy for reproductive purposes may be the best choice, if available. Multiple myomas can be removed through an amazingly small incision, and the interval of healing until attempts to conceive are made is as short as three months. Delivery rates of about 70% are expected in well chosen patients following myomectomy.

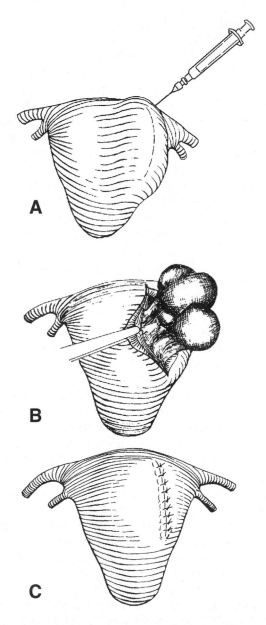

FIGURE 10.5   Removal of uterine myomas (myomectomy). (A) Injection of Pitressin along intended incision to reduce bleeding, (B) Multilobulated myomas "shelled out" through incision, (C) Closure of incision in layers.

Repair of Uterine Structural Abnormalities

Congenital structural uterine abnormalities were discussed in chapter 2 and illustrated in figure 2.5. No attempt to repair a bicornate uterus should be made in the absence of an adverse reproductive history. Even a severely misshapen uterus can produce a healthy newborn. Surgery generally is reserved for cases with repeated pregnancy loss, usually at least two consecutive failures, unless the age of the patient with at least one loss dictates a more aggressive approach. Figure 10.6 shows the steps involved in removal of an intrauterine septum. The hysteroscopic approach has almost completely replaced laparotomy for repair of the septated uterus. Performed on an out-patient basis, pregnancy can be initiated in the next menstrual cycle. In our experience a septate uterus is found in a ratio of 8:l to bicornate uterus. The differential diagnosis between the two entities cannot be made by the appearance of the HSG or by hysteroscopy. Ultrasound in the non pregnant state is fairly accurate, and MRI has the highest degree of accuracy. Additionally, and of great importance, the HSG appearance is in no way predictive of the future reproductive performance of that uterus; reliance must be based on the previous obstetrical history. Neither condition is a cause of infertility. The septate variety is more often associated with early (first trimester and early 2nd trimester) loss than the bicornate malformation. Bicornate uterus, on the other hand, is more likely to cause immature delivery, is approached by laparotomy, needs three months to heal, and dictates delivery by cesarean section after plastic reunification of the two cavities. Surgery for either of these two conditions carries with it a 70%-80% success rate for leaving the hospital with a healthy newborn in the next pregnancy. The procedure for dealing with the bicornate uterus is schematically illustrated in figure 10.7. Bicornate uterus is frequently associated with some degree of cervical incompetence. Therefore, even after repair of the cavity, cervical cerclage at about the 12th week of pregnancy, as a prophylactic measure, should be considered.

A typical case is that of a 29 year old woman referred because of losing four pregnancies in a row between 8 and 14 weeks. Her x-ray picture showed two uterine cavities. Laparoscopy and hysteroscopy confirmed the diagnosis of septate uterus. The septum (figure 10.8) was cut via hysteroscopy as an outpatient procedure. She has since delivered two babies at term. This septum went undetected in spite of the fact that she had three dilatation and evacuation (D&E) procedures performed at the time of pregnancy losses. Therefore patients with pregnancy wastage should be screened with hysteroscopy, ultrasound, or an HSG for uterine structural abnormality.

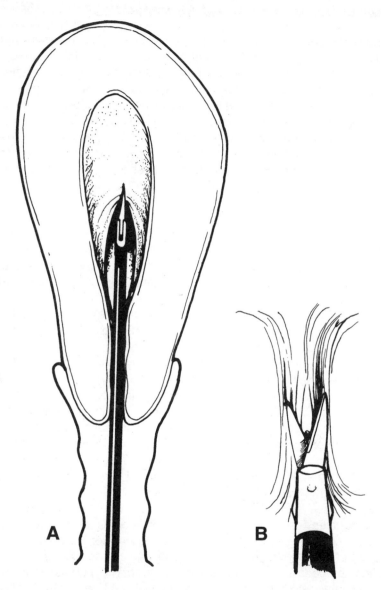

FIGURE 10.6   (A) Hysteroscopy has indicated a septate uterus. Scissors are inserted
through an operating channel, (B) A close-up view of the septum showing
the scissors being used to cut the septum. The septum is composed
mainly of fibroelastic tissue which separates easily when cut.

The unicollate uterus, which represents failure of one of the lateral halves of the uterus to develop is not associated with infertility, but because of its small sized cavity, may cause premature labor and delivery. Bed rest and sometimes cervical cerclage are helpful. There is no specific surgical repair for this condition, but about 70% of pregnancies will achieve success defined as a newborn of sufficient maturity for normal development. True double uterus, with two separate cavities, two cervices, and often a vaginal septum as total duplication of the reproductive tract, has an excellent prognosis without the need for any surgical intervention. Uteri with a small, atrophic "blind horn" may come to surgery because of pain caused by the blockage of menstrual flow from the area without connection to the cervix.

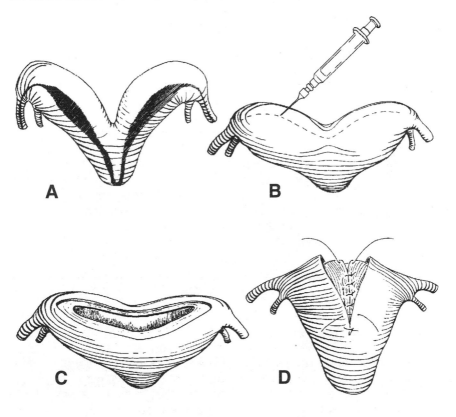

FIGURE 10.7   Steps in repair of bicornuate uterus. (A) Appearance before surgery with two small separate cavities, (B) Injection of Pitressin along incision to control bleeding, (C) Appearance after cavities united, (D) Closure of incision in layers.

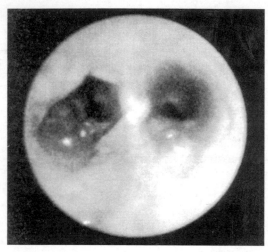

FIGURE 10.8
Picture of uterine septum

Adenomyosis

Adenomyosis is a condition in which endometrial tissue grows into the muscle fibers of the uterine wall. It frequently causes symptoms of **dysmenorrhea** (painful menses), menorrhagia, and **dyspareunia** (painful intercourse). Since adenomyosis occurs most frequently in women over 35, its effects on reproduction have not been widely appreciated. The exact mechanisms by which it exerts a negative influence on pregnancy is unknown, but since this is a form of endometriosis involving the uterus, there may be some parallels. Medical treatment is similar to that of endometriosis which will be discussed later. Surgical treatment is that of removal of discrete **adenomyomas,** similar to myomectomy, sometimes more easily said than done. Because the clinical symptoms and signs overlap with myoma, diagnosis can be difficult. A pelvic MRI is the only pre-operative diagnostic test with consistent high accuracy.

Luteal Phase Defect

As we mentioned previously, luteal phase deficiency (LPD) may result from inadequate production of estrogen in the follicular phase and/or less than normal progesterone synthesis from the ovary in the luteal phase, with the ovary as the culprit. On the other hand, the problem may be the ability of the endometrium to respond to normal levels of hormonal stimulation based on reduced or altered receptor sites. Hormonal supplementation can be tried and the effect monitored by serial ultrasonic evaluation of the endometrial pattern and thickness rather than with endometrial biopsies.

11

Endometriosis,
The Enigmatic Disease

Endometriosis is defined as the presence of endometrial glands and supporting stroma outside the endometrial cavity. This tissue, most commonly found implanted on the pelvic organs, can be anywhere in the body including the central nervous system, lungs, colon, and urinary system. Symptoms usually arise because the implants respond to hormonal stimulation in a fashion similar to normal endometrium which results in cyclical bleeding into surrounding structures causing inflammation and scarring. Diagnosis is made at the time of laparoscopy or laparotomy, although the ultrasound picture of endometriosis of the ovary can be quite suggestive. Biopsy of suspicious areas is recommended for confirmation because the gross appearance of the lesions is quite varied. Implants can be non pigmented, red, yellow- brown, or deep purple-black in color according to how much bleeding has occurred and the duration of the process. Most begin as surface lesions but may spread laterally or deeply into the tissue. The areas most commonly affected are the broad ligaments and uterosacral ligaments which flank the uterus, the ovaries, and the space between the uterus and the colon known as the posterior cul-de-sac. Figures 11.1-11.3 schematically illustrate these areas. How does this happen? The original theory put forth by Samson in 1927 explained pelvic endometriosis on the basis of retrograde menstruation with viable pieces of endometrium regurgitated from the end of the tubes and implanting on nearby adjacent structures. Subsequent theories also allowed for endometriosis to arise directly from changes in the cells which line the

153

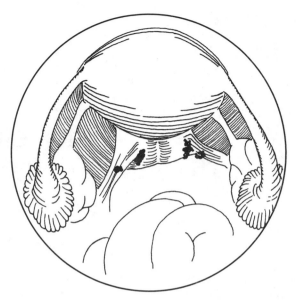

FIGURE 11.1   Small endometriotic implants along uterosacral ligaments supporting the uterus.

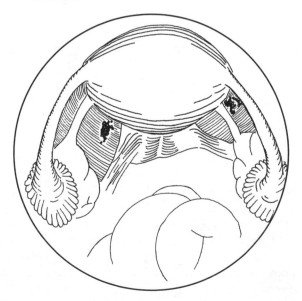

FIGURE 11.2   Endometriotic implants on broad ligament on either side of the uterus.

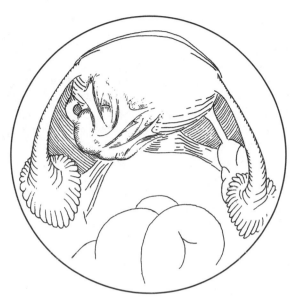

FIGURE 11.3 Left ovary adherent to back of uterus as a consequence of endometriosis.

peritoneal cavity. Neither of these explanations covers the finding of endometriosis in distant sites. Therefore, routes of spread through the vascular system and lymphatic system were postulated. Since laparoscopy performed during menses demonstrates that in at least 90% of cases some menstrual blood and tissue can be seen leaking from the tubes, the question is why don't all women get endometriosis. It seems as though endometriosis is more common in women who have had incessant ovulation without interruption by pregnancy or use of birth control pills. Remember that as we pointed out before, effective contraception by any means has a short history in human evolution; women were bioengineered to be pregnant or breast feeding, and not ovulating for long, uninterrupted intervals.

Prevalence and Heredity

It used to be taught in medical schools that endometriosis was an affliction of white, thin, "high strung" career women in their 30s. Not so. First of all, laparoscopy in teenagers complaining of severe dysmenorrhea (painful periods) not relieved with the usual analgesics or birth control pills demonstrates the presence of biopsy-proven endometriosis. Endometriosis is found in all ethnic groups, although less commonly in African-Americans than Caucasians and somewhat more frequently in Asians.

Endometriosis can be found in normally fertile populations as a silent entity seen, for instance, at the time of elective tubal ligation for sterilization, with studies showing ranges from 2%-18%. Most studies of unselected "normal" populations report about a 1%-3% prevalence. Having said that, let me emphasize that in many of the studies the extent of the process was extremely limited. When the question of prevalence is raised in an infertile population, the range runs from 5%-33% depending on socio-economic status. That there is a genetic pre-disposition has been documented by studies on first-degree relatives with 7%-10% positive findings in sisters of patients with endometriosis. In a study of identical twins, symptomatic endometriosis was concordant in six of eight.

Clinical Presentation: Symptoms, Signs and Diagnosis

In 1992 I wrote a book entitled "Endometriosis, the Enigmatic Disease", and it remains puzzling, at least to me, seven years later. This pathologic process has remained baffling to patients and physcians because of its protean symptoms, and the well-known fact that the amount of pain often cannot be correlated with the extent of abnormal tissue. Pelvic pain usually is most marked just before the onset of menses probably because the endometriotic lesions start to bleed at that time. But some patients have pain daily with accentuation at ovulation and through the entire luteal phase. But large endometriotic cysts of the ovaries containing deposits of old blood, known as "chocolate cysts" because of the appearance of the material, can be without any symptoms. Dyspareunia (painful intercourse) is most common with endometrial implants in the posterior cul-de-sac and uterosacral ligaments. With deep lesions rather than superficial implants penetration during coitus may cause excruciating pain. There is little correlation between the amount of pain and degree of infertility. Implants on the bladder wall will cause pain when urine is passed. We have found that many women with endometriosis of the bladder have been treated for chronic urinary infections that were not present. Implants on the bowel wall may cause either diarrhea or constipation marked during or just before the menses. If endometriosis invades the bowel wall, rectal bleeding will occur, and surgery consisting of removal (resection) of the affected segment with re-anastomosis of the colon (not a colostomy) may be needed. Endometriosis, perhaps because of its inflammatory nature, is often associated with heavy menses. During the physical examination the pelvic tissues often impart a sensation of being "rubbery" and deep palpation may cause exquisite pain. A combined vaginal/rectal examination may disclose deep implants in the septum which separates them presenting as small lumps that feel like BB shot pellets.

Ultrasonic examination will detect or at least suggest ovarian endometriomas as cystic areas filled with old blood but will not define small implants elsewhere. The MRI techniques are neither cost-effective nor accurate in diagnosis of small lesions, and the definitive diagnosis is almost always made by laparoscopy. The Ca 125 blood test sometimes used to monitor patients treated for ovarian cancer also is elevated in most cases of endometriosis. Ca 125 levels tend to be raised with any pelvic inflammation and when myomas are present. Therefore, its lack of sensitivity detracts from using it as a primary diagnostic tool, although it has a place as follow-up after treatment. If the levels fall and then rise again concomitant with return of symptoms, recurrence is quite likely. Endometriosis has been termed a "recrudescent" process, which means it has the nasty habit of returning. Eventually, hysterectomy with ovarian removal may be the only permanent cure.

Endometriosis is the great chameleon of pelvic pathology. It is often confused with pelvic inflammatory disease because of the similarity of symptoms. It is also misdiagnosed as acute appendicitis and ectopic pregnancy. Many patients with a preoperative diagnosis of simple ovarian cysts are found to have endometriomas instead. Less commonly colitis and other inflammatory bowel disorders are confused with endometriosis. Malignant transformation of these implants is rare, but does occur. About 80% of women with laparoscopic proven endometriosis have dysmenorrhea; about 40% have some pelvic pain not associated with menses; 30% have dyspareunia. There are a number of different scoring systems to grade the severity of the process. The last revision (1996) of the American Society for Reproductive Medicine classification is shown in figure 11.4a along with examples of staging (figure 11.4b). Note that staging is based not only on the amount of endometriosis present, but additionally on the amount of adhesions it provokes. There's general agreement that none of the currently used grading systems correlates well with either pain or infertility except in the most advanced stages.

AMERICAN SOCIETY FOR REPRODUCTIVE MEDICINE
REVISED CLASSIFICATION OF ENDOMETRIOSIS

Patient's Name _____ Date_____

Stage I (Minimal) · 1-5
Stage II (Mild) · 6-15
Stage III (Moderate) · 16-40
Stage IV (Severe) · >40
Total_____

Laparoscopy_____ Laparotomy_____ Photography_____
Recommended Treatment_____

Prognosis_____

	ENDOMETRIOSIS	<1cm	1-3cm	>3cm
PERITONEUM	Superficial	1	2	4
	Deep	2	4	6
OVARY	R Superficial	1	2	4
	Deep	4	16	20
	L Superficial	1	2	4
	Deep	4	16	20

POSTERIOR CULDESAC OBLITERATION	Partial	Complete
	4	40

	ADHESIONS	<1/3 Enclosure	1/3-2/3 Enclosure	>2/3 Enclosure
OVARY	R Filmy	1	2	4
	Dense	4	8	16
	L Filmy	1	2	4
	Dense	4	8	16
TUBE	R Filmy	1	2	4
	Dense	4*	8*	16
	L Filmy	1	2	4
	Dense	4*	8*	16

*If the fimbriated end of the fallopian tube is completely enclosed, change the point assignment to 16.

Denote appearance of superficial implant types as red [(R), red, red-pink, flamelike, vesicular blobs, clear vesicles], white [(W), opacifications, peritoneal defects, yellow-brown], or black [(B) black, hemosiderin deposits, blue]. Denote percent of total described as R___%, W___% and B___%. Total should equal 100%.

Additional Endometriosis: _____   Associated Pathology: _____
_____   _____
_____   _____

To Be Used with Normal
Tubes and Ovaries

To Be Used with Abnormal
Tubes and/or Ovaries

L   R   L   R

FIGURE 11.4a ASRM endometriosis scores and examples

EXAMPLES & GUIDELINES

STAGE I (MINIMAL) STAGE II (MILD) STAGE III (MODERATE)

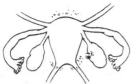

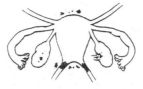

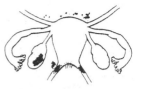

PERITONEUM		
Superficial Endo – 1-3cm	· 2	
R. OVARY		
Superficial Endo – < 1cm	· 1	
Filmy Adhesions – < 1/3	· 1	
TOTAL POINTS	4	

PERITONEUM		
Deep Endo – >3cm	· 6	
R. OVARY		
Superficial Endo – < 1cm	· 1	
Filmy Adhesions – < 1/3	· 1	
L. OVARY		
Superficial Endo – < 1cm	· 1	
TOTAL POINTS	9	

PERITONEUM		
Deep Endo – >3cm	· 6	
CULDESAC		
Partial Obliteration	· 4	
L. OVARY		
Deep Endo – 1-3cm	· 16	
TOTAL POINTS	26	

STAGE III (MODERATE) STAGE IV (SEVERE) STAGE IV (SEVERE)

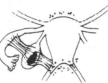

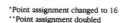

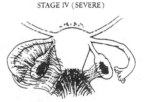

PERITONEUM		
Superficial Endo – >3cm	-4	
R. TUBE		
Filmy Adhesions – < 1/3	· 1	
R. OVARY		
Filmy Adhesions – < 1/3	· 1	
L. TUBE		
Dense Adhesions – < 1/3	· 16	
L. OVARY		
Deep Endo – < 1 cm	-4	
Dense Adhesions – < 1/3	-4	
TOTAL POINTS	30	

PERITONEUM		
Superficial Endo – >3cm	· 4	
L. OVARY		
Deep Endo – 1-3cm	· 32**	
Dense Adhesions – < 1/3	· 8**	
L. TUBE		
Dense Adhesions – < 1/3	8**	
TOTAL POINTS	52	

*Point assignment changed to 16
**Point assignment doubled

PERITONEUM		
Deep Endo – >3cm	· 6	
CULDESAC		
Complete Obliteration	· 40	
R. OVARY		
Deep Endo – 1-3cm	· 16	
Dense Adhesions – < 1/3	· 4	
L. TUBE		
Dense Adhesions – >2/3	· 16	
L. OVARY		
Deep Endo – 1-3cm	· 16	
Dense Adhesions – >2/3	· 16	
TOTAL POINTS	114	

Determination of the stage or degree of endometrial involvement is based on a weighted point system. Distribution of points has been arbitrarily determined and may require further revision or refinement as knowledge of the disease increases.

To ensure complete evaluation, inspection of the pelvis in a clockwise or counterclockwise fashion is encouraged. Number, size and location of endometrial implants, plaques, endometriomas and/or adhesions are noted. For example, five separate 0.5cm superficial implants on the peritoneum (2.5 cm total) would be assigned 2 points. (The surface of the uterus should be considered peritoneum.) The severity of the endometriosis or adhesions should be assigned the highest score only for peritoneum, ovary, tube or culdesac. For example, a 4cm superficial and a 2cm deep implant of the peritoneum should be given a score of 6 (not 8). A 4cm

deep endometrioma of the ovary associated with more than 3cm of superficial disease should be scored 20 (not 24).

In those patients with only one adenexa, points applied to disease of the remaining tube and ovary should be multipled by two. **Points assigned may be circled and totaled. Aggregation of points indicates stage of disease (minimal, mild, moderate, or severe).

The presence of endometriosis of the bowel, urinary tract, fallopian tube, vagina, cervix, skin etc., should be documented under "additional endometriosis." Other pathology such as tubal occlusion, leiomyomata, uterine anomaly, etc., should be documented under "associated pathology." All pathology should be depicted as specifically as possible on the sketch of pelvic organs, and means of observation (laparoscopy or laparotomy) should be noted.

FIGURE 11.4b

How Does Endometriosis Cause Infertility?

As you might have guessed, the literature dealing with diagnosis and treatment of endometriosis, a poorly understood process, is vast, often contradictory, and many times burdened by the lack of a group of patients picked at random who agree to serve as untreated controls. Almost anything you can think of which bears on the reproductive process has been studied and shown to be adversely affected by endometriosis. When tubes and ovaries become entrapped in dense adhesions caused by the inflammatory response to endometriosis seen in severe cases, it is easy to explain the mechanism of infertility, at least in part, on a mechanical basis. But, explaining infertility in apparently mild cases remains an exercise in frustration. Obviously, there is some differentiating factor, some measurable marker, still unknown to us, which could be used as an indicator of fertility potential in these circumstances. In many respects endometriosis can be viewed from the perspective of an immunodeficiency etiology. This would explain the familial increased prevalence as an inherited trait, the low efficiency with which retrograde menstrual flow actually causes endometriosis, and the tendency for it to return even after apparently successful treatment. Although we have the concept that endometriosis is a relentlessly progressive process, this is not always the case. Studies have been done with patients who had laparoscopy either as a diagnostic or therapeutic procedure. Repeat inspection six months later in the group that had no actual surgical treatment directed against endometriosis except visual diagnosis, showed that the extent of the disease was the same in 25%, somewhat reduced in 25%, and increased in the other 50%. In almost all cases the arrival of menopause has a quieting influence on endometriosis because of the drop in estrogen levels. Some care must be taken if hormonal replacement therapy is initiated with respect to estrogen dose lest the process of endometriod proliferation be stimulated.

The fluid in the peritoneal cavity contains many different cell types, some of which act as "killer cells", to protect us against invading organisms. Many studies have demonstrated that the activity of these cells is decreased in patients with endometriosis. The same type of tests done with cells in the bloodstream have shown similar results, suggesting an immunologic alteration as part of the process. Different studies have focused on the presence of inflammatory cells in the peritoneal fluid. Generally speaking, these studies find that there's an increase in the population of these types of cells probably as a result, rather than as a cause of endometriosis. The inflammatory response is associated both with pain and infertility. In some cases, it seems to be disproportionately greater than expected for the amount of endometriosis present. As part of the inflammatory response there are released local inflammatory compounds- prostaglandins, cytokines and interleukins, among others. Perhaps one of these will prove to be the much sought after marker. Attention has been paid as well to behavior of sperm suspended in peritoneal fluid from patients with endometriosis vs. controls. While there's no complete agreement, the majority of studies show inhibition of sperm motility and the acrosome reaction necessary for sperm fertilizing activation. Antibodies directed against the endometrium have been detected in infertile women with endometriosis. Integrins are naturally occurring compounds which play a role In the Implantatlon process between the early embryo and uterine wall. Some patients with endometriosis have low levels of these compounds which rise after successful treatment. Preliminary work suggests that there's a correlation between the integrin level in the uterus and pregnancy rate. The serum of infertile endometriotic patients has been shown to have a deleterious effect on development of mice embryos in an in vitro fertilization test system. In some, but not all studies, human embryos in endometriosis patients have a lower implantation rate after IVF transfer to the uterus than other IVF patients. When patients with endometriosis become pregnant, the miscarriage rate seems to be increased in those patients pregnant without active treatment compared with patients who conceive shortly after medical or surgical therapy.

Treatment

The form of treatment chosen for endometriosis is often dependent on whether the primary goal is relief of pain or establishment of pregnancy; of course, the situation becomes sticky when both are desired. As a prelude to treatment protocols, we must first address the issue of whether minimal (Stage I) and/or (Stage II) endometriosis truly reduces fecundity, and if therapy is warranted. If one looks at studies on patients having donor insemination and who have laparoscopically proven but untreated mild endometriosis, the conclusion is that compared with laparoscopically normal insemination patients, fecundity rates were reduced by about 60% for the patients with an apparently mild process.

I still see many infertile patients with proven endometriosis who have been treated with suppressive medical therapy such as danazol or the GnRH analogs (Lupron or Synarel). There's no question that this form of treatment does not increase pregnancy potential. Even after the three to six months of amennorrhea during which pregnancy is obviously impossible, the fecundity rates after menstrual function has been restarted are no better than no treatment at all. The rationale of this therapy is to create a low estrogen, pseudomenopausal state which leads to regression of the lesions. True, but while the beneficial effect on pain may be sustained for some time after the usual three to six month drug course, there is no beneficial effect on fertility. GnRH analogs given as once monthly or once every three months injections, or as daily nasal sprays are associated with the usual side effects of estrogen deprivation—hot flashes, vaginal dryness, poor sleep habits, bone mineral loss (usually reversible) and sometimes migratory joint pain. Danazol, an orally administered medication which has androgenic qualities, can lead to substantial weight gain, edema, acne, hair growth, oily skin, and rarely, permanent deepening of the voice. Because of the last potential, singers should avoid using it.

An excellent study was done by Toma and associates (Obstet Gynecol 80:253, 1992). Women undergoing donor insemination also had diagnostic laparoscopy. Figure 11.5 shows the cumulative pregnancy rates for patients with minimal or mild endometriosis compared with those patients who had normal laparoscopic findings. Obviously, at the end of six cycles of insemination, the rates for the normal patients were about double those for the endometriotic patients. Of equal interest were the findings shown in figure 11.6 which illustrate that neither surgical nor danazol treatment made any difference in the fecundity rate compared with no treatment. This last conclusion was at odds with that reached by Tulandi and Mouchawar (Fertil Steril 56: 790,1991) whose results appear in figure 11.7. They found that patients who had surgical treatment at laparoscopy for mild endometriosis had a much greater pregnancy yield at 36 months compared with those who had only laparoscopic inspection. Perhaps the best single study on this issue appeared in the New England Journal of Medicine (337:217, 1997) representing the results of a Canadian collaborative multi-centric study. Women were randomly assigned to treatment vs. no treatment at the time of laparoscopy, and then observed for up to 36 weeks or 20 weeks into a pregnancy, with the positive end point being that of a pregnancy reaching at least 20 weeks. The cumulative probability of pregnancy for the 172 women surgically treated was 30.7% compared with 17.1% for the 169 women having diagnosis only.

FIGURE 11.5 The effect of minimal mild endometriosis on donor insemination pregnancy rates

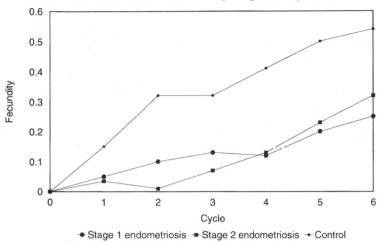

Cumulative conception rates of patients treated with donor insemination who have stage I, stage II, and no endometriosis. (Toma SK, Stovall DW, Hammond MG. Obstet Gynecol 1992;80:253-56)

FIGURE 11.6 The fecundity rates with endometriosis: Treatment versus no treatment

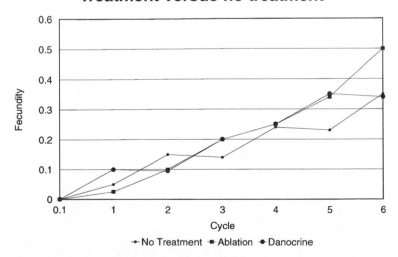

Cumulative conception rates for donor insemination patients with stage I and stage II endometriosis subdivided into different treatment groups. (Toma SK, Stovall DW, Hammond MG. Obstet Gynecol 1992;80:253-56)

FIGURE 11.7
Pregnancy after treatment of mild endometriosis.

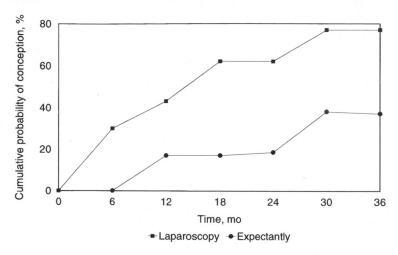

Cumulative probability of conception of women with mild endometriosis who were treated electrosurgically by laparoscopy and those who were treated expectantly (observation only). (Tulandi T, Mouchawar M. Fertil Steril 1991;56:790-91)

If one were to review the literature dealing with the issue of treatment /no treatment, it would not be difficult to support observant management only for some reasonable duration of time, especially considering the complexity, costs, logistics and risks of treatment. Putting that philosophy into every day practice is another matter. Patients argue, with considerable logic, that by the time they see a fertility doctor, they often have exercised the no treatment option. Outside of a study situation, there's little reason not to treat endometriosis at the time of laparoscopic diagnosis since the risks associated with the surgery are mostly those of laparoscopy itself separate from the surgical approach to endometriosis, except in severe cases when bladder and/or bowel is involved. Another conclusion based on personal experience and literature consensus is that ovarian endometriosis in the form of a presumed cystic endometrioma is almost always an indication for surgical rather than medical therapy.

Moderate to severe endometriosis is a different story, and when fertility rather than pain control is the goal, surgery is always indicated. Patients who conceive after ovarian suppression would probably have done so with no intervention of any kind. In spite of the fact that the presently utilized scoring systems are not accurate predictors of fertility potential, the more advanced stages of endometriosis are associated with greater degrees of long-term infertility. While laparoscopy is more convenient and less invasive for the patient, even the most skillful laparoscopic surgeon will occasionally have to resort to laparotomy in order to deal effectively with the pathology which is encountered. For that reason, our patients are counseled that a laparoscopic procedure may be extended to a laparotomy, and the operating room is set up for quick and easy conversion. Pregnancy rates with stages III and IV endometriosis following laparoscopy or laparotomy average 40%-60% and 25%-40%, respectively, by 36 months. Considering the tools used during surgery, there's now general agreement that lasers are not magic wands; pregnancy rates following surgical sharp excision of endometriosis, electrosurgical eradication of lesions or laser ablation and destruction of implants show no difference. The magic is in the hands of the surgeon.

Medical therapy, sometimes given as repetitive courses of danazol or Lupron, or long-term treatment with Depo Provera has a definite role in control of recurrent endometriosis-induced pain. The only real place for these agents when fertility is at stake is to use them as a preoperative adjunct to reduce the inflammatory response in order to facilitate surgical procedures.

Indirect Fertility Treatment for Endometriosis

Sometimes nonspecific treatments for endometriosis-associated infertility either before surgery or after surgery may increase the pregnancy yield. Gonadotropin ovulation stimulation increases fecundity compared with what has been called "expectant management " which is a fancy euphemism for doing nothing. If insemination is added to the stimulation cycle pregnancy rates jump from about 2%-5% with observation only to 12%-16%. Why should this approach work? First, there are more fertilizable oocytes per cycle. Higher estrogen levels favor better endometrial development (up to a point) and receptivity. Some of the minimal ovulatory defects and altered hormonal patterns sometimes seen in the presence of endometriosis are obviated with this approach. Insemination, even with normal seminal parameters, places hundreds of times more sperm into the tubes than can be achieved with intercourse, perhaps overwhelming any putative adverse effect of endometriosis on sperm migration or the fertilization process.

When all else fails, assisted reproductive technology (ART) may come to the rescue. In our own series, combined laser treatment for endometriosis at the time of gamete intrafallopian transfer (GIFT) produced a 45% pregnancy rate. Provided that tubal function is normal, this is an excellent approach to the problem since it employs the double barrel of achieving pregnancy on one hand and simultaneously treating the endometriosis on the other. IVF data suggest that results may be improved by pre-treating with analogs for one to three months prior to actual stimulation. This duration of suppression may allow some regression of the inflammatory response to endometriotic implants, thus improving egg quality and yield. The literature remains somewhat mixed concerning the issue of pregnancy and liveborn rates with IVF for endometriosis patients compared with other groups having IVF. While a few studies indicate that there is a decrease in egg quality and embryo implantation rate, the majority of reports from successful programs show no such differences.

By now you may have a feel for the problems that physicians encounter when counseling and treating patients with this still mysterious disorder. Past the basics, there is little in the way of treatment which cannot be debated. The most reasonable sequential approach seems to be diagnostic laparoscopy coupled with simultaneous surgical eradication of all visible lesions followed by an interval of watchful waiting with the time frame dependent upon the age of the patient and whether or not additional fertility factors are present. The next step should probably be that of gonadotropic ovarian stimulation with IUI for up to three or four cycles, reserving IVF or GIFT as a last resort. This algorithm is based on an increasing degree of complexity and nuisance logistically to the patient. If, however, this is viewed from a cost basis, the argument can be made that going directly from diagnosis to IVF is more cost-effective and time-saving. If the insurance carriers would fund the combination of diagnostic laparoscopy and GIFT for low risk patients (not those suspected of having advanced endometriosis) the cost per baby would be less, and pregnancy for some couples would be more immediate. As currently practiced, both IVF and GIFT are associated with high multiple pregnancy rates which need to be substantially lowered in order for these technologies to become more attractive as first line therapies.

12

A Sojourn Through the Fallopian Tubes

To make its contribution to fertility, a fallopian tube must catch an egg cast adrift in the pelvis and move it toward the uterus while secreting the fluid which nourishes the egg and capacitates the sperm. The structures that enable the tube to accomplish its mission – the sweeping fimbria, the waving cilia, the secretory cells in the endosalpinx which line the tube – are perhaps the most delicate and least resilient in the female reproductive tract.

Disorders of the Fallopian Tubes

Damaged fallopian tubes are a major cause of infertility. Some women are born with tubes that are abnormal as a consequence of developmental failures during intrauterine life, while others have congenital tubal changes brought about by exposure in utero to a toxic agent such as DES. An inherited genetic disease can be another cause of abnormal tubal development or function. With improved medical care women with cystic fibrosis now are reaching reproductive age. The same cilial defect present in the lungs is also active in the tubes which prevents the egg from reaching the uterus even though the tube is open. Most cases of infertility on a tubal basis, however, result from the aftermath of an infectious insult. Tubal infections can be treated effectively with antibiotics, but even with expeditious diagnosis and management the inflammation which occurs may cause permanent damage to the specialized cells which line the tube, and in severe cases the end result is tubal closure from scar tissue formation.

DES

Thus far we have learned that exposure to DES during fetal life can result in major structural changes in the cervix and uterine body. We now must ask if the reproductive effects extend to the tube. Depending upon socio-economic levels, the ectopic pregnancy rate in the population at-large is somewhere between 1.25% and 2%. In women with a DES exposure sufficient enough to cause a change visible on the HSG in the uterine contour, that rate approachs 10%. These tubes appear to be normal but have alteration of the normal mechanisms controlling propagation of a smooth contractile wave necessary for the egg to reach the uterus. Some women with DES exposure do not conceive even with insemination and ovulation induction, probably because of the malfunction of the tubes, but become pregnant when IVF is employed.

Tubal Infections

Pelvic inflammatory disease (PID), is a catch-all term used to describe pelvic infection in the tubes, and sometimes the surrounding tissues including the ovaries. In its most severe form this leads to formation of an abscess involving the tube and ovary which usually has to be surgically or ultrasonically drained even after vigorous intravenous antibiotic therapy is given. The infectious process can spill over into the bloodstream causing death from septic shock in cases which are neglected or which involve organisms resistant to the antibiotics used. Almost any bacterial organism can be responsible, although most cases follow contact with chlamydia trachomatis, a sexually transmitted infectious agent.

Acute PID may be difficult to diagnose with the differential list including appendicitis, ectopic pregnancy, endometriosis, ovarian cysts, and inflammatory bowel disorders such as colitis. White cell count elevation in the bloodstream, fever and pelvic pain constitute the triad used for many years to make the diagnosis, but all three may not be present. In its chronic form, the infection may smolder, causing chronic pain in the pelvis with a chance of a flare of symptoms years later occurring spontaneously or provoked by a hysterosalpingogram, laparoscopy or even following intercourse. Once the tubal lining has been damaged it becomes vulnerable to secondary invaders even though the original organisms have been cleared.

For many years the organism giving rise to gonorrhea was the major cause of infectious tubal infertility. Diagnosis can be made with a special culture from the cervix, or urethra/anus/pharynx in either sex, depending on the port of entry. Most cases can be treated with oral antibiotics but some patients need injections or intravenous routes. Even with good care 12% to 15% of patients with infection sufficient to cause symptoms will become sterile as a consequence of tubal closure. The chance for sterility increases with each infection since there is no immunity which results from contact. Infected male partners must be treated concomitantly to avoid re-infection of the female. Cultures in the heterosexual male are taken from the urethra. A discharge may or may not be present in acute cases. Cultures must be repeated until negative to be certain that the organism has been eradicated especially now that antibiotic-resistant strains have appeared.

Chlamydia is now seen more commonly in sexually transmitted disease clinics than gonorrhea. It, too, is sexually transmitted. In some ways it is more insidious than infection with the gonococcus. Symptoms are usually milder and commonly are completely absent, with the diagnosis made solely by cervical cultures or cervical swab examination for specific DNA of the organism. Cases of tubal closure may have resulted from a long forgotten single sexual exposure many years ago. Past exposure to the organism can be detected with antibody testing of the serum. Different strains of chlamydia exist, with one causing pneumonia as a potential source of confusion. The antibody test is supposed to be specific for each strain but this does not always hold true since there is some cross reactivity. Because of the social implications, we're careful in explaining to the couple that there is a margin of error in making a diagnosis of previous exposure. Infection with chlamydia does not always produce tubal damage, especially if the process does not extend past the cervix. In general, the appearance of the tube following infection is less dramatic than with gonorrhea. The tube may look normal grossly but microscopic inspection reveals cilial damage. Acute infections are easily treated with tetracycline derivatives with other drugs as second line choices in case of allergy. Both partners need to be treated simultaneously, and cultures need to be repeated until negative. Chlamydia can be harbored for years in the tube after cervical cultures turn negative. Therefore, to be safe, we will usually treat anyone with a positive antibody even though the original infection may have occurred in the distant past. A history of infection with either of these two organisms is more common in the population with ectopic pregnancy than in a control group. The extent of the damage may be moderate, allowing the egg to enter the tube but subsequently to be caught in adhesions on its path to the uterus.

A positive antibody level can be detected in about 10% of the general North American female population, rising to approximately 20% for the general subfertile population, and 35% for the subgroup of infertile women with demonstrable tubal damage. Women with chlamydial antibodies are four times as likely to have an ectopic pregnancy compared with negative controls. Streptococcus and Staphylococcus strains are common bacteria normally found on skin and sometimes in the vagina. They are capable of causing tubal damage under certain circumstances. These infections usually occur in conjunction with delivery or miscarriage. About 20% of secondary infertility is a result of tubal infection acquired at delivery. Fever is not always an accompanying sign. Escherichia coli is a family of bacteria found normally in the colon. Vaginal contamination because of poor bathroom hygiene or anal/vaginal intercourse may lead to ascending pelvic infection. Tuberculosis of the uterus and tubes is rather rare in North America, but we see it in people who have grown up in underdeveloped countries who have been infected by drinking non pasteurized milk from infected cows. This causes damage to both organs which even IVF rarely solves. The tubes can become infected secondarily during acute appendicitis and other primary bowel infections. Infection following abdominal surgery for any reason can result in permanent tubal damage. There is an association between intrauterine device use and tubal infection, usually as a consequence of infection acquired during the insertion.

Tubal Inflammation

Salpingitis isthmica nodosa (SIN) is an inflammatory disease of the tubes not resulting from an infectious process. It affects the proximal portion of the tube at the junction of the isthmus and the intramural portion of the tube as it passes through the muscular tunnel of the uterus (figure 12.1). Like other inflammatory conditions of a chronic nature such as arthritis and colitis, SIN waxes and wanes. Eventually, however, most affected tubes become rigid, fibrotic, and closed. Frequently there is an association with the presence of active endometriosis, but the two can exist independently of each other.

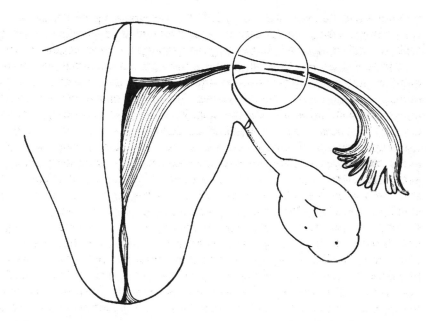

FIGURE 12.1 Point of blockage in salpingitis isthmica nodosa.

Repair of Damaged Tubes

No medication can restore severely damaged tubes. Donor tubal transplants are technically possible but are not done because the drugs used to prevent rejection are potentially dangerous. A synthetic substitute for the tube has not been invented, and probably never will be. I have practiced long enough to witness the rise and fall of tubal surgery. Up until the 1970s, tubal surgery was performed by laparotomy with dismal results. The advent of tubal micro-surgery dramatically improved pregnancy yield but still had the drawbacks of invasiveness and cost. Laparoscopic techniques were also applied to the problem with results that equaled those achieved with a microscope but with much less operative insult and with a decidedly shorter recovery period. The love affair with lasers was short lived when it became obvious that results are no better than when surgery is performed mechanically or with electrosurgical techniques. Almost any tube can be opened, but remaining open is another matter, and function is always the bottom line. Although scar tissue causing a tube to become closed is obvious at the time of surgery, microscopic inspection of the entire tube almost always documents scattered areas of damage from previous infection, explaining in large part the relatively poor pregnancy yield following even expertly performed tubal surgery. Surgical batting averages depend on the skill of the surgeon and the usual ancillary factors that we have mentioned before, but especially on the degree of severity of tubal damage. Thus, a surgeon who operates on severe cases may have a lower success rate than a less skillful surgeon who is more likely to reject as a surgical candidate a woman with horrendous tubal pathology. Introduction of IVF in the United States in the 1980s gave doctors and patients at least a theoretical choice of therapies. But insurance coverage for IVF continues to be poor despite numerous independent demonstrations that IVF is a more cost-effective primary path for all but the mildest forms of tubal damage.

Although infectious organisms can cause damage anywhere along the tube, fimbrial damage with closure of the distal end of the tube is most common as shown in figure 12.2. In its most mild form infection will form adhesions around a tube which can be cut at laparoscopy with the expectation of a 50% pregnancy rate. If the fimbria are damaged and adherent to each other, that rate is dramatically reduced. Tubal damage can

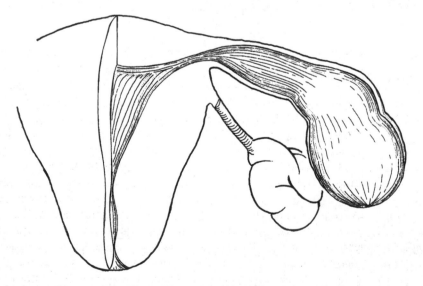

FIGURE 12.2   Dilated hydrosalpinx caused by blockage of the distal end of the tube producing a collection of tubal secretions.

be staged similar to the system employed to assess endometriosis. While pregnancy rates are fairly good for stages I and II, stages III and IV, which have poor prognosis, are usually encountered in 80% of patients operated for tubal disease. Factors influencing success include the health of the mucosa, the rigidity of the tube, the degree of inflammation, the thickness of the wall, whether fimbria remain, and whether the ciliated cells have been obliterated. Because the tubal lining has been damaged the ectopic pregnancy rate following tubal repair is substantially elevated.

Opening a closed tube is known as a **salpingostomy**. Usually, there is a small pucker at the point where the tube's natural fimbriated opening had been. The idea is to find this, trim away scar tissue and evert the normal mucosa, almost like turning a cuff. The problem is that the amount of diseased tubal tissue may not allow the surgeon to remove all of the scar tissue lest there be virtually no tube remaining.

Intrauterine pregnancy rates following surgery for tubal disease are usually in the vicinity of 20%-30% overall, but less than 15% for the two most severe grades. Ectopic pregnancy can be expected in an additional 5%-8% over an 18 month duration. The majority of pregnancies are observed between months 6 and 12. The argument over the proper course of action to be followed when an HSG shows closed tubes filled with fluid, hydrosalpinx, — laparoscopy for tubal repair or direct entry to an IVF program — may be a moot point.

In the last few years reports from all over the world have indicated that IVF results are significantly adversely affected by the presence of hydrosalpinx. This effect is eliminated when the tubes are removed. In some studies the fluid contained within these chronically damaged tubes has been demonstrated to be toxic to mice embryos grown in IVF conditions. The mechanism postulated is that the trapped tubal fluid intermittently leaks into the uterus. Our current philosophy is to perform laparoscopy as a procedure to either repair or remove the tube(s) with the decision made by the surgeon according to the appearance of the tubes after appropriate discussion with the patient. This assumes that the couple is willing and able to proceed with IVF in the event that the tubes are deemed to be irreparably damaged. By three or four months postoperatively, an HSG should give a fairly good idea of whether a surgically repaired tube has remained open, and whether some time should be given to allow pregnancy to occur, or whether IVF should be strongly considered sooner rather than later.

The outlook for patients with proximal blockage is a lot brighter provided that the distal end of the tube is normal and especially if the obstruction is localized as a consequence of inflammation rather than infection. Older approaches to the problem were surgical with micro-surgical removal of the segment and re-establishment of continuity (anastomosis) just as with colon resection, or re-implanting the tube in the uterus. Today these operations are performed less frequently. The usual first approach is to employ hysteroscopy and laparoscopy to pass a small diameter guidewire and catheter through the uterus and into the tube to clear the obstruction similar to some coronary artery procedures— a medical roto-rooter. The laparoscopy allows the surgeon to inspect the entire length of the tube, but if this is not necessary, the procedure can be done with equal results using x-ray dye in the radiology department. Pregnancy rates at the end of one year are in the 40% range, and ectopic pregnancy is only about 2%-4%. Here again, IVF can serve as a fall back position.

Ectopic Pregnancy

Ectopic pregnancy is a term applied to any pregnancy implanting outside of the uterine cavity. This includes abdominal structures such as the ovary, bladder and bowel wall, but is almost always limited to the fallopian tube. In most cases, the tube has been damaged previously by some infectious or inflammatory insult. Scar tissue forms inside the tube creating blind pockets which can trap the fertilized egg. The high rate of ectopic pregnancy (EP) seen with the DES syndrome is more a consequence of anatomical changes and perhaps altered patterns of tubal contractile waves than anything else. Most commonly the site of implantation is in the outermost region of the tube in the ampulla, especially near the fimbria, but the isthmus may be involved, and rarely the intramural portion of the tube at the cornual area of the uterus.

Symptoms may include bleeding or spotting from the uterine cavity, and pelvic pain and the usual symptoms of early pregnancy. Often, however, no symptoms are noted until the pregnancy within the tube progresses to the point of tubal rupture with intra-abdominal bleeding and symptoms of shock caused by internal loss of blood. Among the indigent, EP is a leading cause of maternal mortality because of delayed medical care. The last menstrual period frequently is described as late and light. Women at increased risk for EP are those with a history of previous surgery on the tube, prior EP, pelvic infection in the past, and present IUD use, because the intrauterine device protects well against intrauterine pregnancy but not against pregnancy elsewhere. Approximately half of all pregnancies which occur as failures of female sterilization are ectopic.

Diagnosis can be exceedingly difficult, especially when there are no known risk factors that raise the index of suspicion. Progesterone levels are often low. The diagnosis is frequently one made by exclusion. When the pregnancy test of ß hCG reaches a level somewhere between 1000 and 2000 mIU/mL, a sac should be seen within the uterus on ultrasonic examination. Sometimes the pregnancy sac can be seen outside the uterus in the region of the tube and ovary, making the diagnosis quite obvious. Normally, in early pregnancy, the ß hCG levels double every two or three days for the first 30 days after ovulation. Failure to double on this time schedule is common in ectopic pregnancy, but much more often is associated with an intrauterine pregnancy which is destined for miscarriage. Therefore, neither the magnitude of hCG levels nor the rate of rise can be used with any reasonable degree of assurance to rule in or out an ectopic pregnancy. Provided that a minimal level of hCG is present as mentioned above, the ultrasound is the best diagnostic tool to employ considering its accuracy, cost, and ease of performance.

An older method of diagnosis known as culdocentesis involves placing a needle through the top of the vagina into the pelvic cavity in order to test for the presence of non clotting blood as an indication of ectopic pregnancy. False positive tests include intra-abdominal bleeding from any source, and false negative results will be obtained if the tube has not ruptured or if bleeding from the end of the tube into the pelvic cavity has not occurred. Frequently tissue is taken from the uterus with a suction device in order to microscopically search for the presence of pregnancy specific tissue from the early placenta called the trophoblast. The presence of this tissue means that the implantation site has been biopsied. But in many cases if the patient has had some bleeding vaginally, she may have already passed this small volume of trophoblastic material causing the biopsy to be negative and leading to the assumption that the pregnancy was not in the uterus. Even laparoscopy can fail to diagnose an ectopic pregnancy which usually is visualized as a blue swelling of the tube. Passage of blood from the end of a tube may represent retrograde bleeding from the uterus rather than a pregnancy in that tube. Frequently the ectopic pregnancy is ejected by the tube into the pelvic cavity through its natural opening as a tubal abortion. If the tissue does not implant secondarily in the pelvis, the entire process may come to a spontaneous cure without any medical intervention. The pregnancy test, if negative, rules out EP as a diagnosis, and consideration should be paid to entities such as appendicitis, bleeding ovarian cyst, pelvic infection, or pain from endometriosis among others.

Classically, surgery has been employed to deal with the problem. We have come full circle in the philosophy of what to do with the affected tube. Before the 1970s, the standard of care was to remove the tube. With the increased popularity of first micro-surgery and then laparoscopy, coupled with earlier diagnosis, tubes that looked reasonably good, and not demolished by tubal rupture, were salvaged rather than removed. Many studies agreed that the risk of repeat ectopic pregnancy was not really increased with this maneuver compared with taking the tube out. Sometimes the patient had gotten pregnant in the better rather than the worse of the two tubes. IVF has taken the pressure off the patient and surgeon to save tubes hopelessly damaged before and during the ectopic pregnancy process. So you see, the pendulum has begun to swing back to removal. After the first ectopic pregnancy, 60% to 80% of patients can expect a normal next pregnancy. Repeat EP in the next pregnancy is seen in 8% to 15% with this figure rising after two episodes of EP.

Figure 12.3 depicts schematically an ectopic pregnancy removed from the fimbriated end of the tube laparoscopically in one case, and extracted from the ampulla portion of the tube in another (a **salpingotomy**). Almost all ectopic pregnancies can be approached laparoscopically, with laparotomy reserved for those that for one reason or another cannot be handled in this fashion. If the tube is salvaged, there is an increased risk of leaving viable trophoblast behind whose presence is made known by failure of the hCG levels to reach zero over the next few weeks. Follow-up blood testing is a must. When ß hCG levels persist, secondary treatment with methotrexate can begin or surgery can be repeated. Alternatively, when ultrasound shows the presence of ectopic pregnancy, or if the diagnosis is made by exclusion early in the pregnancy, methotrexate as a single injection can be given as primary therapy without any surgery. In about 85% of cases the hCG titers over the next few weeks fall satisfactorily and the issue is solved in that fashion. Surgery can be reserved as a fallback position. Intuitively one would think that the medical approach is associated with less chance for additional tubal damage than any surgical approach, but proof for this assertion is lacking. If the EP is viewed through the laparoscope, the surgeon should assess both tubes before making a decision on repair vs. removal of the involved tube. Usually a second EP in the same tube is indication for its removal, especially now that IVF can serve as a reproductive rescue in the future.

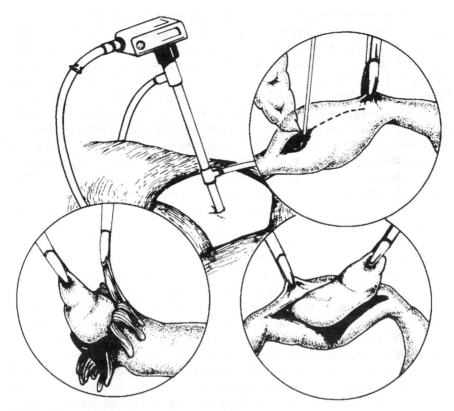

FIGURE 12.3   A fimbrial ectopic pregnancy is shown on the lower left, and an ectopic
pregnancy located at the ampullary-isthmic junction on the lower right.
The fimbrial ectopic pregnancy can be removed easily with laparoscopic
forceps. A laser can be used under laparoscopic guidance to make an
incision in the tube over the implantation site of the ectopic pregnancy
(upper right). The pregnancy sac can then be extracted using forceps.
The tube heals without the need for suture.

Sterilization Reversal

Close to one million women yearly choose sterilization as permanent
contraception. In spite of preoperative counseling, about one percent have
a change of heart sufficient enough to inquire about a reversal procedure,
usually because of divorce and remarriage, death of a child or husband,
and sometimes for various other reasons. Prior to laparoscopy, the Pomeroy
method of sterilization was most widely used, and is still popular today as a

postpartum procedure. Through a small abdominal incision the surgeon forms a small loop in each tube and ties it at the base (figure 12.4a). The portion of the tube above the tie is cut and removed. Weeks later when the suture material has been absorbed, the severed ends separate. Reversal consists of cutting the scar tissue from each stump, bringing the ends together, and reuniting them. Microsurgery with its use of small instruments, fine suture, and careful handling of tissue has brought high rates of success to sterilization reversal. The difference between this approach and the older less sophisticated techniques is greater than that seen with repair of damaged tubes, because in most cases the tube closed by sterilization was healthy to begin with. In all cases success hinges on the amount of tube remaining, especially the ampulla. Figure 12.4b shows the appearance of the tube after fimbriectomy, in which the end of the tube is removed, frequently through a small vaginal incision. With the fimbria permanently gone, restoration of tubal patency can be accomplished, but pregnancy rates are quite low because of inefficient ovum capture. IVF is a better first choice. Figure 12.5 depicts three methods of sterilization performed laparoscopically. The first (figure A) is with destruction of the tube using electrosurgical energy. The length of tube destroyed is variable depending upon surgical technique. Properly performed, damage is limited to the isthmus, but quite often the ampulla is involved. The second (figure B) method shown involves placing a clip across the tube in the isthmic portion. This produces the least amount of tubal damage and scar tissue, making it the most easily reversed. Figure C shows the tube after an elastic band has been applied. The portion of tube trapped above the band loses its blood supply, becomes atrophic, and withers away over the course of the next few weeks. This also is easily reversed.

Preoperative sterilization reversal counseling and testing should include assessment of ovarian function, particularly in patients beyond 35, and a semen analysis. A preliminary HSG will give information about the proximal portion of the tubes upstream of the block. This is important since in some cases a fibrous reaction sets in as a response to suture material or the band used for sterilization. The next step is that of laparoscopy to inspect the tubes for general appearance and to gauge length. The actual repair can be done at that time. Figure 12.6 shows the various anastomoses usually performed. Isthmus to isthmus is the most desirable, because the diameters of the lumens are equal, and no ampullary portion of the tube has been lost. Isthmus to ampulla has the problem of dealing with disparate diameters, and plastic surgical techniques are used to make the smaller one larger,

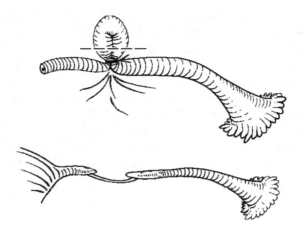

FIGURE 12.4a Pomeroy method of sterilization

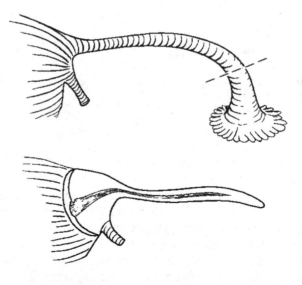

FIGURE 12.4b Fimbriectomy sterilization.

and the larger one smaller. Ampulla to ampulla as shown in figure C is quite easy to perform because the diameters, especially under the microscope, are relatively large, but pregnancy rates are not so good as with isthmic procedures because some of the critical ampulla has been lost.

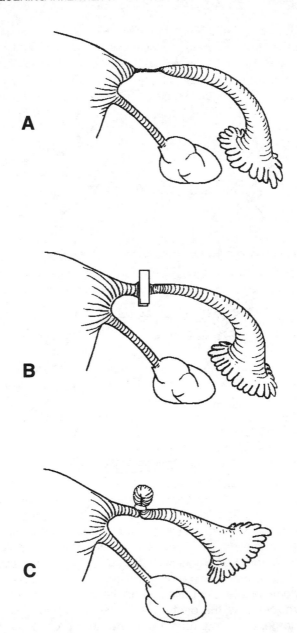

FIGURE 12.5   Laparoscopic sterilizations. (A) Electrofulguration, (B) Clip application, (C) Ring application.

Sometimes the scar tissue on the proximal portion extends into the intramural portion of the tube at shown in figures D and E. This is technically the most challenging of the procedures. When reversal is done under an operating microscope, pregnancy rates between 50% and 90% are expected depending upon the amount of normal tube remaining (especially the ampulla), the status of the fimbria, and the other ancillary factors that you already know.

Years ago I dealt with a newly married couple each of whom had been quite fertile in the first marriage. Because the woman was almost 41, I was reluctant to proceed with surgery. She insisted that she had always conceived in the past within a month or two after stopping contraception, and that she would do this same thing following sterilization reversal. She finally wore me down, and with some reluctance I performed the reversal. Her prediction was correct, and within three months she had conceived. As I subsequently learned with greater experience, the population of sterilized women who previously had conceived easily, continue to do so often well into the 40s and constitute a completely different subset of patients than those usually seen in a fertility practice. A few surgeons have a series of patients with sterilization reversal performed laparoscopically using techniques borrowed from microsurgery. The results are almost as good, and the patient usually returns home on the same day. Microsurgical repair of the tubes can be accomplished through a small abdominal incision with the patient discharged the next day, or in some cases in the evening following surgery. Tubal healing is rapid, and the pregnancy curve over time is much steeper than with surgical treatment of damaged tubes. Most pregnancies occur within six months, and the curve flattens by 15 months. One of my patients conceived at the time of her first postoperative sexual intercourse (23 days). If pregnancy has not been achieved by six months postoperatively, a HSG can be done to check on tubal patency. Ectopic pregnancy rates are surprisingly low, in the 2%-4% range, probably because the tube being operated is basically healthy. If the diagnostic laparoscopy shows that neither tube is amenable to repair, the patient is discharged and IVF offered as an alternative. There's nothing wrong about choosing IVF initially as a less invasive process, particularly if a single pregnancy is desired rather than unlimited potential fertility following successful tubal repair.

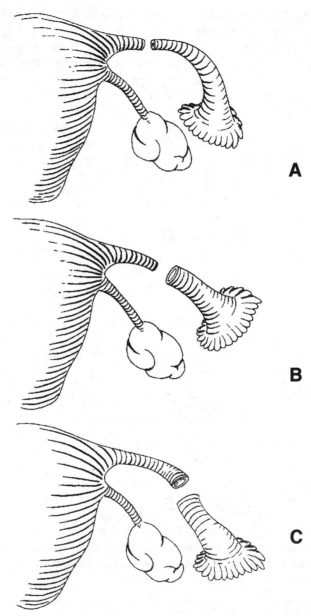

FIGURE 12.6   Sites of tubal anastomosis for sterilization reversal. (A) Isthmus-to-isthmus,
(B) Isthmus-to-ampulla, (C) Ampulla-to-ampulla, (D) Isthmus-to-intramural,
(E) Ampulla-to-intramural.

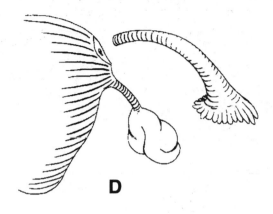

D

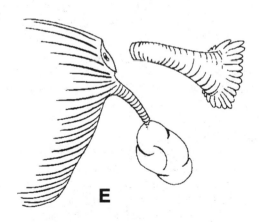

E

13

Male Infertility: When the Little Guys Don't Work

In an unscreened subfertile population some seminal problem can be uncovered in about 40% of cases as the sole abnormality possibly responsible for the couple's inability to conceive. In an additional 10%-15% seminal issues co-exist with a diagnosed female problem. Because pregnancy can occur with even tremendous reduction of sperm numbers, the count is the least important part of the semen analysis. Motility is the most important with morphology as an intermediary factor. Additionally, there's great variation in sperm count on a day-to-day basis, and that says nothing about the variation from laboratory to laboratory. The percentage of variation of sperm concentration is most marked at the lower end of the scale. Men with oligospermia are likely to have a range which could easily be two million per mL one day and 12 million with the next analysis. Table 13.1 lists the major causes of male infertility. Varicocele tops the list and will be discussed shortly. Infection has at least two deleterious results. The first has to do with infection and the inflammatory response in the prostate and other accessory glands causing release of substances known collectively as "reactive oxygen species" which are somewhat toxic to sperm. The other effect has to do with the response to chronic infection leading to closure of the ejaculatory ducts similar to the situation following tubal infection. Congenital problems include failure of testicular development or descent into the scrotum and anatomic abnormalities which interfere with production or delivery of sperm, some of which may be genetic as with the cystic fibrosis gene and deletion of a small part of the Y chromosome. Pharmacologic factors include all the medications which interfere with

Table 13.1
Causes of Male Infertility

Variococele	Endocrine
Infection	Iatrogenic
Congenital	Acquired Testicular Disease
Genetic	
Pharmacologic	Immunological
Sexual Dysfunction	Environmental

erection, ejaculation and libido and include nicotine and alcohol. Sexual dysfunction can also be present as a psychological factor. Endocrine disorders include hypothyroidism and diabetes mellitus, with the latter causing retrograde ejaculation. Iatrogenic infertility follows some medical procedure, such as surgery on the genito- urinary system which could not be performed in such a fashion as to prevent subsequent fertility problems. Also included in this category is inadvertent damage during hernia repair to the abdominal portion of the vas deferens. Trauma may lead to testicular damage, and immunological malfunction may result in production of antibodies directed against sperm. Environmental causes include those occupations associated with high temperatures and voluntary exposure to heat in recreational activities — saunas and steam rooms. At the end of the day, however, less than half of male infertility can be traced to a specific event or illness.

Anatomical Factors

Cryptorchidism is a term used to describe the absence of testes within the scrotal sacs. Since the testes must be maintained at about 4°F lower than body temperature for normal function, their continued presence in the abdominal cavity even up to early childhood can lead to permanent damage. Cryptorchidism should be corrected soon after birth, but prompt surgical treatment does not necessarily ensure normal adult function, since failure to descend may be a sign of some fault in testicular development. Another reason for prompt treatment is that testes which remain undescended are at increased risk for development of malignancy. While we are considering the effects of temperature on sperm production, let me add a comment on the time-honored recommendation to switch from jockey shorts to boxers as an aid to sperm production. To the best of my knowledge this has never been proven to be helpful, although reduction of obesity and a lessened exposure to extreme heat as with saunas, hot baths and certain occupations will make a difference. There is marketed an ice pack scrotal supporter which is purported to improve semen quality, but scientific documentation of this claim is sparse.

The Varicocele

The veins in the scrotum have valves just as do those in the legs, which when competent, prevent gravity-induced backflow. When these valves fail, the veins become dilated, and temperature rises within the scrotal sac. This is the usual explanation for the association between varicocele and reduction of sperm count, motility and percentage of normal morphology. A popular theory some years ago, which has lost support, is that there is leakage of blood containing high levels of steroid hormones from the adrenal gland to the testes as a consequence of failure to prevent retrograde flow down the venous system. Actually, we're not talking about one vein, but a network or cluster of veins. The venous collecting system is asymmetric in the human, and varicocele is usually found as a left-sided only problem (95%); occasionally there is an additional right-sided varicocele (5%), but a right varicocele alone is quite rare (<1%).

What seems to be on the surface a straightforward cause and effect relationship actually is complicated and has sparked a continued controversy for half a century, which is still unsettled. Varicoceles can be diagnosed, when large, by simply looking at the scrotum with the patient standing, or by palpating the dilated veins on physical examination (see figure 13.1), also in the standing position with the man straining. More subtle cases are diagnosed by placing a Doppler microphone on the scrotum and determining whether there is any downward flow in the veins during standing.

Varicocele can be found in about 10% of the general population, but is increased to about 20% in the subfertile group and to at least 30% in patients with any seminal abnormality. Students of logic would correctly conclude that one can have a varicocele and be perfectly fertile, that infertility in general, and male infertility in particular, is associated with

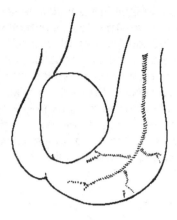

FIGURE 13.1 A left scrotal varicose vein.

an increase in varicocele prevalence, but the third conclusion is the one that causes the problems. That is, the finding of seminal problems associated with varicocele presence is not necessarily a cause and effect relationship. Repair of this anatomic abnormality is simple, and consists of tying off the cluster of veins through a small incision in the groin rather than the scrotum. This can be done under local, regional, or general anesthesia as an outpatient or one night stay. The risk of doing anything deleterious is low, and the operation is not at all technically difficult. Because of the 72 day sperm developmental cycle, improved semen quality may not be apparent for three months. The question is, does this surgery have any benefit on pregnancy rate, rather than seminal quality, as the bottom-line, compared with no surgery. Alternative methods of occluding the veins include injection with tissue adhesives or insertion of blocking balloons or umbrella-like valvular devices which remain in place, all done under radiographic guidance in the x-ray department or small surgical suite. Medical therapies include hormonal stimulation of sperm production and (indirectly), artificial insemination techniques.

Let's state what is generally agreed; the size of the varicocele has no relation to seminal parameters or establishment of pregnancy. Second, patients who have a diagnosed varicocele and who agree to follow-up care without surgery generally have a progressive diminution of sperm count and decreased testicular volume but neither of these two measurements correlates well with initiation of pregnancy.

By now I'm sure you know the study which is necessary. We need a population infertile for least three years in which the only finding is abnormal semen quality in conjunction with the presence of a varicocele. Men would be chosen completely at random to have surgical repair or observation only for a sufficiently long duration of time to see if there were a difference in pregnancy rate between the groups. As simple as this sounds, very few studies with valid protocols have been performed. There are many reports in the literature on pregnancy rates following varicocele repair— varicocelectomy – but few with a true control group. Of the studies which are properly formulated, the results are mixed.

Our group addressed the issue of whether insemination techniques would be helpful, dependent upon the results of the hamster egg penetration assay (SPA). We found that the pregnancy rate was 21% (9% monthly), for insemination performed in couples in which the SPA was normal, but no pregnancies occurred in 121 cycles of insemination in 43 varicocele patients with abnormal penetration results or defects in all three areas of the semen analysis. An attempt to improve sperm quality with use of stimulating agents such as clomiphene citrate or tamoxifen rarely produces positive benefit unless FSH or testosterone levels are low. The usual recommendation is to proceed with either insemination first or direct treatment of the varicocele first, reserving the other if the first choice fails, and holding IVF/ICSI as the ultimate solution.

Other Anatomical Problems

Hypospadias (figure 13.2), the opening of the urethra on the underside of the penis rather than at the end, usually can be surgically repaired so that sperm can be effectively delivered to the vagina; if not, insemination techniques should suffice as a method of treatment.

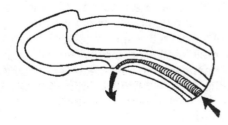

FIGURE 13.2 Hypospadias with urethral opening on the underside of the penis.

Retrograde ejaculation of sperm into the bladder occurs when a sphincter muscle fails to contract. This is seen most commonly with diabetes, but can also result from bladder surgery, prostate surgery, urethral procedures, and the use of some drugs. Diagnosis is made by microscopic inspection of urine passed immediately after ejaculation. In some cases medications can improve the function of the sphincter. Otherwise sperm can be collected if the patient voids soon after ejaculation. The sperm can be concentrated by centrifugation and processed for intrauterine insemination (IUI). Because the urine is hypertonic and has an osmotic gradient, it is important to drink a great deal of water for 24 hours in advance in order to make the urine dilute. Additionally, urine is normally acidic, an environment poorly tolerated by sperm. Therefore for the two or three days prior to anticipated sperm collection these men alkalinize the urine by taking 600 mg of sodium bicarbonate three times daily. Men with spinal cord injuries are functionally sterile even though they continue, in most cases, to produce sperm. Sperm can be collected with vibratory or electrical stimulation with rectal probes. Close medical supervision is necessary because one of the side effects in these patients with neurologic injury is transient blood pressure elevation from the stimulation.

Blockage of the ejaculatory ductal system at any point can be approached surgically if the problem is a localized one rather than failure to develop. Scar tissue formation following sexually acquired infection may produce this end result. The blocked segment can be removed and the ends united, analogous to tubal surgery. Again, we see a parallel with female tubal surgery; microsurgical techniques give the best results. Even with skillful surgery, the inflammatory process may cause the duct to close down postoperatively. For that reason, a small testicular biopsy is often taken during surgery, so that tissue can be processed and sperm extracted and frozen for possible later IVF/ICSI. Congenital absence of the vas does not lend itself to surgical repair. The diagnosis is suspected when azoospermia exists but the fructose test is negative. Physical examination confirms the absence of the vas. In vitro fertilization techniques with direct insertion of sperm into the egg will bypass this problem with the sperm being collected either by needle aspiration or a small testicular biopsy under local anesthesia. In all cases of congenital absence of the vas, the patient should be screened for the carrier state of cystic fibrosis. If positive, the wife needs to be screened as well.

Infections

We have already mentioned both short-term and long-term effects of genital infection on male infertility, but other systemic infections can also cause problems. Mumps acquired after puberty may leave the victim permanently sterile as a direct effect of the virus on the testes. Sustained high fevers seen with malaria can also cause permanent testicular damage. Any systemic illness with inflammation such as ulcerative colitis, regional enteritis, rheumatoid arthritis, and systemic lupus erythematosis can interfere with sperm quality. The semen picture usually improves during periods of remission. One of the drugs commonly used for inflammatory bowel disorders, azulfadine, has an adverse effect on sperm production.

Trauma

It is the rare man who has never suffered physical trauma to the scrotum from sports or accident. The truth is these injuries rarely produce any long-term effects on testicular function. Severe injury may require drainage of a blood collection within the scrotal sac (a hematoma). Testicular torsion is another matter and must be surgically corrected quickly in order to avoid losing the testicle.

Hormonal

Hormonal deficiencies are rarely causes of male infertility. Problems with the thyroid or adrenal glands sufficient enough to interfere with sperm production usually are diagnosed because of systemic symptoms long before the visit to an infertility office. The Kallman Syndrome causes a deficiency in FSH and LH release as a consequence of hypothalamic failure to release adequate amounts of GnRH. A related symptom is inability to detect odors (anosmia). The treatment is to use gonadotropins such as Humegon, analogous to ovulation induction in the female, but with the course of treatment sustained daily over many months. Prolactin elevation in the male is unlikely to cause milky breast discharge as in the female, and is often unsuspected. Prolactin excess leads to suppression of testosterone production with decreased well-being and sex drive. The treatment is the same as in the female using oral agents.

Low dose testosterone as a stimulating agent has no place in treatment of male infertility. The effect is similar to that of giving birth control pills to women. Testosterone is helpful, however, as a supplement for men whose testosterone levels are low with associated symptoms and where fertility is not an issue. Although small doses of daily clomiphene citrate or tamoxifen have been used for years as a testicular stimulant, almost all well controlled studies fail to show a significant beneficial effect. But within the groups, there usually are a few individuals with a phenomenal change in seminal quality. Unfortunately we have no test which would identify the small percentage of men with poor semen quality who respond so well to this treatment. For that reason it is still used empirically, at a dose of 25 mg daily for three to six months. Men whose FSH levels are already elevated are least likely to have a positive response. Small doses of hCG, used as an LH surrogate have also been employed as treatment for seminal problems. The typical program is twice weekly injections for ten weeks. Results are not startling. Elevation of FSH levels in the blood is a sign of incipient testicular failure of sperm production, slightly different than the reservoir effect in the female, but with the same poor prognosis.

Genetic and Developmental Factors

The Klinefelter syndrome describes a man who has 47 chromosomes rather than 46 with an XXY instead of the normal male XY sex chromosome complement. These individuals frequently have poorly developed genital structures, slow beard growth and non muscular body build. In some cases there is minimal sperm production within the testes, although sperm are rarely found in the ejaculate. IVF with ICSI has achieved pregnancy in these cases. There are a number of related inherited syndromes involving hormonal receptor defects in which the target tissues cannot bind testosterone and similar hormones. At the moment there's no known treatment for this, but in the future gene insertion therapy to correct the chromosomal change may be helpful. We've talked about cystic fibrosis before but a related disorder of a milder nature is **Kartagener** syndrome which affects cilia throughout the body. High power microscopy demonstrates the defects in the structure of the sperm tail (flagellum). IVF with ICSI is the answer to this problem as well.

We now understand that there are certain sites on the Y chromosome which must be present and active in order for normal spermatogenesis to take place. If one or more of these specific areas is deleted as a consequence of a genetic error occurring after fertilization, that man in his adulthood will probably be azoospermic, but may have some minimal sperm production within the tubules of the testes. Even though the sperm are extremely immature, IVF with ICSI has been amazingly successful in bringing about pregnancy. The downside, however, is that this chromosomal problem which arose during fetal development can now be passed on from the affected father to son.

Drugs

Sustained, heavy use of marijuana has a negative effect on testosterone levels, sex drive and semen quality. Cocaine, thought to heighten sexual enjoyment, actually reduces sexual function when used regularly. Tranquilizers, anti-hypertensive drugs and mood altering agents can interfere with sex drive, erectile potency and ejaculation. Often a substitute drug can be found. The family of calcium channel blockers used for treatment of cardiovascular disorders affects male fertility by interfering with the acrosome-capacitation reaction. Nitrofurantoin, a urinary antibiotic, also adversely affects sperm quality. Just as with the female, treatment of life-threatening malignant disorders with radiation and/or chemotherapy can bring about temporary or permanent failure of sperm production. Although semen quality is frequently poor at the time diagnosis is made because of the systemic effects of the illness, banking a few sperm specimens for possible later use with IVF/ICSI prior to treatment is a good policy if there is a desire to maintain potential fertility. Cigarette smoking has been shown to have an adverse effect on semen quality. In most cases this is probably not of clinical significance, but is important for those men who have borderline or low sperm function.

Immunologic Infertility

Autoimmune diseases are actually not rare, with thyroiditis, regional enteritis, ulcerative colitis, systemic lupus erythematosis, and rheumatoid arthritis representing but a few of these disorders. Antibodies directed toward sperm can arise in a man as a consequence of entry of sperm material into the vascular system where contact is made with white blood cells. The sperm protein is perceived as foreign material and serves as the antigenic stimulus for antibody production. While this is understandable following testicular trauma or surgery, most men with documented anti-sperm antibodies have no such history. Direct treatment could be use of agents such as cortisone-like steroids to suppress antibody production in general. Besides leaving the individual more prone to infections because the defense mechanisms have been blunted, use of these agents is associated with the potential for some major side effects such as induction of diabetes, activation of ulcer, psychosis, and most feared —aseptic necrosis of the hip necessitating replacement with an artificial hip joint. IVF with ICSI eliminates the need for this potentially dangerous therapy if insemination techniques are not successful in establishing pregnancy.

Vasectomy Reversal

Men seek reversal of sterilization for the same reasons as women. Sterilization by vasectomy is the most popular and effective method of permanent contraception. Severing and sealing the vas is a simple procedure which can be performed quickly in an office or operating room. But as with the female, reversal is more complicated. Figure 13.3 schematically shows the steps in this process. The first line of stitches brings together the vas after the scar tissue has been trimmed away. The second row of stitches serves as a buttressing support. Here too, microsurgical technique gives results far superior to surgery unaided by magnification. Sperm will re-appear in the ejaculate in about 90% of cases, although six months may go by before this takes place. The pregnancy rate, however, is in the 50% zone with the differential a function of associated female fertility factors which might be present and because formation of anti-sperm antibodies originating from the vasectomy interferes with sperm motility or egg penetration. Unlike female sterilization reversal, there is a definite time factor. If sterilization was performed more than five years prior to reversal, results are definitely decreased. Just as with any ductal surgery in the testis, fluid at the point of the blockage should be taken and inspected for the presence of sperm which can be frozen in case the vas scars down postoperatively. The sperm present in the testis further upstream are more immature, but are healthier than those collected at the point of blockage, and therefore a small testicular biopsy should be taken. I counsel patients that an antibody study should be done prior to surgery; if positive, the success rate following anastomosis is decreased even if sperm re-appear in the ejaculate. Under those circumstances, IVF/ICSI might be a better first choice. The first sperm which appear after successful repair are usually poorly motile, and up to two years may be necessary before specimens demonstrate normal motility characteristics.

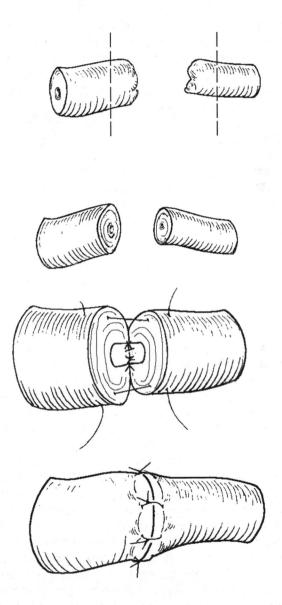

FIGURE 13.3 Vasectomy reversal. Top to bottom, trimming of scarred ends, alignment and anastomosis of the two segments.

14

Artificial Insemination

Artificial insemination is a technique of delivering sperm produced by masturbation to the vagina, cervix, uterus, tubes, and/or peritoneal cavity. The sperm may be from the patient's partner or from a donor; the sperm may be used soon after ejaculation as a fresh specimen or after frozen sperm have been thawed. Various methods of preparation may be used. The indications for artificial insemination, husband (AIH) are broad, and as you already may have guessed, the results are quite varied and dependent on the problem which AIH is thought to address. When is AIH indicated? How is it best timed? How many inseminations per cycle are necessary? Over how many cycles should AIH be used before going on to different solutions? The following paragraphs will address these questions, and then we will consider artificial insemination, donor (AID).

Indications and Timing

Table 14.1 shows the usual indications for artificial insemination with husband's sperm. Male anatomical problems usually relate to hypospadias not satisfactorily corrected, to extreme obesity, or to inability to deliver sperm to the vagina because of extreme penile shortness. Retrograde ejaculation has already been mentioned and discussed in the previous chapter. Inability to erect whether caused by drug effects, previous surgery, or sexual dysfunction on a psychologic basis can be a reason to employ AIH so long as the patient is able to ejaculate a specimen. An increasing indication for AIH is that of

Table 14.1
Indication for Artificial Insemination, Husband

Male	Female
Anatomic	Anatomical
Retrograde Ejaculation	Dyspareunia, Physiologic or Psychologic
Physiologic Impotence	Sexual Dysfunction
Cryopreserved Semen	
Sexual Dysfunction	

cryopreservation of semen stored because of impending chemotherapy or radiation. The sperm can be stored in liquid nitrogen indefinitely. There's always some loss of motility over the entire freeze — thaw cycle. Therefore, a specimen should be processed in the laboratory after the thaw to regain motility.

Female anatomical factors include the congenital abnormalities of the vagina and cervix as well as those acquired by trauma, disease or surgery. Dyspareunia may be so severe with endometriosis in spite of treatment that sexual intercourse becomes a dreared event; under those circumstances AIH becomes an attractive option.

Table 14.2 lists some of the methods most commonly used to time the inseminations. The BBT chart as we know is convenient, inexpensive and non-invasive. The problem is that it is a much better indicator of ovulation in the past tense rather than the future, and inseminations should be done just before ovulation in order to achieve best results. Sperm, even when subpar, probably have more hours of activity after insemination than the egg has for normal fertilization after ovulation. Blood tests, which would have to be done serially in order to detect the LH surge, constitute an unattractive package of expense and travel. We use this approach only for those patients who, for some reason, can

Table 14.2
Methods of Timing Insemination

Basal Body Temperature Chart

Serum Luteinizing Hormone (LH) Determination

Urinary Luteinizing Hormone Detection Kits

Serial Ultrasound Examinations

Ovulation Triggering with human Chorionic Gonadotropin (hCG)

not read consistently the urinary LH kits, which are the most cost-effective and accurate method of timing insemination. Because follicles mature at different diameters, the high-tech ultrasound approach for insemination timing has the same drawbacks as blood tests for LH levels. Additionally it has decreased accuracy as a predictor, rather than as a confirmer of ovulation. Of course, if agents such as Humegon are used for ovulation induction, ultrasound becomes a necessity. Even in a natural menstrual cycle, ovulation can be triggered by administering hCG when the single follicle is ripe. The drug is expensive and its use is usually limited to situations in which the woman ovulates irregularly or when an upcoming weekend promises to spoil the best laid plans for insemination because of laboratory closure.

The procedure which we follow in our office is for the patient to call on the afternoon in which her urinary LH kit first turns positive. Although the risk of infection from a well prepared specimen used for IUI is probably 1-2/1000 according to literature results, we have our patients take a single 100 mg doxycycline capsule on the night before, the morning of, and the evening following insemination (or an equivalent if she has an allergy to tetracycline antibiotics) as a prophylactic measure against infection. At 8 a.m. the husband or wife drops off a semen specimen which has been collected at home and transported to the office in a shirt pocket within two hours of collection in order to maintain temperature. The laboratory processing (for us) takes about 2-3 hours, after which insemination is performed, usually as IUI.

Great care is taken in the laboratory to double label all specimen jars, tubes and final syringes so that a disaster of mistaken identity does not occur.

Processing and Techniques

The human ejaculate normally contains a mixture of live motile sperm, live non-motile sperm, dead sperm, chemical crystals, urinary tract cells and often some white blood cells constituting a great deal of unwanted debris. The goals of specimen preparation include; (1) removal of material not contributing to fertilization, (2) isolation and collection of the most motile sperm, and; (3) obtaining as high a yield of total motile sperm as possible. At the same time the processing must not injure or harm the sperm in any way.

Still widely practiced is the technique of placing the seminal specimen in a high-powered centrifuge, and spinning down until a pellet of solid material is at the bottom of the tube. This pellet contains all the items mentioned above. Live motile sperm over time will disengage themselves from this trap and "swim up" into the medium. After a time the liquid medium is transferred to another tube, centrifugation repeated, the liquid poured off, and the secondary pellet re-suspended in a small volume of fluid ready for insemination. This sounds like a reasonable process, but it is not. First, this process results in a low yield of "total motile sperm", that is, the total number of sperm showing motility which will be used for the insemination, not a concentration as in the semen analysis. Second, the force of the centrifugation used in the first step is sufficient to cause damage to the sperm and evokes release of the dreaded "reactive oxygen species" known to be injurious to sperm.

If one of the goals is to separate live, swimming sperm from the rest of the junk, it makes some sense to construct a separation system based on sperm motility. One of the first systems used with this philosophy in mind was composed of a glass wool filter similar to that used in ventilation systems. This worked fine with respect to yield, but the sperm heads seemed to be damaged in the process. Currently inert small particles made of silica or other non-reactive material are used in layers in a tube into which the sperm have been placed. The sperm can be collected in a more gentle fashion and with excellent percentage yield at the end of the procedure. Sometimes we put special medium into the container used to collect the sperm which may increase the number of sperm not bound in cases of antibody formation. Pentoxyfillene is an interesting agent with properties similar to caffeine. Biochemically, it inhibits the enzyme which breaks down the energy source in intermediate metabolism. Some sperm specimens with poor motility characteristics even after laboratory processing have a dramatic boost of motility when this agent is added to the medium.

The insemination is performed with a syringe and a small volume of medium in which the sperm are suspended. There's little or no place for intra-vaginal insemination in a medical office. This can be done at home with semen collected by masturbation if intercourse cannot be accomplished. For many years all inseminations were done as intra-cervical deposits. For the last ten years, however, intrauterine insemination (IUI) has been the mainstay. The consensus is that pregnancy rates are higher with IUI than with cervical insemination. When sperm are placed within the uterine cavity, it is important that all the seminal plasma has been removed from the specimen. Semen contains large quantities of prostaglandins, which cause intense uterine contraction, nausea, vomiting and diarrhea — not a pretty picture! From time to time papers appear extolling the virtues of tubal insemination performed with a catheter passed through the cervix and uterus into the tube. Additionally, there has been fleeting enthusiasm for placing sperm directly into the posterior cul-de-sac via a needle puncture at the top of the uterus (not a pleasant procedure). Neither of these two approaches appear to offer any improvement in pregnancy rate compared with IUI.

Our technique for IUI begins with insertion of a speculum to visualize the cervix. Next, the cervix is wiped with a cotton ball so that that vaginal material will not be transmitted upwards by the insemination. A soft plastic catheter is introduced into the cervix and upwards into the uterine cavity. This is usually accomplished without the need for a cervical tenaculum (which hurts) or any cervical dilators. The small volume of suspended sperm, usually 0.5 mL is delivered with a syringe, and that's all folks. Because the sperm are in the uterus, the patient does not need to maintain a reclining position. If there is any regurgitation of fluid through the cervix as a consequence of uterine contractions, a small plastic coated foam rubber tampon can be placed against the cervix, to be removed by the patient hours later. Some patients experience significant uterine cramps just from the catheter alone; administration of drugs such as Motrin before the insemination is very helpful in avoiding any discomfort.

Results

The two major indications for IUI are poor postcoital tests with normal semen analyses, called a cervical factor and poor postcoital tests in the presence of abnormal seminal characteristics. Additionally, IUI is frequently used coupled with gonadotropin ovulation induction for unexplained infertility and infertility associated with minimal to mild endometriosis. The usual spread of results for IUI performed when semen quality is poor ranges from 0% through 23% depending on the quality of sperm. If, after processing, <3 million motile sperm are recovered, the procedure is probably not worthwhile. Total motile count seems to be the most important prognosticator, with morphology also somewhat predictive. Pregnancy yield with IUI performed because of a cervical factor is significantly greater, with a pregnancy rate somewhere between 16% and 43% as reported in various studies.

A study which we did produced results which generally reflect the role for IUI as a treatment for infertility. We measured monthly fecundity in 302 couples treated in 991 cycles of IUI compared with 255 couples untreated in 2668 cycles. The overall results showed a 10% monthly pregnancy for IUI coupled with hMG (human menopausal gonadotropin), three percent monthly with IUI alone, and one percent spontaneous pregnancy monthly without therapy. The yield for the combination therapy was 16% monthly for patients with unexplained infertility, 12% for minimal endometriosis, 11% for pure cervical factor and six percent for male factor. As with other fertility treatments which are influenced greatly by individual laboratory or physician skill levels, there is little consensus concerning the role for IUI, but in some areas there is general agreement. First, male factor infertility responds less well to IUI than pure cervical factor and has the lowest pregnancy rate (PR) of all the diagnostic categories treated with insemination. Second, almost every study has concluded that 90% of all pregnancies achieved with hmG/IUI occur by the end of the fourth cycle and that continuation of therapy beyond six cycles is probably unwarranted. The combination of clomiphene citrate and IUI has little to offer to the normally ovulating patient. By contrast, the combination of gonadotropins and IUI seems to be synergistic with PR greater than the sum of the two when used alone.

Artificial Insemination, Donor

Indications for donor insemination appear in table 14.3. Although the possibility of pregnancy always exists when any number, no matter how small, of motile sperm can be placed into the female reproductive tract by intercourse or insemination, there comes a point where frustration, expense and unfavorable odds point to consideration of AID as a solution. Of course, if no sperm are present or if they cannot be collected, that individual is considered to be functionally sterile. IVF, and particularly ICSI, have revolutionized the approach to the couple infertile because of severe seminal problems. Nevertheless, at this time we cannot solve all of the seminally related infertility problems with these techniques.

Table 14.3
Indications for Artificial Insemination, Donor

Male Factor Infertility

Azoospermia   Other Semen Abnormalities

Oligospermia   Previous Male Sterilization

Paternal Genetic Disease

Physiologic Impotence

Psychologic Impotence

Absence of a Male Partner

Severe Female Rh Disease

Many of the genetically well identified disorders can be diagnosed early in pregnancy with great accuracy. In cases where the genetic defect is one that will lead to early childhood death or a life of severe handicaps and pain, the diagnosis can be used as a reason for pregnancy termination. For many couples at risk, this is a devastating process, and for some, totally unacceptable under any circumstances. Even pre-implantation genetic testing of an embryo may fail to diagnose a serious inherited problem. As an example, Huntington's chorea, which does not strike its victims until adulthood is carried as a male autosomal dominant factor. Most of the time couples do not know that they are at risk until they or someone in the family have had an affected pregnancy. AID with a donor properly genetically screened can eliminate this risk. For some people with physiologic or psychologic impotence with ejaculatory failure, obtaining a semen specimen may be not only a psychologic hassle, but an actual physical risk such as seen with the use of electroejaculation in spinal cord injury patients who may suffer rectal burns from the probe and/or significant hypertension during the process. Over the past few years we have seen an increase in single parent requests for a sperm donor. These usually emanate from an executive or professional career woman, who, in some respects, has become married to her profession but who very much wants to parent. Remember that there are many single parent families in our country, some by design, but many through death or divorce. In spite of the fact that Rh incompatibility as a cause of fetal loss is almost totally preventable with a single injection of immune globulin at the completion of the first pregnancy, thus safeguarding the next, mistakes or lapses happen and Rh negative women become sensitized after the initial pregnancy with an Rh positive fetus. In the vast majority of cases Rh sensitized pregnancy can be managed with fetal transfusion and early delivery. But for those cases in which maternal antibodies cross the placenta causing fetal anemia and heart failure so severe that in spite of good treatment intrauterine death occurs, donor insemination using an Rh negative donor becomes the answer.

The first successful donor insemination was performed in 1884 by Dr. William Pancoast at Thomas Jefferson University in Philadelphia. Today, the best guess is that there are between 30,000 and 50,000 births annually as a result of AID. This is a guesstimate because in our country the process is usually cloaked in secrecy and there is no national registry for egg or sperm donors as there is in some other countries.

Counseling and Work-Up

In many cases a complete fertility survey already has been performed so that the female needs no additional testing. Otherwise, her ovulatory status should be determined. All the screening tests discussed earlier as part of the general fertility evaluation should be done with inclusion of any special screening based on ethnic background. She should be tested for all of the common sexually transmitted diseases prior to exposure to donor semen. This list includes gonorrhea, syphilis, chlamydia, hepatitis, and HIV. Unless there is a history of tubal infection or pelvic surgery, we will usually initiate therapy without a HSG since many pregnancies occur quite quickly. If, after three inseminations pregnancy has not been established, the tubal evaluation is done at that time. Some programs perform screening HSG in all patients as a prelude to AID. We do not believe that this is desirable as a routine because of cost, discomfort and radiation exposure.

The decision to undergo AID should be made with great thought. It is quite normal initially for there to be considerable ambivalence, since this is, at best, a second reproductive choice. In our practice, we find that it is the husband who usually initiates consideration of AID. Regardless of which partner is the driving force, it is important that both accept this method of reproduction and that one of the partners is not being dragged along against his or her will. For that reason we insist that every couple in our practice, or single woman candidate for AID, be interviewed by our reproductive psychologist. AID is not the best answer in all cases; sometimes adoption is more easily accepted by one partner or the other as an equalizing factor. Long-term psychologic studies of the family unit show that properly counseled couples are quite happy with the decision to have AID.

A special situation can exist when a family member such as a brother or father is considered as the sperm donor. In the United States AID was begun with anonymous sperm donation and until very recently this was the exclusive method of treatment. Not so in the rest of the world where family values and family units are stronger. In India, for instance, the father is the first choice as a donor if he is still fertile. Otherwise, two or more of the brothers, who usually live in close proximity, will donate semen specimens which are then pooled for the actual insemination. With proper psychologic counseling, which includes the semen donor relative and his wife, if married, this can be an excellent pathway to follow. Family feuds, however, can be vicious, and as many as possible of the "what if" scenarios should be explored. Geography is no longer an impediment because sperm can be collected, frozen and stored in liquid nitrogen indefinitely for shipment when and where needed.

The couple needs to formulate a plan to handle the question of what to tell the child or family. Less than 20% state that they will at some point disclose to the child, although this percentage seems to be increasing. There is no right or wrong answer to this question. It is up to the couple, and their plan today may change years from now. This is only one of the important points which a good psychologist will bring to the couple's attention for consideration.

In our practice the psychologist reviews the donor list with the couple so that they can select a donor. Today all anonymous donor insemination is done with frozen —thawed sperm usually obtained from a sperm bank. The reason for the change from fresh sperm had to do with the risk of HIV transmission as part of the insemination process. Although this was true for all the other sexually transmitted diseases, and appreciated for years, the other pathologies were less likely to result in death. One advantage of banked sperm is that the donor is never on vacation, a problem that we faced yearly when our medical student donor population scattered to the four corners of the globe in the summer. An additional advantage of using frozen-thawed sperm is that once pregnant, the couple can choose to purchase additional supply of that particular donor to be used in the future for a sibling pregnancy. The donor lists usually include information on ethnic background, height, weight, hair and eye color, general appearance, educational background, family history, profession and general interests. In some programs, pictures may be available, but few donors give permission for this. Rarely, donors have given permission for the offspring to contact them upon reaching adulthood; it is too soon to tell if this social experiment will have positive benefits.

Donor Screening and Selection

The goal of a sperm bank is to recruit healthy suitable donors, with high fertility potential, who are free from sexually transmitted diseases (STD's). Guidelines exist from ASRM which apply to donor selection. First, donors should be below the age of 40 in order to lessen the risk of age-related chromosomal abnormalities in the offspring. Semen criteria include volume > 1 mL, count > 50 million per mL and progressive motility > 60%. A test freeze-thaw should demonstrate at least 50% of the initial motility. Not so long ago, sperm banking was somewhat of a cottage industry. Most fertility practices had ten or fewer donors as a nucleus group. Today consumers are more demanding in donor choice, and the suggested guidelines for testing, and the need for cryopreservation have tended to solidify sperm banking in the hands of a few large commercial sources which are capable of shipping frozen samples just about anywhere in the world. The potential advantage for the patient is one of having a greater choice of donors, allowing for a better match with the husband; on our side we have concerns about the adequacy of the screening process regarding personality type and character, which we used to do personally.

A complete medical history should be obtained. The prospective donor must be free of major disorders such as hemophilia. According to his ethnic background he should be screened for those autosomal recessive genes known to be prevalent in that population, sickle cell trait as an example. All Caucasian donors should be screened for cystic fibrosis. A strong family history of diabetes, hypertension, schizophrenia or alcoholism should be reason for disqualification. Most programs do not obtain a full chromosomal analysis on prospective donors because of cost considerations and the expected low yield (< 2%). A thorough family history of first-degree relatives is probably the most important item in the check off list. There should be no history of major malformations, and no suspicion of autosomal dominant or x-linked disease. Some programs administer standardized psychologic tests. At the least, a thorough interview with a health professional should be performed.

A detailed sexual history must be obtained in order to exclude donors at increased risk for STD, and HIV in particular. This disqualifies one with any use of intravenous drugs in the past, homosexual relationships, and current multiple sexual partners. The American Association of Tissue Banks published standards for semen banking in 1997. Table 14.4 lists testing requirements. The

Table 14.4
Donor Testing Requirements

Test	Initial	6-Month Release
Genetic (Tay-Sachs, thalassemia, sickle cell, cystic fibrosis)	Recommended when donor's family history or genetic background indicates increased risk	
Anti-HIV-1/Anti-HIV-2	Yes	Yes
Hepatitis B surface antigen	Yes	No (hepatitis B infection will be detected by anti-HBc)
Anti-HBc	Yes	Yes*
Anti-HCV	Yes	Yes
Anti-HTLV-I	Yes	Yes
Syphilis	Yes	Yes
Neisseria gonorrhoeae	Yes	Yes
Chlamydia trachomatis	Yes	Yes
Semen Analysis	Yes	

Note: Anti- = antibody to; HBc = hepatitis B core antigen; HBs = hepatitis B surface antigen; HCV = hepatitis C virus; HTLV-I = human T-lymphotropic virus type I. *Anti-HBc positive donors may be accepted if they also test positive for anti-HBs.

Linden JV, Centola G. Fertil Steril 1997;68:597-600

standard protocol for sperm banking around the world is for the frozen sperm to be in quarantine, and to be released when the repeat STD tests continue to be negative at least six months after the last collection. This interval is based on the time necessary for antibody detection in the bloodstream following exposure to one of these infectious agents. Cytomegalovirus is a problem. Antibody can be detected in approximately 40% of the prospective donor population, potentially disqualifying a large number of otherwise suitable candidates. If the recipient is also positive, the donor can be used. A special urine test can be used to document that the infection is old, and that live virus is not being shed. As you might imagine, the entire screening process is extensive and expensive. It requires considerable commitment from the donor and the bank. Compensation for the donor's time and expenses may be given, but not so great as to make monetary incentive the prime consideration to be a donor. In many European countries, donors are not compensated over and above transportation costs. In France donor sperm comes from one source, which makes for marvelous records and scientific data collection. In all cases the donor should sign a consent form disavowing any paternal rights. The general recommendation is that each donor have no more than 10 offspring with the number reduced for small rural communities. The actual risk of two individuals subsequently marrying who had the same biological father (the donor) has been computed and is somewhere in the range of one in many millions.

Specimen Preparation and Insemination Technique

The frozen sperm is kept in liquid nitrogen tanks in canisters which hold small vials called "straws" each of which is usually sufficient for one insemination. There are a number of different protocols for thawing, some in room air and some in a water bath. The sperm are suspended in a physiologic culture medium. Insemination is almost always as an IUI because of the loss of motility associated with the freeze-thaw process. Insemination timing is the same as with AIH. The abortion rate and congenital abnormality rates in the offspring are no different from fresh sperm inseminations or in the general population. Multiple inseminations per cycle add nothing but cost, provided that timing is accurate.

Results

A study which we did a few years ago reflects the results achieved in most established programs of AID. One IUI per cycle using frozen-thawed sperm was performed in 796 AID treatments in 143 women. There were 112 pregnancies, or a 53.1% pregnancy rate per patient (some had more than one pregnancy). Cycle fecundity was 13.1%, 18.4%, and 13.0% in cycles one through three, respectively, with overall cycle fecundity 14.1%. The 50% cumulative pregnancy mark was reached by the sixth cycle, and no pregnancies occurred after cycle 12. If all the women who did not conceive had continued in the program for 12 cycles, the projected pregnancy rate for the entire group would have been 86.9%. For the first pregnancy, the median time to conceive was 2.5 months versus the mean of 3.9, SD 2.9. With the median less than the mean, conception was very quick for the majority of those conceiving. The mean age of our patients was 34.8, SD 4.5 years with the oldest patient 46. Concomitant female fertility factors included ovulatory dysfunction in 42.5%, endometriosis in 12.9% and other factors in 10.2%. We were most interested in analysis of the seminal data which could be predictive of success. For instance, we wondered if the total number of motile sperm used in the insemination, an important factor for AIH, made any difference in an AID situation. When we were all finished with statistical gyrations, we found that the total motile count either before or after laboratory processing of the specimen made no difference in the outcome. The only seminal parameter that was statistically associated with outcome for AID was the motility of the specimen after processing. When the data were bracketed into quartiles, of 35%-60%, 61%-74%, 75%-80%, and 81%-95% motility, fecundity rates were 9.8%, 12.6%, 13.5%, and 24.7%. The findings were of some practical importance because in some programs a lower limit may be set on the total number of motile sperm satisfactory for insemination, which means if that threshold is not crossed, an extra specimen will be used, which will double the cost of the procedure without increasing chances for pregnancy. A few paragraphs back we mentioned the advantages of frozen compared with fresh sperm insemination. The disadvantage was that until recently, when we learned how to deal with the motility issue, cycle fecundity rates remained higher for insemination with fresh sperm compared with frozen. Now, we are achieving better results in shorter time frames than mentioned above. Not everyone can get pregnant in the first month of treatment. I counsel my patients that if normal fertility is defined by pregnancy within a year, they should be prepared for the same interval with AID, although the truth is that the majority will be pregnant by six months.

15

Immunological Infertility

Our bodies' immune systems protect us against invasion by microorganisms in a double-barrel fashion. Specialized white cells rise to mount an instant attack on the foreign intruder. At the same time a process is initiated in which, if this is a first time exposure, circulating antibodies specific to the external antigen, usually the outer protein coat, will be manufactured. This antigen-antibody response is then filed away in our immune system repository, so that continued exposure, or a repeat contact even years later will be greeted with a quick production of millions of antibody molecules circulating in the bloodstream or produced locally as with cervical mucus. As many of us know, nasal mucus is also involved in the classic response to inhaled pollen perceived as allergens during rosefever and hayfever seasons. Allergic responses to latex (natural rubber) is becoming an increasing problem to patients and medical personnel. Thus, what started out as an excellent defense mechanism can become a nuisance or even a life-threatening inappropriate response. To those allergic to shellfish, entrance into a restaurant serving lobster or clams may be sufficient to provoke a serious respiratory attack from just breathing the air. In another area, the surgical technical ability to transplant organs from one person to another exceeds our ability to cope with immune rejection of these transplants even when powerful immunosuppresive drugs are used.

We may also manufacture antibodies against our own tissues as is the case with rheumatoid arthritis, rheumatic fever, and glomerulonephritis, with the latter two often triggered by infection with streptococcus. Normally the sperm manufacturing and delivery systems are completely separate from the vascular

211

system. Through injury, disease, surgery, or sometimes for no obvious reason, sperm protein coatings enter the vascular system and provoke production of anti sperm antibodies. These antibodies are categorized as immunoglobulins of three types—IgG, IgA, and IgM. Only the first two are of clinical importance. The first, IgG, is more easily measured in blood, while IgA tends to be a more locally important antibody. Depending on which part of the sperm protein coating served as the antigenic stimulus, the antibodies may be directed against the head, neck or tail of the sperm. The antibodies usually have more than one attachment site per molecule, so that one molecule of antibody can bind to multiple sperm. This causes the sperm to appear to clump or agglutinate when viewed microscopically. Figure 15.1 demonstrates the head-to-head agglutination phenomenon, and Figure 15.2 shows primarily a tail-to-tail pattern; both can occur within the same individual. Understandably, these antibodies can affect the ability of the sperm to swim, attach to the egg and/or to penetrate the outer membranes of the egg.

Considering that sperm are foreign material, absorbed from the vagina, uterus, tubes and peritoneal cavity, all women should manufacture antibodies active against sperm. In fact, few do. Nature has allowed for a compensatory mechanism to deal with this. Blocking antibodies are produced, which have no deleterious action on the sperm, and which inhibit production of the active type of antibodies. So in effect, the production of anti-sperm antibodies by the female represents a failure of her immune system to be normally tolerant to the sperm. Usually these antibodies are against all sperm, but rarely they may be directed against the husband's sperm only.

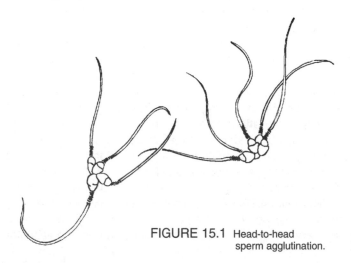

FIGURE 15.1 Head-to-head sperm agglutination.

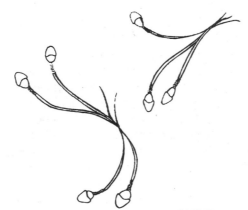

FIGURE 15.2 Tail-to-tail
sperm agglutination.

Diagnosis

By now, we've learned how to ask the proper questions, but obtaining lucid answers is another issue. How does one test for the presence of sperm antibodies in males and females? Are the tests reliable and reproducible from one laboratory to another? More importantly, does a positive finding have any reproductive significance? How many normally fertile couples can be demonstrated to have these antibodies, and are there any clues as to their presence?

There are many different systems of tests designed to indicate the presence of anti-sperm antibodies. Most involve testing blood and/or portions of serum and white blood cells against sperm, but cervical mucus tests are also used to a lesser extent. Positive results in one system may be negative in another. Many of these systems are difficult to set up and run, requiring a great deal of expertise and actual hands-on time. The immunobead test, devised by Dr. Richard Bronson, has emerged as the most widely employed because of its ease of performance, consistency of results and reasonable cost compared with the other methods. Blood from both partners and a semen specimen are required. The test is based on the following sequence of events. Rabbits are injected with human immunoglobulins in order to produce antibodies against the human antibodies, which act as an antigen under these circumstances. The rabbit antibodies are then isolated and used to coat plastic microspheres. Sperm and blood specimens are mixed and the coated microspheres added. Under the microscope one can see sperm to which the microspheres have become attached, because the sperm are coated with human antibody to which the coated microspheres bind. Sometimes, only the head or tail is involved, sometimes both. The spheres are coated with rabbit antibody specific to one of the three human immunoglobulins. A positive end point is not easily missed, and the test is reproducible between laboratories.

In a general fertile population, male or female produced antibodies should be found in less than 1%-2%. The prevalence in the infertile population ranges from 3% -10%, but may rise to 15% in the so called unexplained infertile group. These figures tell us that infertility on an immunologic basis is not common, except when other causes have not been found (although certainly two or more causes may coexist). John Collins, an excellent biostatistician and clinician at McMaster University in Hamilton, Ontario, whose works were mentioned in previous chapters has come to our rescue again with another fine study (Hum Repro 8:592, 1993). In 471 infertile couples, antibody testing with three different systems produced positive results in at least one test in 8.1% of males and 1.3% of the females. The immunobead test (IBT) was positive in 31 cases, versus 14 and 3 for the older methods used to test the males, with comparable figures for female testing of 4, 2, and 1. In the older methods, there was one couple with both partners testing positive. Repeat IBT testing 6-24 months later showed 85% of original positives still testing the same. What have we learned so far from these results? First, the IBT had either increased sensitivity or a higher degree of false positives compared with the tray and gelatin older methods. Second, female produced antibody response is significantly less common that auto-antibodies in the male. Finally, the IBT seems to give consistent results, regardless of questions concerning its prognostic value. The prevalence of abnormal results was not higher in the unexplained infertile group in this study. Male auto-antibodies were more commonly encountered in men with some abnormal semen analysis finding. There were nine pregnancies (23.7%) among the male antibody group and one pregnancy in the female produced anti-sperm antibody group. In the Collins study, the presence of antibodies could not be shown to correlate with time to pregnancy. But within that report, a literature review and statistical analysis concluded that the presence of anti-sperm antibodies was associated with a 40% reduction of fertility. To quote Dr. Collins, "...the case remains unproven, as judged by present day standards of evaluation" and not much has changed since publication of that paper.

Sometimes an abnormal postcoital test gives a clue that antibodies may be present. Sperm that are agglutinated, or shaking in place with little or no progressive forward motion, suggest the need for antibody screening. The presence of virtually no sperm on the microscopic examination, especially when the semen analysis has been normal, points to antibody screening as the next step. Keep in mind that the female is an unlikely source of antibody production, and the postcoital test may appear to be normal in the face of documented antibody production. In the latter case, the test results may have lessened clinical relevance.

Treatment

Interpreting the results of treating a laboratory finding which may or may not be a causative factor for infertility in a given couple is enough to make a biostatistician cry. Over a 30 year period of time, starting in the 1960's, steroid therapy for either partner had some popularity. Drugs such as prednisone and prednisolone were employed based on the premise that all antibody production would be suppressed in that individual. The original glowing reports in the literature could not be duplicated as measured by increased PR when tested in larger number of patients in multiple fertility practices. Nuisance side effects were common—altered sleep habits, fatigue, joint pain after stopping medication, and rashes. Induction of diabetes, gastric ulcer and psychosis in those with previous psychologic diagnoses, was more than trivial. But the most feared side effect was induction of aseptic necrosis of the hip, necessitating hip joint replacement as a consequence of steroid-induced spasm of the single artery servicing the head of the femur. This usually was not clinically apparent until a year or more after therapy had been stopped and hip pain lead to an x-ray of the joint. For all these reasons, this form of treatment is rarely used today.

Artificial insemination seems like a logical approach since it deposits many more sperm closer to the egg than can be achieved with intercourse. In any one practice the number of patients treated with this approach is too small to draw conclusions, and even a review of the world's literature doesn't add much. Over the years, we have gained an impression that IUI with special preparation may be helpful in cases of auto antibody production in the male, but is useless for female produced antibodies.

In vitro fertilization, with direct insertion of sperm into the egg under microscopic guidance (ICSI) is the last alternative, and apparently a highly successful one, although no single clinic has a great number of cases to support this conclusion, which is based on overall experience. The immunologic contribution of recurrent pregnancy loss will be discussed separately in the chapter on reproductive wastage.

16

Unexplained Infertility

Even after an assiduous investigation, somewhere between 5%-15% of infertile couples remain undiagnosed. As we learned earlier, the spontaneous PR drops off considerably after three years of infertility. When to initiate therapy, and what types of treatments to provide have been debated for some time. Guzick and a number of collaborators (Fertil Steril, 70:207, 1998) performed a meta-analysis of this subject, which is a statistical method of reviewing previous reports and weighting individual studies according to the number of patients, protocols employed, and other similar factors. Based on 45 studies, the estimated monthly spontaneous pregnancy rate without treatment in this population group was 1.3% overall. But if only studies that randomized couples to treatment or no treatment were considered, the fecundity rate was 4.1%. The authors acknowledge that this rate probably overstates reality, because, as we already have learned, the rates drop off with increased time of observation.

Intrauterine insemination (IUI), alone, in this clinical situation offers nothing; a fecundity rate of 3.8 was observed. Clomiphene citrate alone gave a rate of 5.6 pregnancies per cycle, which was increased to 8.3% when combined with IUI. The small additional increase with the combination may reflect the benefit of IUI in those patients whose cervical mucus quality/quantity may have decreased as a drug effect, but in any case, the results are not astounding. Gonadotropins alone, given by injection, produced a rate of 7.7% but had a 17.1% rate when combined with IUI. Humegon or Pergonal alone (these studies pre-dated wide-spread use of the newer agents such as Follistim (Puregon) and Gonal-F) were not really an improvement over clomiphene citrate alone, but

217

there is a subtle selection bias at work. In most cases, there was a step-wise treatment approach, in which patients were given clomiphene citrate first, and then moved on to the more costly and complicated forms of therapy if they had failed to conceive. The reason(s) for the jump in success rates seen with gonadotropins/IUI, remains unclear, but has been validated in many studies. Rates with IVF and GIFT were 20.7% and 27.0%, respectively, but once again may reflect the bias of waiting until less costly and invasive therapies had proved to be ineffective. Remember that these data are taken from group studies, and the results may not be applicable to you, especially if you have been infertile for a long duration and the female partner is beyond 35 years of age.

In reviewing the literature, not unsurprisingly, one finds varying definitions for "unexplained infertility". What is the minimal work-up necessary to reach this conclusion? Most fertility specialists would insist on documentation of normal ovulation with a BBT, or urinary kit indication of an LH surge, a normal luteal phase progesterone level and probably an in-phase endometrial biopsy, a normal semen analysis and postcoital test, normal hysterosalpingogram and finally a normal laparoscopic examination. Findings during laparoscopic examination in a patient with no symptoms and with a normal HSG are significant in about 40%-60% of patients, who up to that point have no apparent reason for infertility, which is why it is said that no work-up for infertility is complete without laparoscopy. Even when another factor is found, laparoscopy may disclose additional pertinent information. I would argue that some second level tests be performed before the term "unexplained" is applied. Among these should be a genetic screen on both partners, an ovarian challenge test, screen for sperm antibodies and a hamster egg penetration assay. Properly performed and interpreted, the clomiphene citrate challenge test has excellent predictive value; the antibody screen and the hamster test certainly are less strongly correlated with reproductive outcome, but are still helpful in directing the path of therapy.

An interesting study was performed in Israel (Simon et al, Hum Repro 6: 222, 1991) in which 87 couples with unexplained infertility were treated with gonadotropins in 446 cycles with PR compared with 72 similar couples who had 108 IVF cycles as the primary treatment (skipping the ovulation stimulation). Pregnancy rates were 34% and 28% (per couple, not per cycle), respectively. The cumulative PR (remember that?) after three office cycles was 23% compared with one IVF cycle of 22%. Reading the fine print, we discover that some (exact number unknown) of the stimulated patients had IUI, so we may conclude that the final PR might have been higher if all had been inseminated. Mean ages were 31 and 33 (certainly younger than our average patient) respectively, and duration of infertility was 5.8 and 9.0 years, respectively. The groups were not chosen in a randomized prospective fashion, and obviously the IVF group started out with a poorer prognosis than the other group. Additionally, IVF results in 1991 were not as high as present levels. The per cycle PR with stimulation ± IUI was 6.7%, which we would now consider to be on the low side, and the PR curve flattened after seven cycles (we now use three or four). Still, the data give us food for thought. The economics of treatment are at play for us whereas in Israel the socialized medical system gives doctor and patients almost a free choice of treatment options. In the United States, three office ovulation stimulation-IUI cycles have a total cost about that of one IVF cycle, with less chance for severe hyperstimulation because the goal is not one of maximizing the total number of mature oocytes present at ovulation. Additionally, the expected multiple pregnancy rate with the former treatment of about 10%-20% is about half that seen in most IVF programs. Therefore, most of the fertility therapists will recommend the office approach first, reserving IVF for cases of unexplained infertility, especially if insurance coverage of some sort is available for the former and not the latter.

Back in chapter 6, the Collins' study of live births in observed but untreated infertile couples was discussed. For the unexplained group the projected rate was 33% at 36 months. In our medical system this option is not considered to be reasonable by those who seek an instant cure for their lack of conception, especially if the female is beyond 35 years of age.

If we consider only couples with at least three years of unexplained fertility, clomiphene citrate seems to increase the monthly fecundity from about three percent to eight or nine percent, but the effect wanes after the sixth cycle of use. This is inexpensive (relatively) therapy with little risk of severe ovarian hyperstimulation syndrome, and only a 6% or so multiple PR with very few triplets or more, so this is a reasonable empiric therapy. The next logical step is the combination of injected gonadotropins coupled with IUI. As was stated before, this combination exhibits synergy, with expected pregnancy rates between 10% and 22%, depending on female age, up through the fourth cycle. I would urge you not to opt out of the IUI part of the program even if the semen analysis and the postcoital test are excellent; almost all of the studies support the conclusion that this is a useful addition. My personal bias is to alternate cycles of gonadotropic stimulation with non treatment cycles. First, this allows the ovary to recovery from any residual cysts which may have formed during stimulation; second, the patient needs a month off from blood tests, ultrasounds and the general stress of the treatment cycle.

Direct insertion of eggs and sperm into the tube (GIFT) rather than IVF may be the best next move when pregnancy does not occur with gonadotropin stimulation/IUI. Because the gametes (eggs and sperm) are deposited via laparoscopy, this has the benefit of a diagnostic look in the pelvis, even if a previous laparoscopic examination has been recorded as normal. In our program GIFT performed for unexplained infertility failing the treatments mentioned above, gave a 57% pregnancy yield. The other aspect of this double barrel approach is that pathology, such as adhesions or endometriotic implants can be corrected at the same time. Many programs do not offer GIFT, for many different reasons, one of which is inability to schedule operating room time on demand, seven days weekly. The costs are greater than those associated with IVF because of operating room and anesthesia costs, although local anesthesia with intravenous sedation can be used in lieu of general inhalational anesthesia. Second, many insurance carriers refuse to cover GIFT, even when the case for the diagnostic portion of the procedure is valid. Last, some programs never achieved a PR with GIFT equal to or better than IVF which would justify the added costs and invasiveness.

IVF, then, for many reasons, is usually the next modality employed for continued unexplained infertility, especially now that PR in most programs has risen to a level close to that seen with GIFT (see statistics in the ART chapter). Although one might think a priori that PR with IVF should be greater for this group than for other diagnoses such as tubal disease or endometriosis, this has not been the general experience. One reason for this may be the inclusion of patients in this category who have some major defect in sperm or egg, but one which can not be diagnosed with presently available methods. Because IVF involves days of laboratory observation there can be documentation of fertilization, which is not possible with GIFT. True, some of the eggs can be kept out for IVF fertilization attempts during a GIFT cycle, but since the best looking mature eggs are immediately transferred to the tube(s), failure to observe fertilization in the remaining second tier of eggs has no strong prognostic significance. Failure of the entire cluster of eggs to achieve even one fertilization in an IVF cycle may be an indication of sperm or egg problems. BUT as a number of studies have shown, regardless of the cause, this often is a result specific to that cycle, because in the next cycle, without any changes in the stimulation protocol or laboratory technique, over 50% of those failing to have any fertilization in the preceding cycle, do so in the next.

17

Pregnancy Wastage – Repeated Spontaneous Abortion (RSA)

I believe that this is the hardest chapter for me to write, and perhaps for you to read. First, the emotional aspect of subfertility or infertility pales when compared with the anger, frustration and despair associated with repeated miscarriage. Second, the truth is that diagnosis and therapy of RSA is probably the most confused area in treatment of reproductive problems. Let's see if we can make any progress in understanding this beast. We know by now that spontaneous abortion increases with age. Therefore any statement referable to a normal or control population must reflect an age distribution similar to that which exists in the geographic area under study. Additionally, we know that pregnancy loss is high early in pregnancy during the first two weeks following the missed menses, which leads to problems in definition of whether a pregnancy is represented by a positive pregnancy test alone or whether ultrasonic evidence of a gestational sac is necessary. An excellent study done in England almost 20 years ago followed 197 women who wished to conceive. Pregnancy testing was done with a sensitive urinary test starting in the mid-luteal phase. As defined by a positive test at any time, there were 152 conceptions in 623 cycles with a pregnancy loss of 43%. Fifty pregnancies were clinically non apparent, and only 14 could be diagnosed clinically as spontaneous abortions (Miller et al, Lancet, September 13, 1980). Therefore, on clinical evidence alone the miscarriage rate would have been said to be nine percent. The miscarriage rate in the general population of North America at the present time is usually quoted as ranging from 10% to 16% which reflects the demographics of postponing pregnancy. At most, the chances of having two pregnancy failures in a row is .16x.16, or just less than three percent. Striking out three times in a row by chance rather than because of a repetitive cause is 0.4% or four per thousand (.16x.16x.16). It is generally accepted that infertile patients have higher spontaneous loss rates. The definition of chronic abortion, RSA, classically was that of three consecutive pregnancy failures before the 20th week of pregnancy. Definition or not, we now are under great pressure to treat women in their late 30s who have had two consecutive losses and who are under considerable stress as they embark on the third try. Recurrent pregnancy loss affects 2% to 5% of the general population, which tells us that since this is much greater than the 0.41% predicted by non repetitive factors, there must be some couples with an ongoing problem likely to cause pregnancy loss unless diagnosed and successfully treated. There is some general agreement on the work-up, but the tests used, particularly for immunologic screening are non standardized with respect both to methodology and interpretation. In many cases (about 40%) no apparent cause can be isolated. Spontaneous resolution in the next pregnancy without any therapeutic intervention is relatively high. While this is good news for the couple, it raises havoc with evaluation of any treatment compared with a control group. In general, success in the next pregnancy is inversely correlated with the number of previous miscarriages. For instance, after three consecutive losses, the risk in the next pregnancy in cases of unexplained RSA is somewhere around 40%, rising to over 50% with six or more previous losses.

The Investigation

The Chromosomes

Chromosomes are rod-shaped structures that contain the individual genes which determine our physical features, pre-disposition to disease, and to some extent, intelligence. The building blocks of the genes are segments of deoxyribonucleic acid (DNA). The DNA itself is determined by long sequences of nucleotides. Every somatic cell in the human body normally contains 46 chromosomes existing as 22 pairs of autosomes and two sex chromosomes, XX in the female and XY in the male. Sperm and eggs, however, contain half that number with 22 single autosomes and one sex chromosome. Eggs always have a single X (normally) while sperm can have either X or Y, and thus determine the sex of the embryo. The full complement of chromosomes is restored when the nucleus of the sperm and the nucleus of the egg fuse. Chromosomes can be studied with special staining techniques called banding. Figure 17.1 illustrates the chromosomal pattern of a normal male white blood cell. Most genetic

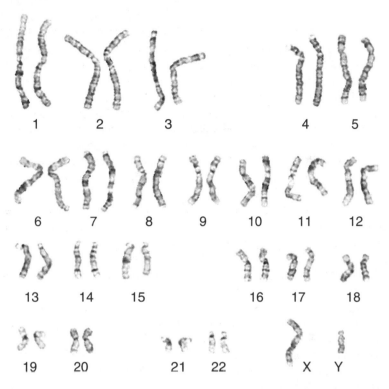

FIGURE 17.1   A normal karyotype analysis of a male patient. (Courtesy of Dr. Albert Yuzpe.)

diseases are a result of minute disturbances in the DNA building block sequence rather than abnormal distribution of the chromosomes. A giant project is underway to completely map the human genome, so that each gene can be identified, defined and studied with the hope that in the near future an abnormal genetic code can be detected and normal DNA substituted either in fetal life or shortly after birth.

Errors do occur in chromosomal distribution at the time of fertilization and early cleavage. One of these errors is known as trisomy, which means that one of the chromosome pairs is actually represented by three rather than two structures. This can arise from "non-disjunction" or "anaphase lag" at the time of division, causing one daughter cell to have three copies of a chromosome and the other daughter cell to have one rather than two. A fetus with trisomy usually does not progress into a liveborn delivery. The major exception to this rule is trisomy 21, the Down syndrome of mental retardation and physical deformities.

Another common genetic error, triploidy, occurs when three rather than two sets of chromosomes are present. This usually results from two sperm fertilizing an egg, giving rise to a cell with 69 chromosomes, incompatible with normal development. Absence of chromosomal material is called deletion and can occur as part of a chromosome not present, or an entire chromosome lost. If the amount of DNA absent is more than minute especially in an autosome, fetal demise will occur. Sex chromosome deletion as in Turner's syndrome (XO) is compatable with life. Human reproduction permits few genetic errors; all but the most subtle will result in early miscarriage. Chromosomal testing of early miscarriage fetal tissue shows in about 50% a chromosomal imbalance usually as an egg phenomenon or initiated at the time of fertilization.

But apparently normal people can have a chromosomal structural basis for repeated pregnancy loss. Some people carry the proper amount of chromosomal material, but arranged in an abnormal distribution. These re-arrangements are known collectively as translocations. Figure 17.2 illustrates the most common types of translocation. A **reciprocal translocation** is one in which genes crossover from one chromosome to another. This process can result in a normal offspring, a balanced translocation carrier like the parent with the chromosomal exchange, or a fetus with too much or not enough genetic material. Nearly all unbalanced translocations abort. The **Robertsonian**, or fusion, translocation involves the attachment of one chromosome to another, with loss of small fragments from each. As shown in figure 17.2, this can result in cells having not enough or too much genetic material, both of which are usually lethal, or a balanced state.

Couples can be screened for chromosomal abnormalities with karyotyping, using a sophisticated banding technique. Since this is expensive, it should not be performed except in cases of repeated wastage. One great advantage of diagnosing translocations in either partner is the elimination of unnecessary and fruitless hormonal support for subsequent pregnancy. There is currently no direct treatment for pregnancies with abnormal chromosomal distribution. Couples with this problem need to know that given time a healthy combination of genetic material will result in a normal child, or a child with a balanced translocation who will function normally. Unfortunately, since this is somewhat of a random event, the couple may have to go through a series of pregnancy losses before eventually reaching success. Most demographic studies of couples experiencing at least three consecutive losses find a chromosomal abnormality in one partner or the other in 3%-6% of those screened.

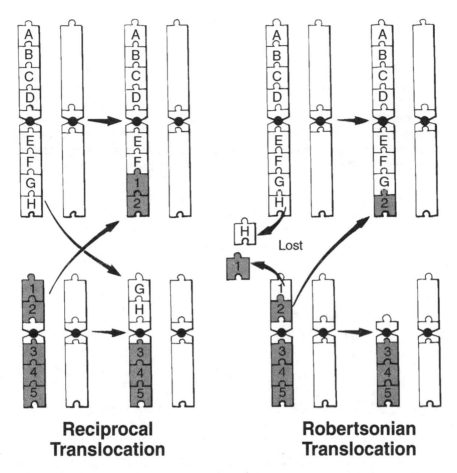

Reciprocal Translocation

Robertsonian Translocation

FIGURE 17.2 Two types of translocation causing imbalance of genetic material

Genetic Screening During Pregnancy

Sampling the fetal tissues or amniotic fluid during pregnancy is recommended for all women who will be over 35 years of age at the time of delivery, and in some women who have given birth to an abnormal child in the past. A family history of children with genetic disorders is another indication.

Amniocentesis

The classic approach to genetic diagnosis during pregnancy is amniocentesis as shown in figure 17.3, which is done at about 16 weeks after the last menstrual period. With this method the fetus is located and examined with ultrasound. Under local anesthesia, a needle is passed through the abdominal wall, uterus, and into the pregnancy sac. A small amount of fluid is withdrawn. The cells contained in the fluid are grown in tissue culture and examined for genetic content in two or three weeks. Amniocentesis is both safe and accurate, but has the disadvantage of time with respect to when it can be performed and the interval before information is available. Terminating a pregnancy because of a major fetal abnormality at 18 weeks is not a simple procedure. Additionally sometimes the tissue culture fails, and the test must be repeated. Direct loss of pregnancy as a consequence of this test procedure is somewhere around 2-4/1000.

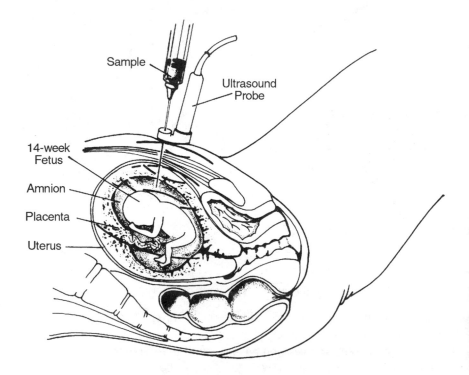

FIGURE 17.3 Amniocentesis. Under ultrasonic guidance amniotic fluid is withdrawn for chromosomal evaluation and biochemical testing.

Chorionic Villus Biopsy

The chorionic villi which surround the fetus represent placental tissue with the same genetic construction as the fetus itself. As shown in figure 17.4, it is possible with ultrasonic guidance to place a small biopsy needle through the cervix or uterine wall in order to obtain a small piece of this tissue. The test is usually done about the 10th week of pregnancy, and results are available within days. While chorionic villus sampling (CVS) has the advantage of earlier performance and faster acquisition of results, amniocentesis indirectly provides more information than CVS because the accompanying ultrasound examination is conducted later in pregnancy. Non-genetic defects in the fetus such as hydrocephaly and spina bifida can be diagnosed at 16 weeks but not at 8. As greater experience has been achieved with CVS, and with better ultrasound imaging, the safety factor differential between CVS and amniocentesis has narrowed so that there is now little to choose in that area. Some early reports of congenital abnormalities of bony development of the upper limbs and chin following CVS were technique related, and are not increased compared with control groups in good hands. Most prenatal diagnostic units offer both and have well-trained counselors to explain the pros and cons of each technique.

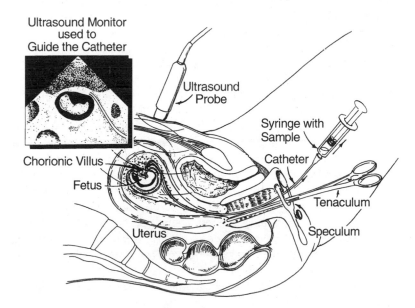

FIGURE 17.4 Chorionic villus sampling. Under ultrasonic guidance chorionic villi are obtained for rapid genetic assessment.

Fetal Abortion Genetic Sampling

Because infertility patients who become pregnant are followed early in pregnancy, and usually more closely than others, falling ß hCG titers and/or ultrasound demonstration of failure of fetal growth accurately predict impending miscarriage before the actual event. Therefore, armed with this knowledge it is possible to obtain a biopsy of fetal tissue or villi before the tissue becomes so necrotic that genetic studies are unsuccessful. In a general population, about half of all miscarriage tissue submitted for chromosomal evaluation is abnormal. Frequently these genetic maldistributions of too much or not enough specific chromosomal material arise during early embryonic or fetal development with no correlation with chromosomal content of either parent. Individual sperm or eggs may carry an abnormal complement of chromosomes, and this is more common in eggs than sperm, and the defect is not present in every gamete. In some cases the presence of trisomy 21 or a translocation points to the need for testing of both parents to rule out the presence of a chromosomal distribution that might be responsible for repetitive loss and which is present in every cell. Another benefit which can accrue from the study is the knowledge that the pregnancy loss was not a consequence of inadequate hormonal production, endometrial response, or anything that the mother might have done or not done. Emotionally, this is of great importance, and is sufficient enough to justify the study.

The Effect of Maternal Age on Fetal Chromosomal Abnormality

Fetal abnormality related to abnormal chromosomal content as expressed at delivery of a liveborn appears as a rate per 1000 in table 17.1. Remember that amniocentesis or CVS, if performed, will identify almost all of these and that elective termination of the pregnancy will occur in the majority of cases. Moreover, the spontaneous abortion rate in these cases is very high. Therefore the end result represents cases where genetic testing was not performed, or where the parents elected not to intervene even though the information was available early in the pregnancy. At age 34 and beyond, the Down syndrome is the most common abnormality among liveborns, not only because of its frequency, but also because the associated abnormalities are not so incompatible with continued fetal development as some of the other altered chromosomal patterns. But even at age 40, the sum total of genetically related abnormalities is only 15.9 per thousand livebirths—less than 2%.

Table 17.1
Rate of chromosomal abnormalities per 1,000 live births according to maternal age

MATERNAL AGE	DOWN SYNDROME	ALL OTHERS	TOTAL
25	0.8	1.3	2.1
26	0.9	1.3	2.2
27	0.9	1.3	2.2
28	0.9	1.4	2.3
29	1.0	1.4	2.4
30	1.1	1.5	2.6
31	1.2	1.5	2.7
32	1.3	1.8	3.1
33	1.6	1.9	3.5
34	2.2	1.9	4.1
35	3.2	2.5	5.7
36	4.1	2.5	6.6
37	5.2	3.0	8.2
38	6.7	3.2	9.9
39	8.6	3.7	12.3
40	10.8	5.1	15.9
41	14.3	6.3	20.6
42	18.4	8.1	26.5
43	25.1	8.1	33.2
44	32	10	42
45	40	15	55
46	52	17	69
47	70	21	91
48	90	26	116
49	112	38	150

Source: Compiled by the author.

Newer Methods of Genetic Analysis

The majority of genetic heritable disorders are not a consequence of chromosomal deletions or excess, but rather a result of subtle changes in the DNA structure at one of the many sites on an individual gene. If the exact nucleotide sequence of the normal gene is known, it is possible to compare it with a sample taken as early as the four cell stage of the embryo prior to implantation within an IVF cycle, thus enlarging the clinical horizon of IVF from a fertility promoting procedure to a genetic screening process. With a technique known as the polymerase chain reaction, (PCR) the DNA content of an individual cell can be rapidly multiplied so that this genetic diagnosis is available within a day or two, permitting placement of only normal embryos in the uterus. Because so many genetic problems are sex—linked, appearing only in the male having a single X chromosome, another technique has become clinically valuable. Fluorescent in situ hybridization (FISH) as the name implies, can sample a single fetal cell, to determine if it contains an X or Y chromosome. It can also be used to determine if there are too many or not enough of an autosomal chromosome (non X or non Y) in the cell, with rapid delivery of results. These techniques are evolving, they are expensive and are not widely available.

Human Leucocyte Antigen (HLA)

We all carry on our tissues histocompatability antigens. White blood cells are used in the laboratory to discern this genetic fingerprint which identifies an individual. It is these genetically determined factors which are important when organ donor tissue transplants are performed. The closer the match, the less chance for rejection. In the case of pregnancy, however, the situation may be reversed, with close fetal-maternal similarities associated with increased pregnancy loss. Studies done in tightly knit population groups, such as the Hutterites, demonstrate increased miscarriage proportional to the number of HLA sites held in common between husband and wife. Animal studies suggested that immunizing the mother with white blood cells from the father could overcome the deleterious effect of too similar genetic endowment. It was reasoned that this finding was proof of a natural mechanism to counteract inbreeding. Over the past two decades a debate has raged over whether immunizing women with white cells from their husbands really alters the outcome. Considering that the background success rate with no treatment is relatively high, it becomes very difficult to prove the point. The test groups studied varied with respect to age, the number of previous miscarriages and the number of HLA sites held in common. The only way to really study this is to have a double blind placebo study in which neither the patient nor the physician has knowledge of whether an actual immunization is performed.

In 1994 the results of a worldwide collaborative investigation from 15 centers were published. Using two separate teams of statisticians, the live birth ratios were 1.16 (1.01—1.34, p= 0.031) and 1.21 (1.04—1.37, p= 0.024) respectively comparing treatment and no treatment. With the confidence limits over one, and the p values < 0.05, the results are statistically significant, but the clinical effect in terms of increased births is quite small with only a 10% increased yield at most. The study comprised 449 patients, and results were similar in all the clinics. The immunization was not totally without clinical symptoms, with viral infections such as hepatitis and CMV being transmitted from husband to wife along with some transfusion type reactions. A small number of patients developed autoimmune problems including rheumatoid arthritis. If only patients with no previous live births were studied, the ratio became 1.46. A significant statistical problem was posed by the finding that in about half of the pregnancies that failed during the study, genetic analysis demonstrated abnormal chromosomal content, which is called a confounding variable since it would not have been expected to be influenced by the treatment protocol.

Since the HLA pattern is inherited from both parents, all fetuses should act as antigenic stimuli to the mother. Although the actual anatomy in the uterus is designed to limit direct communication between fetus and the maternal bloodstream, the presence of fetal cells in maternal blood samples and clinically, Rh sensitization, document leakage in both directions. A new method of treatment is that of recurrent doses of intravenously administered immunoglobulin which will be discussed below.

Anatomic Factors—The Uterus

The uterus is expected to serve as a hospitable nurturing environment for the developing fetus. Anatomic changes either present at birth or acquired can adversely influence the ability of the uterus to adequately perform what really is its sole purpose in life. Women with a true double uterus usually do fairly well reproductively. A bicornate uterus with two horns frequently has associated with it some degree of cervical incompetence leading to premature or immature (<28 weeks) delivery, but is not considered to be a cause for RSA. The septate uterus, however, is thought to be responsible for pregnancy wastage in some cases near the end of the first trimester. The usual reason given as an explanation is that the placenta implants totally or in part on the septum which has a poor blood supply. Women having a hysteroscopic septal incision have a 70% success rate in the next pregnancy. But since close to two percent of the general population has a septum to some degree, many women with a septum experience no adverse effect on pregnancy continuation. Therefore, the decision to operate should be made on the obstetric history. The unicollate uterus, which is actually half a uterus, is associated with premature labor but not miscarriage. Scar tissue forming in the uterus usually after dilatation and evacuation of retained placental fragments can cause both infertility and early miscarriage as a result of reduced blood supply to the area of placental implantation. Polyps are not thought to predispose to RSA, but myomas, which under the hormonal stimulation of pregnancy can grow quickly, may very well cause pregnancy loss by pressure effects on the uterine cavity and increased uterine irritability. The uterine abnormalities brought about by exposure to DES can cause infertility, RSA and premature delivery. Remember that these changes in uterine structure and function can occur as a spontaneous, non drug related event.

When the hormonal environment is normal, the uterus may still be less than normally responsive to the stimulation if cells of the endometrial lining lack receptor sites. Molecular biology dealing with human implantation is in its infancy, and we're just starting to learn the basics of what is normal.

Infectious Organisms

While certain infections contracted during a specific pregnancy can cause abortion or severe fetal developmental abnormalities, there's no literature support for an infectious agent responsible for RSA.

Endocrine Factors

Luteal phase deficiency can be defined according to serum progesterone levels or the microscopic appearance of the endometrium and perhaps according to ultrasound measurements of thickness and pattern. The trouble with this neat package is that a single progesterone measurement may show a 40% variation if measured one hour later. Usually a low progesterone level is seen in a pregnancy which has already started to fail and is an effect rather than a cause. Three separate studies were unable to prove that routine progesterone supplementation in pregnancy improved miscarriage rates over controls—but this does not apply to pregnancy in cycles where pituitary down regulation with GnRH analogs has been employed. Endometrial biopsy is not done purposely in a pregnancy cycle, therefore, previous biopsy findings may not apply. Additionally, as stated before, there are many variables involved in reading these biopsies, 30% of which will be read as normal when repeated in the next cycle without any treatment. Some normally fertile women acting as controls in these studies also had biopsies which were read as out of phase. The ultrasound measurements of endometrial thickness at specific times in the menstrual cycle probably correlate better with pregnancy outcome than the traditional endometrial biopsy.

Diabetic patients do not have an increase in early miscarriage unless they are in poor control. I hyroid disease is not cause for RSA unless there is an auto immune component with additional self-directed antibody formation. Polycystic ovarian syndrome (PCOS) not only causes anovulation and infertility, but additionally seems to increase the miscarriage rate. Somewhere between 25% and 40% of pregnancies in the PCOS population will abort in the first trimester. Based on animal studies it was thought that high levels of LH might be the culprit because of a deleterious effect on egg quality. If this were true, lowering the LH levels by using GnRH analogs should have a beneficial effect, but the literature on this remains mixed.

Immunologic RSA

The hot topic in RSA is immunologic factors. Antibodies directed against one's own tissues can have a multiplicity of actions. The class of antibodies known as antiphospholipids encompasses many different antibodies but the subclass of most importance are the anticardiolipins, and the lupus anticoagulant factor with antinuclear antibodies playing a lesser role. These antibodies are active in the small vessels of the body, particularly in the placenta during pregnancy where they cause localized clotting. Women with these antibodies are also more susceptible to early stroke and heart disease. In most cases of cardiolipin antibody formation, an initial fetal heartbeat can be seen on the ultrasound prior to miscarriage. The laboratory assays are not standardized, and some patients will have low levels of positive results which are not consistent and probably not of clinical significance. There's no question that high titers of antiphospholipid antibodies impact in a negative fashion on reproduction, not only in the first trimester but later on as well, causing intrauterine growth retardation, and an increase in the incidence of pre-eclampsia.

A specific type of white blood cell known as "CD 56+ natural killer cells" (sounds like something that Darth Vader would enjoy) have been implicated in RSA because they are found in high concentrations in some of these patients. Whether or not they are elevated as part of the autoimmune process, a cause or effect, is not known. Once again we are confronted with the problem of proving that an association is a causation.

The lupus anticoagulant is somewhat of a misnomer. In the laboratory, serum from patients with this circulating antibody takes longer to clot than normal, but the effect in the body is the opposite with promotion of thrombosis causing stroke, heart attack, high blood pressure and pulmonary embolus. Patients with this factor usually **do not** have the disease known as lupus erythematosis. Studies of patients with RSA show a prevalence of 3% to 14 % for the lupus anticoagulant and a range of 8% to 22% for anticardiolipin antibodies (ACA), compared with less than 1% and 2%, respectively in a population of normally pregnant women. Repetitive testing in a number of studies has demonstrated that an initial positive result may not be duplicated in subsequent samplings. This adds to the confusion; which result should we rely on? The miscarriage rate for the next pregnancy in RSA patients having ACA is about 50% in most studies. However, there are dissenters, and a recent collaborative NIH sponsored study (Simpson et al. Fertil Steril 69:814, 1998) could find no association with pregnancy loss and antiphospholipid antibodies or ACA. Nevertheless the consensus is that women with RSA and demonstrable antibodies be treated. Treated how?

One of the early treatments for RSA was low dose (one 80 mg tablet) of aspirin daily. The rationale is a reduction of thromboxane locally in the placenta thereby reversing, at least in part, the heightened coagulation tendency. This is the same reasoning which has led to many people taking aspirin at this dose for prevention of heart attack. In most of the studies success rates in the next pregnancy were in the neighborhood of 50% to 70%, impressive with such simple and safe therapy, but often not different from the untreated patients. Steroid drugs such as prednisolone which have the general effect of reducing antibody formation also have been employed alone or in combination with aspirin. There's little added benefit and there seems to be an increase in premature births when steroids are used. We also know from a previous discussion that long term use of steroids is far from innocuous. Heparin, a widely used injectable anticoagulant has been used to reverse the clotting tendency in the small placental vessels involved at the site of the antigen—antibody reaction. The usual combination is aspirin and 5,000 to 10,000 units of heparin injected twice daily subcutaneously. This usually produces a pregnancy yield of about 70% success, even in patients unsuccessful previously with aspirin alone.

In the last decade intravenous administration of immunoglobulin has been used to treat immunologic RSA when antibodies are detected, in the presence of HLA problems and for unexplained continued pregnancy wastage. Immunoglobulins are used clinically to prevent or treat viral or bacterial infection in patients whose immune systems are compromised. Within the context of RSA, use of immunoglobulin treatment has been demonstrated to reduce the natural killer cell activity. There is no standard protocol for dose or frequency of administration but early studies with small numbers of patients were promising. There are only four well controlled studies with randomized double blind placebo protocols which have been published. Two of the trials showed a benefit from this treatment; the other two did not. Combining all the data the absolute treatment effect was 10% above no treatment. A course of treatment will cost over $7,000 for the immunoglobulin alone. That's a great deal to spend for an unproven treatment. A major problem in evaluating all of these studies is that the mechanism behind an individual miscarriage may not be the same in each case for each individual. For example treating a patient with documented antibodies with any pharmacologic agent will not have a beneficial effect when that particular fetus has a chromosomal abnormality. Patients with RSA want treatment and often press the physician to do something, anything, that might bring about success. As physicians, we lean towards treating, often empirically, but treatments are not always benign, as is the case of steroids. With a high background rate of non-treated success, prying out what really works can be difficult if not impossible. Our frustration with the current state of affairs is second only to yours.

Metabolic Disease

We have already mentioned that diabetes, unless it is poorly controlled, is not responsible for RSA. Wilson's disease results in high copper levels in the tissues of the body. It is associated with RSA but is extremely rare. Less rare is an autosomal recessive inherited metabolic alteration called homocysteinuria, which results from inability to metabolize methionine in the diet. A single study has suggested a relatively high percentage of elevated levels of homocysteine in the serum of RSA patients. Large doses of high folic acid containing prenatal vitamins will reverse the metabolic abnormality, but it is not known as yet whether this also will be a valid treatment for RSA.

18

Assisted Reproductive Technology: In Vitro Fertilization-Embryo Replacement

In vitro fertilization (IVF) and its associated technologies is the last form of active therapy to be presented in this book for two reasons. First, it is the most complicated and most expensive form of therapy, requiring the input of a number of professionals with special skills, and a commitment on the part of the patient to go through an arduous treatment schedule. Second, since IVF is frequently the court of last resort for those with reproductive problems, this is the most logical place for its description.

Please indulge this writer who believes that you might find a bit of history interesting, especially since he was around at the time and one of the main characters was a friend.

In vitro fertilization and embryo replacement leading to successful delivery of healthy animals in a number of species on a regular basis had become established by the 1970's. Human research was dramatically hampered by conservative attitudes of institutional review boards subjected to great pressure by various groups with strong restrictive views and by theoretical objections voiced by often self appointed ethicists. Robert Edwards, a well respected British reproductive physiologist was looking for a skilled laparoscopic surgeon interested in the project of human IVF, since ultrasonic methods of approaching the ovary for egg retrieval had not yet been invented. Patrick Steptoe was equally famous in the world of laparoscopy as one who had introduced the procedure in the English speaking world. No funds were available from the English equivalent of our National Institutes of Health, and a major portion of the shoestring budget was funded from the proceeds of a clinic which Mr. Steptoe (in the UK surgeons are known as "Mr.") opened in Oldham in order to generate money for their research.

After almost a decade of trial and effort a pregnancy was achieved, but it was ectopic. A lesser team might well have quit at this point, but persistence paid off with the birth of Louise Brown in 1978. These early cycles were conducted without any ovarian stimulation, and accurate timing of laparoscopic retrieval of the single egg was quite difficult. Success achieved outside the pillars of the academic community was a hard pill for some to swallow, and Edwards and Steptoe were accused of faking the results and numerous other scientific improprieties. No matter, for within a few months their accusers were making the pilgrimage to Bourn Hall in England, a country estate that served as the world's first IVF center, in order to learn the technique. Clomiphene citrate was the next step in evolution and eventually it was replaced by menopausal gonadotropins in order to achieve development and maturation of more than one egg per cycle.

Bourn Hall was a lovely country estate with the main house having many French doors. Parked against these doors were the English equivalent of our Gulfstream sleek aluminum house trailers, which I believe are called "Porta-Cabins". The overall view resembled an airport with multiple terminals. These each housed about six women during the treatment cycle; husbands were at a nearby inn, but meals were served in common in a large dining room. At lunch, Mr. Steptoe would announce the names of those patients having embryo replacement that evening. The roster of names resembled a United Nations roll call vote, because people came from all over the world to this mecca. Even at this shrine to high technology, there was a great deal of clinical intuition and adherence to tradition that entered the treatment protocol. The trailers had hospital beds on wheels that also had bumpers at the foot of the bed below the level of the mattress. Patients having embryo replacement were brought to Mr. Steptoe's office usually about 11 p.m. or even later and the embryos were placed into the uterus via a catheter with the patient in a knee-chest position with her knees on the bumper and her shoulders on the mattress— all of this with illumination supplied by Mr. Steptoe's goose-necked desk lamp. The patient was then told to slide forward on her abdomen and to hold that position through the night. Her roommates were responsible to make certain that she did not roll over in her sleep. Today we might chuckle at this ritual, but it was rigidly enforced at that time since there was concern that the early embryo might simply fall out of the uterus with gravity. No amount of credit and honors is excessive for these two men who overcame scientific hurdles with little or no help from any outside source in an atmosphere of skepticism and distrust from the public and even their colleagues.

IVF—The Basics, Indications and Complications

Basically, IVF can be divided into three segments. The first has to do with the stimulation process by which multiple eggs are brought to maturity before retrieval. The philosophy of stimulation is substantially different from that which exists during a cycle of office ovulation induction. In the latter, whether intercourse or insemination is employed during the attempt for pregnancy, one has no control over the fertilization process leading to high order multiple pregnancy in cycles where many eggs have developed. With IVF, on the other hand, there is a desire to produce and retrieve a large number of eggs since not all will fertilize and divide in a normal fashion. The presence of many embryos allows the couple and the therapists to decide on how many will be placed in the uterus, and how many will be frozen for subsequent attempts at pregnancy. Therefore, there is a mechanism by which multiple pregnancy rates can be controlled to some extent, but at the very least, more so than in the former example. Although theoretically sound, in actual practice, because IVF is so expensive, and because clinics often compete for patients, excessive numbers of embryos may be replaced in an attempt to maximize pregnancy rates, leading to an unacceptable rate of associated high order multiple births. Today GnRH agonists such as Lupron and Synarel are used to shut down communications between the pituitary and the ovary so that high levels of estrogen production emanating from multiple follicular development does not lead to early and inappropriate (under these circumstances) release of LH. The GnRH antagonists used in Europe will soon be approved in the United States and will bring with them a number of advantages. First, the onset of suppression is much faster, allowing for the first dose to be given during stimulation rather than during the preceding menstrual cycle. This translates to a substantial reduction and cost of the total dose of gonadotropins used for stimulation. Additionally, since the antagonists have no initial stimulatory action, the induction of ovarian cysts, sometimes seen with use of the agonists, does not occur. Use of the antagonists will almost totally eliminate the inadvertent administration of an agent such as the GnRh agonist in the preceding luteal phase of an unsuspected pregnancy conceived in a non-treatment cycle.

The second phase of IVF starts with the egg retrieval (figure 18.1a). Initially this was performed via laparoscopy in an operating suite. Because hCG is given as the final trigger for egg maturation, the interval between the injection and egg collection is critical with little room for error. Operating rooms frequently have difficulty with schedules designed to accommodate this need. Therefore the development of ultrasonic guided egg retrieval relieved that pressure as well as offering a less invasive and expensive method of approaching the ovary. Early techniques were all performed with transabdominal needles with the necessity of a full bladder to serve as a contrast necessary for ovarian visualization. This was uncomfortable for a number of reasons. Today almost all retrievals are performed with an ultrasonic probe placed in the vagina through which a needle can be inserted. Normally, the ovaries sit just over the top of the vagina, and can be accessed easily by this route without the necessity of a distended bladder. Egg retrievals are usually performed with intravenous sedation and local anesthesia, although other forms of anesthesia such as general and epidural have been used. The average time for egg retrieval in our program is 14 minutes. The drugs used for sedation have quick onset and short duration so that patients are usually ready to leave in an hour following the procedure. The trend has been to move the process out of an expensive

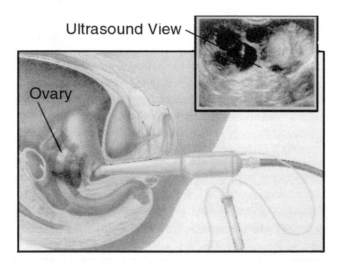

Figure 18.1a   Using ultrasound to view the ovary, the physician inserts the needle through the wall of the vagina into the ovary and removes the egg for use in IVF or GIFT.

hospital environment in favor of an outpatient facility. But great care must be paid to the environment with respect to air quality and the presence of potentially toxic agents in the laboratory. Most IVF labs have elaborate air filtration systems and employ a "clean-room" concept similar to that used in the drug manufacturing and computer chip industry.

During the process of egg retrieval, the physician aspirates from the ovary collections of fluid, which may contain mature follicles, with a needle connected to a suction pump. In fact, only about 40% to 70% of the taps will produce an egg because in some cases the egg has ceased to develop within the surrounding fluid. The biologist examines the fluid under a dissecting microscope, isolates the eggs, and places them in an incubator in small Petri dishes in an environment of constant temperature, humidity and with a special mixture of gases (figure 18.1b). In the usual process, the eggs are then exposed to sperm placed in the dish in order to bring about fertilization. The eggs are inspected the next morning to see if fertilization has occurred. The medium in the dish may be changed a few times over the next two days of observation. Not all the eggs are mature when collected; not all will become mature in culture; not all will become fertilized; and not all of those will continue to divide. Now you begin to understand why there is a premium placed on stimulating in a strong fashion in order to

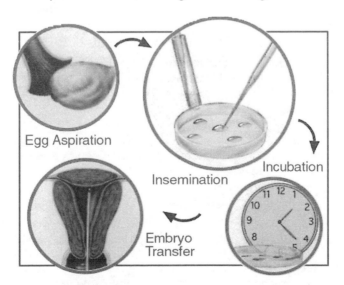

Egg Aspiration

Insemination

Incubation

Embryo Transfer

Figure 18.1b   In IVF, egg harvested from the woman's ovary are placed in a petri dish and fertilized in the laboratory with sperm. The embryos are then transferred into the uterus.

start out with a good number of eggs. That final number is dependent upon the type of stimulation, especially the age of the patient, and the skill of the person performing the retrieval. The downside of a strong stimulation cycle may be development of the most severe form of the hyperstimulation syndrome leading to hospitalization and potentially dangerous complications. The usual interval between egg retrieval and embryo replacement for many years was two days. The early media were not able to support embryo growth for much longer than that. As the media improved, most laboratories have moved to a day 3 replacement. The advantage here is that between days two and three, some of the embryos which appeared to be developing normally on day 2, cease dividing by day 3. Therefore, extending the time of observation in the laboratory allows the biologists to identify those embryos most likely to continue normal development leading to a newborn. Even the most scrupulously designed and prepared medium does not have the same composition as the fluid that normally surrounds the developing embryo in the tube and in the uterus. Therefore these embryos are subjected to some degree of insult related to an absence of certain growth factors during this period of time. There is a move today to extend the laboratory time out to five days in order to allow developing embryos to achieve the blastocyst stage as further evidence of normalcy. The final goal is to be able to replace fewer embryos in order to achieve consistently satisfactory pregnancy rates with a substantial reduction in high order (triplets or more) multiple pregnancy. Remember that implantation normally does not occur until six days after fertilization so that early replacement of the embryo in the uterus also involves the risk that the uterus will expel the embryo(s) through the cervix or up into the tubes, with a possibility of inducing an IVF related ectopic pregnancy. There is diligent constant effort spent in the area of improving the culture medium to allow for longer intervals of embryo observation. The laboratory biologists who care for the embryos during this interval are the unsung and often unseen heroes of the team, whose efforts largely go unnoticed.

The embryo replacement process is usually a simple affair. A thin, soft, pliable plastic catheter is used to place the embryos within the uterine cavity. Some centers use ultrasonic guidance to facilitate this replacement in as atraumatic a fashion as possible. It is not unlike an intrauterine insemination. Although tradition, starting at Bourn Hall, would dictate a prolonged interval in the horizontal position, recent studies show no difference in pregnancy rates between patients who recline following replacement compared with those who get up immediately and leave.

The third phase of the IVF treatment cycle is more relaxed with the

Table 18.1
Indications for IVF

Tubal and Pelvic Adhesions

Male Factor

Endometriosis

Unexplained Infertility

Immunologic

(Anovulation)

(Pre Implantation Genetics)

emphasis on making sure that serum progesterone levels reflect adequate support of the endometrium so that embryo implantation is favored. Most programs supplement the progesterone production coming from the ovulation sites on the ovary with injections, suppositories, vaginal gels, or oral micronized progesterone. Some programs use small doses of hCG boosters. Pregnancy tests are usually done at about 12 days following egg retrieval, and if positive, progesterone supplementation is continued. Pregnancy tests are repeated weekly in a quantitative fashion as an index of following the development of the trophoblast during its early stages of implantation. The trophoblast, which develops into the placenta, is responsible for production of hCG. The ultrasound is employed to diagnose a developing fetal sac(s), and later to document development of a fetus with heart motion. At that point the patient will book an obstetric appointment.

Table 18.1 lists the most frequent indications for IVF. Tubal disease from infection or adhesions surrounding the tubes as a consequence of previous surgery remains a major contributor to the IVF population. Although tubal problems represented the initial and sole indication for IVF, in many programs male factor infertility has surpassed in numbers impaired egg transport as the chief indication for IVF, especially following the astounding success of intracytoplasmic sperm injection (ICSI) as a solution to even the most severe cases of diminished sperm production or transport. Endometriosis associated infertility not yielding to surgical treatment and/or ovulation induction with IUI is another reason for IVF. Immunologic infertility is not common, but has been shown to be successfully treated with this approach. Similarly, long-term infertility in the absence of a diagnosis, treated with the usual step-wise approach without success, has an excellent prognosis when IVF is applied. In many cases there is probably a subtle defect in sperm transport or egg capture and transport which is bypassed with this process. Anovulation appears in parentheses because many patients who are not successful with the usual treatments carried out over a reasonable amount of time find themselves turning to IVF with great success even though an explanation for the big jump in pregnancy rates remains lacking.

All treatment protocols have the risk of associated complications. Table 18.2 lists IVF related complications according to the immediate cause. Strong protocols for stimulation and/or unexpected brisk response by the patient can lead to hyperstimulation with no more than abdominal bloating and ovarian tenderness or to the severe form with serum and electrolyte disturbance, reduced kidney function, liver disorders, collection of fluid in the abdominal cavity and chest cavity, blood clots in the arteries and veins, pulmonary embolism, stroke, and rarely death. Some people have a local reaction to injections while others have an allergic response to the medication or the solution that is used to dissolve the powder. We have already discussed in a previous chapter the issue of ovarian cancer related to ovulation induction with the conclusion that there's no strong evidence for a true cause and effect relationship. Complications related to the egg retrieval center around hemorrhage from the needle causing bleeding from the ovary, the vagina or major blood vessels in the pelvis which are inadvertently entered. Not only does this happen rarely, but most needle sticks are self-sealing. Infection can occur as a consequence of the procedure, first because the vagina cannot be sterilized even with a cleansing solution applied just before the procedure, and second because sometimes the needle may enter the colon and secondarily contaminate the pelvic cavity. Manipulation of previously infected tubes may rekindle a long dormant infection. Many programs use prophylactic antibiotics given at the time of retrieval. Anesthesia problems are very few and far between. First, general anesthesia is uncommonly used. Provided that reasonable doses of intravenous sedative agents are utilized, the margin of safety is great with respiratory depression and a drop in blood pressure easily managed. Replacement usually is the easiest part of the entire IVF process. Infection

Table 18.2
Complications of IVF

Stimulation Related	Retrieval Related
• Hyperstimulation mild-moderate-severe	• Hemorrhage
	• Infection
• Local Reaction to Injections	• Anesthesia or Sedation Related
• Allergic Reaction to Medications	**Replacement Related**
	• Multiple Pregnancy
• (Ovarian Cancer)	• Infection
	• Ectopic Pregnancy

of the uterus can occur with any passage of a catheter through the vagina and cervix into the uterus, but is highly unlikely. Gross contamination of the culture medium containing the embryos is usually obvious to the biologists and would preclude an embryo transfer. Ectopic pregnancy can occur with IVF because the embryos can be pushed into the tubes by uterine contractions and probably by tubal contractions as well, even though the egg normally travels from the ovary toward the uterus. We know this is true because small plastic particles placed in the cervix can be retrieved from the cul-de-sac after transport through the uterus and tubes into the pelvic cavity. Sometimes a combined pregnancy, known as a heterotopic pregnancy can occur with one implantation in the tube and another (s) in the uterus. These are especially difficult to diagnose unless an ultrasonic image suggests the true situation. Finally, multiple pregnancy logically can be included as a complication of embryo replacement since the number of embryos placed in the uterus can be controlled in the decision-making process by doctor and patient.

The American Society for Reproductive Medicine (ASRM) through its Society for Assisted Reproductive Technology (SART) division has voiced its concern regarding multiple gestation by producing guidelines for member clinics. Current recommendations call for replacing a maximum of three embryos in patients below the age of 35 (in Europe this would be two); and a maximum of four in patients 35-39, and possibly more in patients over 40. This last recommendation is extremely safe, since the implantation rate per embryo replaced is low in this age group, and triplets or more are rare in women beyond 40.

High order multiple pregnancy is the most common complication of IVF, and one can view this as a nine-month complication or an 18-year complication. Raising three children who are always at the same stage of development is quite different from dealing with three children of different ages. The most immediate consideration is that of the outcome of triplet or more pregnancy compared with twin gestation. If we review the world's literature on this subject, focused around selective reduction of triplet or more pregnancy reduced to twins, certain truths become apparent. First, the procedure is reasonably safe and pregnancy outcome is better with reduction than attempting to carry triplets or more. The main issue is one of gestational age and weight at the time of delivery. Pregnancies with twins that started out as triplets usually deliver at a point mid way between twin pregnancy and triplet pregnancy (on average, two weeks longer than triplet pregnancies managed without embryo reduction). Maternal complications such as pre-eclampsia are significantly reduced. The two week difference may sound insignificant, but in terms of fetal development leading to a reduction in newborn morbidity and mortality, the actual clinical result is greatly improved. Although the recommendation has been that of reducing triplets to twins, statistics suggest that reduction to a single pregnancy is actually better in terms of fetal outcome. Reductions are usually done at 10 weeks of gestation with injection of a simple salt solution into the cardiac sac of a fetus under ultrasonic guidance. If there is any discrepancy in fetal development, the smallest fetus is usually chosen, or else, the sac most easily accessed. In cases of multiple gestation for reduction in women over 33, a genetic study obtained with villus biopsy should be done first in order to screen all of the fetuses. While the recommendation is for genetic screening of women age 35 and over at the time of delivery of a single fetus, multiple pregnancy, by increasing the overall risk of any fetus having a chromosomal abnormality, calls for lowering of the age limit for suggested genetic sampling. Since a genetic diagnosis can be rendered within days of villus biopsy, a fetal reduction can be done soon thereafter.

"Fetal reduction" is, of course, a euphemism for selective fetal abortion, which is repugnant in general and totally unacceptable to some. For this reason a detailed discussion concerning the philosophy of embryo replacement numbers is necessary before the stimulation process actually begins, so that a decision can be made in a relatively relaxed environment, and not in the heat of battle.

The Statistics of IVF

Most people would not buy a house unseen, and most would insist on an inspection and some guarantees, against leaking roofs and termites, for example, before signing on the dotted line. Would you purchase a car without a test drive? Deciding to embark on an IVF voyage and choosing which ship on which to sail is a major decision. The price differential between clinics is usually small, and is a moot point if the process is insurance covered. Assuming the worst case scenario of no coverage for any part of the process, be prepared to spend between $5,000 and $10,000 for a completed cycle including drugs costs and depending on the extras, such as ICSI. By the time you have arrived at the doorstep of IVF, often after months or years of unsuccessful therapy, you want the procedure TO WORK, almost regardless of the costs. Therefore, it may behoove you to read this section carefully. You will learn that presentation of IVF success rates takes a number of different formats, but you will be able to digest the data for any specific clinic or program by knowing how to ask the right questions.

Each member clinic of the Society for Assisted Reproductive Technology (SART) reports its statistics for a calendar year to a central registry. This was begun in 1985, and in 1997, the Centers for Disease Control became involved in the process of data compilation and verification. Ascertain if the program you are considering is a SART certified clinic, which implies adherence to good laboratory techniques and clinical guidelines in addition to compliance with reporting results. A non-member clinic may be reputable and have a good track record, but certainly an inquiry is indicated. The results of a calendar year furnish a base broad enough to judge a facility, unless the total number of patients serviced is small. Pregnancies initiated in December may not deliver until September, and the clinic's results usually are not tabulated before the end of the year. A few months' work is necessary at the central registry before the final data are available. During this time span, the clinic may have had major personnel or procedural changes; therefore be sure that you scrutinize some recent information. Discount any results over a short interval of time; insist on at least a six month summary. Clinic-specific data are available from the ASRM by writing or visiting the website. Many consumers use this information to compare IVF programs in their geographic area. This was not the intent of those who decided to make the data easily accessible to the general public, and such comparisons may be quite misleading. First of all, different clinics may serve quite dissimilar patient populations, with resultant differences in pregnancy rates. Other factors which impact on pregnancy rates include stimulation philosophies, the number of embryos usually replaced, and especially the mean age of the female patient.

Table 18.3 shows the SART registry data for calendar year 1996. The first column shows the total number of standard IVF cycles for that year in the United States, compared with 30,035 and 26,961 for years 1995 and 1994, respectively, but with the Canadian data included for those prior years. The IVF+ICSI column shows the increasing use over the past few years of this approach to severe male infertility, within an IVF format originally designed to deal with female tubal disease. As IVF laboratories improve culture techniques able to nourish and sustain early embryo development, GIFT procedures are becoming less frequent. Egg donor/recipient cycles, on the other hand, are limited at this point by the number of available donors, and continue to increase in proportion to the overall total. The column for cryopreserved/thawed replacements is limited to cycles not in conjunction with "fresh" embryo replacement and also excludes use of donor eggs.

Now let us consider the rows in table 18.3. The number of cycles refers to the total number of treatments initiated. Immediately below that we see the percentage of cancellations. The stimulation cycle may be canceled prior to retrieval because of poor stimulation in terms of follicular development or estrogen levels, or, conversely, because the response to stimulation was so great that there was legitimate fear of hyperstimulation, causing the cycle to be canceled because of safety reasons. Clinics vary in their philosophy regarding cancellation. Sometimes patients have insurance coverage for only one or two attempts, causing the therapy team to cancel any cycle that looks less than perfect with respect to stimulation response. At the other end of the spectrum, some programs are very sensitive to hyperstimulation risk, and will cancel for this reason. While the patient may be disappointed, usually only a small cost is involved when the cycle is canceled prior to retrieval, and another try can be initiated soon thereafter. The third row shows the actual number of retrievals and the next the actual number of embryo transfers. For IVF, this discrepancy represents the number of cases where no eggs were recovered, fertilization did not occur,

Table 18.3 1996 SART Outcomes

ART Procedure

VARIABLE	STANDARD IVF	IVG + ICSI	GIFT	DONOR	CRYO-PRESERVED
No. Cycles*	30,598	14,049	2,879	3,768	9,610
Cancellations (%)	20.3	NA	11.3	6.6	6.6
No. Retrievals	24,383	14,049	2,409	NA	NA
No. Transfers	22,664	13,195	2,379	3,345	8,661
No. Pregnancies	7,581	4,357	834	1,510	1,783
Pregnancy Loss (%)	15.9	16.6	16.3	13.3	18.3
No. Delivered	6,379	6,632	698	1,309	1,457
Deliveries per retrieval (%)	26.2	25.9	29.0	NA	NA
Singleton Pregnancies (%)	60.3	62.2	66.0	59.7	72.6
No. Ectopic Pregnancies	35	18	3	4	10
Ectopic Pregnancies/Transfer (%)	0.1	0.2	0.1	0.1	0.1
Birth Defects per Neonate (%)	1.8	1.8	1.3	1.3	1.9

*All ages and diagnoses

or embryo development failed, all resulting in the cycle having no embryos placed in the uterus. In a small number of cases, all the embryos may have been frozen because the endometrium was judged not to be receptive at that time or because the patient was at risk for hyperstimulation which would be worsened if she conceived in the fresh cycle. This fourth row shows that the actual risk of non-transfer in a cycle is low. The total number of pregnancies comes next, followed by the pregnancy loss percentage. Note that the agreed definition of pregnancy is one of ultrasonic demonstration of a fetal sac(s), and not just a transient positive pregnancy test. These latter events, known as "biochemical pregnancies" should not be included as documented pregnancies in clinic-specific statistics. The percent of pregnancy loss represents the spontaneous abortion rate in this population of patients. The number of deliveries gets us closer to the bottom line, which is the percentage of deliveries per retrieval, which is a reasonable statistic to keep in mind. Many clinics also state their percentage of deliveries per transfer, which of course, will be slightly higher than the preceding rate. Subtracting the singleton pregnancy rate from the total gives the multiple pregnancy rate, which remains rather high. As you can see, the risk of ectopic pregnancy is generally very low, and ectopics occur most often in those with preexisting tubal disease. Reassuring are the birth defect data, which are no worse than for the general population.

Table 18.4 shows the effect of female age on the IVF process, excluding any male factor diagnosis for the years 1995 and 1996. While the reduction in delivery rate per retrieval is striking for the >39 group, also note the difference between those <35 and the 35-39 population. Additionally, note the increase in cancelation rate with age. Even IVF cannot overcome the effect of age on egg quality.

Table 18.5 shows the usual format for clinic-specific reporting. Information describing the clinic program profile appears in the upper left corner. In this center we see the breakdown of the type of ART actually used. The data on the right describes the mix of patients within that program. If the clinic has sufficient numbers, stratifying the ages as shown can be useful. The age-standardized rate along with the 95% confidence interval attempts to predict the range of expected results using age as the standard. This is somewhat schizophrenic, since although consumers are admonished not to use these tables to compare clinics, data presented in this fashion actually encourage such an exercise. In the example shown, the differential of results according to age above or below 35 is less than usually expected, from which we can infer that most of those patients below

Table 18.4 Standard IVF Procedures (No ICSI) by Female Age and Excluding a Male Factor
SART Data 1995 and 1996

Patient Category	No. Retrievals	Percentage Cycles Canceled	Transfers per Retrieval (%)	No. of Pregnancies	No. of Deliveries	Deliveries per Retrieval (%)
1996						
Women < 35	12,036	12.4	93.5	3,829	3,350	31.8
Women 35-39	10,318	19.2	94.1	2,567	2,102	25.2
Women > 39	4,970	27.2	90.6	610	416	11.6
1995*						
Women < 35	11,949	11.8	91.4	3,826	3,285	27.5
Women 35-39	9,317	17.7	90.5	2,013	2,013	21.6
Women > 39	4,096	25.2	86.8	686	433	10.6

*Includes Canadian data

Table 18.5 Clinic Specific Format N.E.W. University IVF Program

Anytown, New East Wales 1996 Program Profile 1996 ART Pregnancy Success Rates

Program Characteristics		Type of ART Used[a]		ART Patient Diagnosis[a]	
SART member	Yes	IVF	81%	Tubal factor	32%
Single women	Yes	GIFT	19%	Endometriosis	12%
Gestational carrier	yes	ZIFT	<1%	Uterine factor	5%
Donor eggs shared	0%	with ICSI	21.3%	Male factor	26%
				Other factors	9%
				Unexplained	16%

Cycles using fresh empryos from nondonor eggs	Age of woman < 35	Age of woman 35-39	Age of woman > 39	Age-standardized Rate[b] (95% confidence interval)	
Number of cycles	243	229	90		
Pregnancies per cycle[c] (%)	25.3	22.6	11.1	21.5 (18.2-24.9)	
Live births per cycle[c] (%)	18.1	17.5	5.6	15.6 (12.7-18.6)	
Live births per retrieval[c] (%)	20.8	20.7	7.1	18.3 (14.9-21.7)	
Live births per transfer[c] (%)	21.4	21.5	7.3	18.9 (15.4-22.4)	
Cancellations (%)	18.5	18.5	27.5		
Average number embryos transferred	2.8	3	2.8		
Multiple birth rate per transfer					
Twins	8	10.3	1.8		
Triplets or greater	2	1.2	0		
Cycles using frozen embryos from nondonor eggs					
Number of transfers	12	11	6		
Live births per transfer[c] (%)	4/12	3/11	0/6		
Average number embryos transferred	2	2.4	2.3		
Cycles using donor eggs					
Number of fresh transfers	8	4	24		
Live births per transfer[c] (%)	3/8	1/4	41.7		
Average number empryos transferred	2.8	2.9	2.8		

* Includes only cycles using fresh embryos from nondonor eggs.[b] no data given if there were too few cycles to permit age-standardized calculations.[c] Pregnancies resulting in one or more children born alive; therefore, multiple births are counted as one.

35 were closer to 35 than to 30. Data are presented as pregnancies per cycle, live births per cycle, live births per retrieval, and live births per transfer. Note the marked reduction in the yield for patients over 39. In this particular program the number of embryos transferred shows probable adherence to SART guidelines, although because the standard deviation is not included, the actual range could be great, with some patients getting one embryo and others four or five. In the >39 group, the average number of embryos transferred reflects, in part, a reduced number available for transfer, rather than a conscious decision to limit sharply the number. Note also the increased cancellation rate with age, which contributes to a decrease in pregnancies per initiated cycle. If the live birth rate is roughly 21%, and multiple births occur in about 10% per transfer, this means that about half the time a delivery results in filling more than one bassinet. The incidence of multiple births is quite low in the >39 group. In general, the incidence of multiple pregnancies beyond twins also decreases sharply with age. We also see that in this program use of donor eggs results in a live birth of 41.7% per transfer for the older woman, with results in the younger groups expressed as fractions because the numbers are too small to generate meaningful statistics.

Table 18.6 shows another common format with which clinics express current results on an ongoing basis. The record keeping is easier than that necessary for the yearly summary shown in table 18.5, and the computer program is one which most clinics have in place, noting that data shown in table 18.5 are calculated at a central registry. In our example, we see a pyramid format which facilitates interpretation. Row B tells us that of 300 cycles initiated, 211 resulted in a retrieval, 70.33% of the time; therefore, cycles were canceled in 29.67% of cases. In only eight attempts was there failure to obtain at least one egg, for a 95.73% success rate (C). In 184 of those 202 successful retrievals, fertilization of at least one egg was achieved, giving us the 91.09% figure (D) and in 14 of those cases embryos were not replaced, probably because of failure of all of the embryos to show normal division and development (E). This led to 65 pregnancies, representing 38.24% of the replacements, 35.33% of all patients who had at least one egg fertilized, 32.18% of all patients in whom at least one egg was retrieved, 30.81% of all patients who came to retrieval, and 21.67% of all patients who started a cycle (F). This is a straightforward and easily understandable method of presenting IVF data. Row G tells us that 56 of these 65 pregnancies were either delivered or ongoing at the time the data were collected with eight ending as spontaneous abortion (H), and one as an ectopic pregnancy (I). Row J shows that multiple pregnancy occurred in 29 of the cases, which constituted 44.61 % of the clinical pregnancies.

Table 18.6 IVF Clinic-Specific Results
Calendar Year (No ICSI)

	# Total	# Age	Avg Age	%A	%B	%C	%D	%E	%F
Initiated	300	297	34.2						
Retrieved	211	209	34	70.33					
Obtained	202	200	34.1	67.33	95.73				
Fertilization	184	182	34	61.33	87.2	91.09			
Replaced	170	169	33.9	56.67	80.57	84.16	92.39		
Clin Preg	65	65	33.4	21.67	30.81	32.18	35.33	38.24	
Ongoing/ Delivered	56	56	33.5	18.07	26.54	27.72	30.43	32.92	86.15
SAB's	8	8	34.3	2.67	3.79	3.96	4.35	4.71	12.31
Ectopic	1	1	29	0.33	0.47	0.5	0.54	0.59	1.54
Multiples	29	29	33.3	9.67	13.69	14.35	15.76	17.41	44.61

One question which patients always ask is "if I don't get pregnant in the first cycle, what are my chances in the second?" A number of studies have addressed this issue, and although there is not universal agreement, the overwhelming conclusion is that there's no statistical difference in pregnancy and delivery rates when the first cycle is compared with subsequent attempts through the third or fourth cycle. That is to say that if your chances for pregnancy are 45% in the first cycle, but you end up in the 55% unsuccessful group, your chances in the next cycle are essentially what they were starting out at cycle 1. Using SART data from 1994, Meldrum et al (Fertil

Steril 1998; 69:1005-1009) documented this conclusion based on data taken from 54 centers with a total of 4,043 oocyte retrievals. Pregnancy rates were 33.7%, 27.0%, 33.9% and 27.4%, respectively for cycles one through four, with corresponding delivery rates of 23.4%, 25.9%, 16.1% and 21.0%.

We have discussed repeatedly the effect of female age on reproduction. But the data obtained from the IVF program at the Hammersmith hospital in London is stratified in such a clear fashion that looking at it is worthwhile (Hum Repro 1998; 13:403-408). Table 18.7 shows clearly the effect of the age on pregnancy rates even in women less than 31. Table 18.8 demonstrates that the age effect is essentially across the board with respect to increasing amounts of gonadotropins necessary for stimulation with a decrease in estrogen production, the number of oocytes obtained, and the number fertilized.

Table 18.7
Correlation between patient age and pregnancy rate in a first in-vitro fertilization attempt

Age (years)	No. of cycles	Canceled cycles (%)a	No. of pregnancies	Pregnancy rate per cycleb	No. of miscarriages (%)c
20-25	89	8 (12.0)	43	48.3	3 (7.0)
26-30	939	129 (13.7)	311	33.1	37 (11.9)
31-35	2089	331 (15.8)	597	28.6	73 (12.2)
36-40	1632	350 (21.4)	348	21.3	52 (14.9)
≥ 41	324	128 (39.5)	25	7.7	5 (20.0)
Total	5073	946 (18.6)	1324	26.1	170 (12.8)

[a] Cancellation rate is higher in women >35 years old (P < 0.001). [b] Pregnancy rate drops with increasing age (P < 0.01 between each age group). [c] There is no significant difference in miscarriage rates between the age groups. *Croucher et al. Human Reprod 13(2):403-408, 1998*

Table 18.8
Relationship between patient age and ovulation induction response

Age (years)	No. of ampoules of hMG	Serum estradiol concentration (pmol/mL)	Days of hMG	No. of oocytes retrieved	No. of oocytes fertilized
20-25	29.5	7376	12.9	12.3	6.6
26-30	31.6	6961	13.2	10.9	6
31-35	35.6	6625	13.1	9.6	5.2
36-40	46.3	6418	13	9.4	4.5
≥ 41	61.1	5736	13.5	6.9	3.5

hMG = human menopausal gonadotropin. Differences were statistically significant ($P < 0.01$) between all age groups and parameters except for hMG dosage and peak estradiol between the 20-25 and 26-30 year age groups. *Croucher et al. Human Reprod 13(2):403-408, 1998*

Special Methods and Maneuvers

Embryo hatching is a special maneuver utilized in IVF to address the observation that the outer membrane of the embryo (the zona pelucida) sometimes becomes thick and hard when embryos are cultured in the laboratory. Weakening this membrane by placing an acidic solution near the wall of the early embryo for a few moments and then removing it, is thought to facilitate hatching of the embryo at the blastocyst stage. There's general consensus that this is more likely to occur in embryos obtained from older women. Although many programs routinely hatch embryos in women over 37 or 39, data obtained from prospective randomized studies are sparse. There's also experimental interest in performing this procedure with the use of a special laser to create small apertures in the membrane.

Co-culture refers to placing live cells from various sources into the culture dish with the embryos. These live cells can have originated from the patient herself, as ovarian granulosa cells or endometrial cells, or can be from another species with monkey kidney cells or bovine (cow) tubal cells most often employed. The rationale behind this is a very reasonable one. Eggs and embryos in tissue culture are by definition deficient in certain growth factors present in the human tube and uterus which are important at the time of fertilization and early embryo development. Live cells from reproductive tissue from any species may supply these factors needed to support early embryo development, especially if the embryos are kept in the laboratory environment for more than two days in an effort to establish a process of selection for those embryos which appear to be most likely to continue development. Whether the source of the cells is human or another species, issues of viral transmission must be addressed. The co-culture issue has been most controversial, with some reports showing significantly improved results when co-culture is used, while others find no effect. As with hatching, any beneficial effect seems to be limited to the older patient.

Cryopreservation, or freezing, in plain language, is a technique which has been applied for many years to sperm with great success. When many embryos are developed in IVF, there may be more than would be safe to replace in the uterus because of the fear of high order multiple pregnancy. Under the circumstances, embryo freezing affords a margin of safety while at the same time allowing for another attempt at pregnancy if conception has not occurred from the fresh embryos replaced in the uterus. Additionally, the embryos can be stored for quite sometime. The couple can return years later for another pregnancy after delivery has occurred as a consequence of the embryos replaced during the initial cycle of IVF retrieval. How long can embryos remain stored? All I can tell you is that we have reported a successful delivery eight years following embryo storage. The usual success rate with frozen-thawed embryos is about half that for fresh, but there is a subtle selection process at play. Usually, the most rapidly dividing and nicest looking embryos are replaced and the second-tier embryos are chosen for storage. On the other hand, in cycles in which no fresh embryos are replaced, for reasons mentioned previously in this chapter, pregnancy rates with subsequent thaw and replacement are as good as with fresh embryos. Here, there is a different selection process taking place. Since the freeze-thaw process stresses the embryos, and only the embryos which demonstrate renewal of development and division are replaced, pregnancy rates reflect this culling. The congenital abnormality rate with babies born from embryo freezing is no different from fresh replacement.

Freezing of eggs is quite a different matter. The cell division initiated during embryonic life is put on hold until just before ovulation. The chromosomal lineup and the status of the DNA is vulnerable to the effects of ice crystal formation during the process of freezing and thawing, even when special agents are used to discourage formation of ice within the cell. We are only just beginning to reach success with egg freezing, thawing, and subsequent fertilization with embryo development culminating in delivery of a healthy child. Considering the number of women whose ovarian function is impaired at an early age because of surgery on the ovary, or chemotherapy for a variety of malignant diseases, this area of IVF needs to be pursued vigorously. An egg bank would be a truly wonderful advance, and may become a reality shortly. An alternative approach to collecting eggs is to take small pieces of ovary as a biopsy during laparoscopy. The tissue can be frozen intact and thawed later with the immature eggs being isolated and matured in tissue culture. Ovarian tissue removed at laparoscopy can be transplanted back to the patient following radiation or chemotherapy with the eggs being matured in a natural fashion or with gonadotropin stimulation.

Treatment of Male Infertility with IVF

Although tubal infertility was the first, and for years the most frequent indication for IVF, It soon became apparent that many problems of male infertility could be alleviated by placing relatively few sperm in a Petri dish with an oocyte. Many men with **oligospermia** (low count) and **asthenospermia** (poor motility) were helped with this technique as were those with **teratospermia** (poorly formed sperm), but to a lesser extent. Still, there were many patients who repeatedly failed to fertilize under laboratory conditions. In some of these cases, it was thought that the mechanisms governing sperm attachment and/or penetration of the egg were faulty, independent of the usually measured sperm parameters, and that fertilization might be possible if an individual sperm could pass the outer membranes of the oocyte.

Partial zona dissection is a technique in which a small opening is made in the outer membrane— the zona pelucida— so that a sperm might pass through this aperture and successfully fertilize the egg. One immediate problem that comes to mind is that more than one sperm might pass this natural barrier and cause fertilization of a single egg with two sperm, which would lead, of course, to a pregnancy destined to fail. The first recorded birth following intracytoplasmic sperm injection -ICSI was in 1992 (Palermo et al). The major force behind development and maturation of this technique is the group in Brussels headed by Andre Van Steirteghem. As depicted in figure 18.2, the process involves passing a very small, sharp pointed glass canula through the zona and the cytoplasmic membrane into the egg proper in order to deliver a previously loaded single sperm. All this must be done under a microscope with special micromanipulation instruments, and requires excellent hand-eye coordination. Of all the advances made since IVF was first successful in 1978, this is probably the most important in terms of the number of couples who potentially can be helped to have a child, and who would continue to be sterile otherwise. With ICSI, men with sperm counts even below 100 and with sperm having no motility have the potential to become biologic fathers. But this is not the full story. Further research demonstrated that men with even minimal sperm production in the testes who had no sperm in the distal ejaculate could also father a child when sperm was taken directly from the testes by biopsy or needle aspiration. Often, a small testicular biopsy is taken and the tissue examined under the dissecting microscope in an effort to identify sperm within the tubules of the testis. The tissue is then ground and sperm isolated. In some cases, we have more eggs than sperm, and I am reminded of one couple who had 10 eggs and eight sperm after processing; they now have twins.

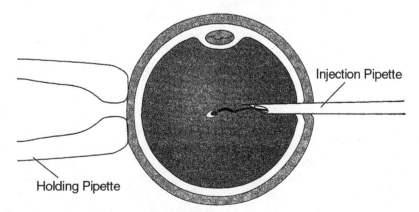

Figure 18.2   Insemination by intra-cytoplasmic sperm injection (ICSI).

Unfortunately, there are some downside issues which must be addressed. First, just to clarify, ICSI cannot compensate for poor egg quality. Sometimes failure of fertilization in the laboratory stems from egg quality, and sometimes from the sperm. In the former case, the egg may not have elaborated the proper receptors on its surface for sperm binding. If this were the only problem, ICSI would certainly circumvent this roadblock to fertilization. Most of the time, however, egg defects are multiple. Even in good hands, the egg is vulnerable to damage from the ICSI process, and about 10% of eggs will be lost in the process. Men who have azoospermia as a consequence of congenital absence of the vas may have a single mutation for cystic fibrosis with little or no other clinical evidence. Since the prevalence of any of the mutant forms of the gene is roughly one in 25 in the Caucasian population, these men who are high-risk must be screened, and the wife must be screened as well. If she is not a carrier, and he is, the worst-case scenario would be a son with the same semen picture as his father. If both are carriers, pre-implantation genetic testing and/or testing during the pregnancy can identify an affected embryo or fetus. Additionally, added experience with men who are azoospermic not because of obstruction, and some of those with severe oligospermia, has shown that there is a 5% to 13% risk for deletion of that part of the Y chromosomal responsible for sperm production. The genes on the Y chromosome involved in coding for sperm production have been identified and their location mapped on the chromosome. Therefore, these men, who are producing small amounts of sperm in the testes, run the risk of producing a son with a similar defect, but with no other known (at this time) problem. The incidence of offspring with sex chromosome deletions or additions is also somewhat higher, with an increase from about 0.2 % to 0.8%, consisting of clinical syndromes such as Turner syndrome, representing a single X chromosome female who will be short and unable to reproduce normally, and men with Kleinfelter syndrome of XXY, who have poor genital organ development and are usually sterile. There is a very small increase in other chromosomal abnormalities after ICSI. For this reason we strongly recommend that patients with azoospermia have a complete genetic work-up including a general chromosomal analysis, a special Y chromosome deletion test and screening for cystic fibrosis so that the actual risk can be determined and discussed with the couple prior to initiation of therapy. There is an alphabet soup of terminology applied to the specific methods of collecting sperm from the testicle or epididymis such as MESA, TESA, and PESA, which we will not bother to define here. Pregnancy rates are just a bit less with ICSI than with conventional IVF, but the miscarriage rate also seems to be slightly increased, probably, in part, related to the genetic discussion above. There is no increase in the rate of major congenital abnormalities aside from those related to the sex chromosomes mentioned above.

IVF and Genetics

The previous discussion leads to consideration of an exciting area on the interface between IVF and clinical genetics. Probably close to 80% of all embryonic chromosomal abnormalities can be attributed to the egg. After the first meiotic division has been completed, a polar body is extruded from the cytoplasm and comes to rest in the space between the cytoplasmic membrane and the zona pelucida (figure 18.3). This organelle contains a haploid complement of chromosomes—23, as should the egg. If the chromosomes have not divided properly, the egg and the polar body will have dissimilar numbers of chromosomes, such as 22 in one and 24 in the other. Thus, the polar body chromosomal content is essentially a reciprocal of the egg picture—if the polar body has an extra, the egg is missing one. Knowledge of this has encouraged polar body analysis for chromosomal content prior to fertilization. Identification of abnormal eggs, none of which could ever develop into a normal embryo, allows for a selective process during exposure of the eggs to sperm, which might both increase pregnancy rates and lead to a reduction in multiple pregnancies since fewer embryos would have to be transferred. Most often genetically balanced embryos at the four or eight cell stage are indistinguishable from

Figure 18.3 First meiosis

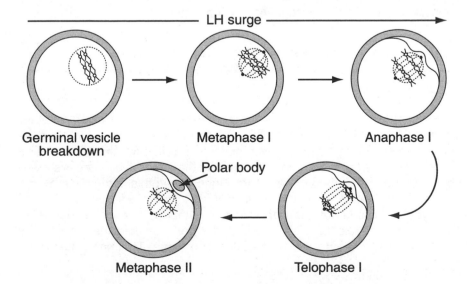

Germinal vesicle breakdown

Metaphase I

Anaphase I

Polar body

Metaphase II

Telophase I

LH surge

unbalanced embryos when viewed under the microscope. If it is known that the mother is a carrier for a genetic abnormality whose DNA code is known, such as cystic fibrosis, or Duchenne muscular dystrophy, a polar body can be subjected to what is known as a "polymerase chain reaction" in which the DNA strand of interest can be rapidly duplicated many times over until sufficient material has accumulated for analysis. In the case of a single mutant gene, if the abnormal copy were found in the polar body, the gene in the egg would be normal, and vice versa.

Biopsy of an early embryo by removing one or two of the individual cells, called blastomeres, can be performed with micromanipulation under the microscope. If done well, the risk to the embryo is minimal. That cell can be investigated with the PCR technique mentioned just above. If the issue is one of proper chromosomal number rather than DNA content, a procedure known as fluorescent in situ hybridization (FISH) can be used to ascertain whether the chromosomes most commonly involved in imbalances— numbers 13, 16, 18, 21, X and Y— are present in the right amount. Whether PCR or FISH is used, identification of abnormal embryos in couples at risk will allow us to replace in the uterus only those embryos which have tested normal. This service, known as "preimplantational genetic diagnosis " is offered in only a few programs on a clinical rather than on an experimental basis and can be prohibitively expensive. With additional experience it may be possible to prove that PGD is actually cost-effective for couples at high-risk for having a child whose total medical bills may run into millions of dollars. The insurance industry is unlikely to move quickly on this question unless pressured by legislation passed as a consequence of consumer lobbying.

SOME IVF SPECIFICS

Tubal Blockage

Patients with tubal disorders have pregnancy rates similar to other women when IVF is chosen as the solution to the problem, unless they happen to have a hydrosalpinx with collection of fluid within the tube. The world's literature is in almost total agreement that pregnancy rates are lower (by about half) and abortion rates are higher when this is the case. Some reports have indicated that this fluid has toxic effects on developing embryos, but this is not a universal finding. Other authors have suggested that intermittent release of this fluid under pressure into the uterus may flush the embryos out by mechanical action alone. Therefore, many IVF clinics will advise patients with hydrosalpinx to strongly consider laparoscopic removal of these tubes prior to initiating therapy. An additional reason to recommend removal is that they constitute a risk factor for IVF-related ectopic pregnancy. In most programs patients at highest risk for this complication are those who have had a previous ectopic pregnancy and who also presently have hydrosalpinx. Finally, during the stimulation process, high estrogen levels may cause an increased fluid collection within the tube leading to pain and difficulty in accessing the ovary for egg collection during the retrieval. A flare-up of previous infection is also possible.

So far as the argument is concerned regarding the merits of tubal surgery for repair of damaged tubes (not sterilization reversal) vs. IVF, the dust has settled, and IVF is the clear winner in terms of cost per baby, reduced ectopic pregnancy rate, and certainly less invasive therapy, except that we must now add laparoscopy for tubal removal in some patients as a pre-IVF treatment. Unfortunately the monolithic insurance carriers, even with their hordes of bean counters, have not yet done their homework. Frequently they will continue to pay for an unlimited number of tubal surgical procedures destined for failure rather than an IVF cycle.

Endometriosis

True to its chameleon nature, endometriosis may or may not have a deleterious effect on IVF results compared with other pathologies. The literature seems to be more or less divided on the question of whether IVF patients with endometriosis fare any worse than other patients, and whether the stage of the process has any bearing on the results. If you believe that the immunologic component of endometriosis is real and important, as I do, then it is not difficult to come to the conclusion that implantation may be adversely affected in endometriosis patients. On the other hand, there are a number of studies from good IVF programs which reach the conclusion that neither the presence nor the stage of endometriosis makes any difference. We seem to have our greatest success in this population when we employ suppression of ovarian function for a few months prior to stimulation. This seems to quiet down the inflammatory process, and may restore the integrin levels within the endometrium which are important for implantation.

Polycystic Ovarian Syndrome

Assessing the pregnancy rate with IVF treatment for patients with PCOS is difficult, first, because there is no real agreement as to what diagnostic criteria must be satisfied in order to reach that diagnosis. PCOS patients usually produce an enormous number of eggs when given the same protocol for stimulation as other patients. However, egg quality is usually low with many eggs either not fertilizing or failing to cleave properly. Although the pregnancy rates are about the same as for other IVF indications, the percentage of eggs showing normal fertilization and development is less. These patients are particularly difficult to stimulate, since they have a real tendency to hyperrespond and to get into trouble with severe hyperstimulation syndrome. We find that we can somewhat control the situation by using an extra long protocol of ovarian suppression prior to stimulation. This makes the patient less susceptible to hyperstimulation and may increase egg quality by reducing endogenous LH levels. Some centers find the abortion rate higher in this group, which also reflects on egg quality.

ART Alternatives to IVF

GIFT is an acronym for gamete intrafallopian transfer. In plain language, this means putting eggs and sperm directly into the fallopian tube(s). The stimulation protocol for GIFT is exactly the same as for IVF. Usually the eggs are retrieved via laparoscopy, mixed with sperm that have been processed, and returned within minutes to the fallopian tubes, as schematically outlined in figure 18.4. This is a quite different physiologic process than IVF because fertilization occurs within the tube, and the early embryo is transported in a normal fashion to the uterus for subsequent implantation. Obviously, patients with tubal disease are not candidates for GIFT. Additionally, while mild seminal defects do not disqualify a couple as GIFT candidates, severe seminal problems are best treated with ICSI. The egg retrieval can be done under local anesthesia as with IVF, using a vaginal approach, and the subsequent laparoscopy for placement of eggs and sperm into the tubes can also be performed with local anesthesia coupled with intravenous sedation. Until just a few years ago there was a wide discrepancy between pregnancy and delivery rates for IVF vs. GIFT. In our program, the delivery rates for GIFT were almost double those for IVF. But as IVF media became more supportive for early embryo development the differential narrowed, and since GIFT is more invasive and more expensive than IVF, fewer cycles of the former now are employed. The difference in pregnancy rate remained

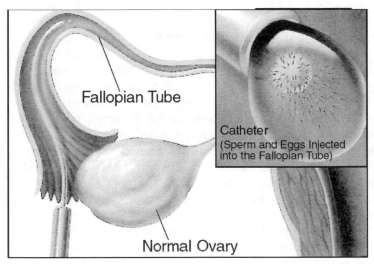

Figure 18.4   After the retrieval of the eggs from the ovary, both sperm and eggs are injected through the catheter directly into the fallopian tube. Fertilization may then take place normally in the fallopian tube.

marked for those patients in the late 30s and early 40s, and for those whose ovarian reserve testing at any age suggested egg quality problems. Since IVF involves keeping eggs and embryos out of the body for a period of days during which there is a deficiency of certain growth factors yet unmatched in our media, GIFT continues to be an attractive alternative for these women whose eggs are best described as "fragile". By pre-selecting a relatively low-yield, population for GIFT, we have driven down our pregnancy rates within this category, but when we compare apples with apples, rather than with oranges, we conclude that this is, indeed, a useful procedure under the circumstances. "Extra" eggs can be fertilized in the laboratory and cryopreserved for later use.

Related procedures are ZIFT and TET, with the former referring to transfer to the tubes of just fertilized eggs in the zygote stage, and the latter standing for "tubal embryo transfer", in which IVF is performed, embryos are created, and then transferred to the tube rather than continuing to develop in the laboratory. First popularized in Australia, these procedures are rarely performed now in the United States, since the fuss and expense of two procedures— IVF plus a later laparoscopy —is not justified by the rather small increase in yield.

Egg Donation

Egg donation has extended the borders of IVF as treatment of egg quantity/quality issues. The number of women conceiving through egg donation has been limited by the availability of suitable donors. First, being an egg donor is a much more complicated process than agreeing to donate sperm. The total commitment is a great one in terms of time, effort and discomfort. Additionally, there is a minor risk of complications arising from the stimulation process and/or the retrieval, which has no parallel for sperm collection. We have not yet found a way around the problem of poor egg quality other than egg donation, although early efforts with adding cytoplasmic material from a younger egg to that of an older woman show promise. For women with a severely compromised egg reservoir, there seems no other biologic choice. Table 18.9 lists some of the major indications for egg donation. Women may be born with no ovaries or with ovaries that contain few, if any, eggs. A minority of women with reduced egg numbers at a relatively young age reach this stage because of loss of ovarian tissue from surgery, and some have had the eggs permanently destroyed by chemotherapy and/or radiation therapy, for life-threatening disease. As a general rule of thumb, the younger the age at the time of treatment, the more likely the ovary is to recover, but this is mostly dependent on the total dose and which specific agent was used. Some women manufacture antibodies directed against their own ovarian tissue, causing an autoimmune premature menopause.

In most cases, however, reduced egg quality, more so than number, results from all of the social and financial pressures which lead to postponement of pregnancy until the late 30s and over. Other reasons for consideration of a donation include the situation where a major life-altering heritable disorder constitutes a risk to the fetus, and when surgery performed previously has made the ovaries totally inaccessible by any route. When patients have had numerous IVF attempts, with cycles being canceled because of poor response to stimulation, or poor fertilization rates and disappointing embryo development, egg donation becomes an alternative. Usually, the egg recipient, if she is still menstruating, is suppressed with GnRH analogs and cycled with exogenous estrogen and progesterone so that her endometrial lining will be receptive for embryo implantation. This requires some degree of synchronization between the egg donor and recipient. In fact, we have about a two or three day window of opportunity, which is usually sufficient to allow for embryo replacement in a fresh cycle. If, for any reason conditions are not quite right, such as the recipient's endometrial pattern or thickness as measured ultrasonically showing

Table 18.9
Indications for Egg Donation

- **Congenital Absence of Eggs**

  Turner Syndrome or Ovarian Dysgenesis
  Ovarian Agenesis

- **Acquired Reduced Egg Number or Quality**

  Surgical Treatment   Autoimmune disease
  Chemotherapy   Premature Menopause
  Radiotherapy   Advance Maternal Age

- **Other**

  Major Heritable disorders
  Repetitive IVF Failure
  Inaccessible Ovaries for Retrieval

unsatisfactory values, the embryos can be frozen and replaced in a subsequent cycle. Because the pregnancy has occurred without ovulation, it is necessary to continue hormonal support through the early part of pregnancy until the placenta becomes sufficiently developed to take over this role. Usually patients are weaned off estrogen and progesterone supplementation by the 80th day of the pregnancy. Weekly hormonal evaluation allows for a smooth transition. At that point, the pregnancy becomes an entirely normal process, with a possible exception of advanced maternal age posing problems later in the pregnancy with respect to development of hypertension, gestational diabetes, and other related problems. For this reason, it is imperative that prospective egg recipients have a thorough physical examination and biochemical testing prior to pregnancy. Because the eggs are usually those of a young woman, genetic testing such as villus biopsy or amniocentesis is unnecessary.

The egg donor may be known to the recipient as a younger relative such as a sister, or good friend but cannot be related to the husband. The majority of donors, however, are recruited by the program, and are anonymous to the recipient. Besides the usual stringent medical and psychologic screening, an attempt is made to match as much as possible for ethnic group, height, eye and hair color, and general appearance. The family history is particularly important, and the donor may need specific testing for ethnically related diseases. The ASRM has guidelines for donor programs. The age of the egg recipient has little to do with the outcome of the pregnancy so long as she is healthy. Specifically, miscarriage rates reflect the age of the egg donor rather than the recipient. Although some programs have no age limitation for the recipient, many programs have upper ceiling of about 48 or 50 years, and most programs will not take known egg donors over 35, and recruited egg donors over 33. A vigorous screening program helps to insure a high yield; most good programs report pregnancy rates in excess of 40% per cycle, with 50% not uncommon. In many cases these young healthy women stimulate easily, and produce a high number of high-quality eggs which leads to many cycles having the option for embryo freezing, which will increase the pregnancy yield per egg retrieval. Thus, a couple has a backup in case of failure to conceive in the fresh cycle, if miscarriage has occurred, or if another child is desired. Great consideration must be given to the number of embryos replaced since the eggs are usually from a population of healthy oocytes, and multiple pregnancy is less well tolerated in a 44 year old woman than would have been the case even five or ten years previously. In many programs psychologic screening for the egg recipient as well as for the donor is mandatory. If it is elective in the program you are considering, by all means take advantage of the opportunity to discuss your anxieties and expectations while at the same time learning how to deal with the frustrations of the process in general and failure in particular.

Some programs offer a financial incentive to patients who are willing to give up some of their eggs to another patient. In general, I am not in favor of this plan. First, the patient, by giving up a proportion of her eggs, decreases her chances for pregnancy, both in the fresh and potential cryopreserved cycle. From the recipient's point of view, she would rather receive eggs from a healthy, young donor than from an infertile patient.

Gestational Carrier Pregnancy

If egg donor pregnancy is one side of a biologic record, then gestational carrier pregnancy is the flip side. In this situation the infertile patient has ovaries which work, but she has no uterus or one which will not reproductively function. She may also have a medical condition of a serious nature which is reasonably stable in the non-pregnant state, but which could become life threatening during pregnancy. The most common examples are shown in table 18.10. The Rokitansky syndrome is one in which the vagina and uterus are absent at birth. A vagina can be surgically created, or the patient may be able to use dilators to produce a functioning pouch sufficient for satisfactory sexual activity, but the uterus is a different matter. Theoretically speaking, presently available surgical techniques will permit transplantation of the uterus from one woman to another, but because immunosuppressants would probably have to be used to avoid rejection, this is entirely unrealistic. The uterus may be lost because of hysterectomy done for cancer, or life-threatening bleeding associated with pregnancy, such as when the placenta does not separate after delivery. The DES syndrome sometimes causes so much uterine distortion that reproduction for these women is impossible. Other women have such extensive myomas, that myomectomy becomes impossible, and hysterectomy needs to be performed. Although most women with cervical incompetence can have the cervix stitched closed during pregnancy, this is not always the case. Uterine scar tissue, usually a consequence of a previous delivery with retained placental tissue and infection, can not always be overcome by corrective surgery.

Serious medical conditions that might lead to the need for a gestational carrier include poorly controlled diabetes mellitus, and the various autoimmune diseases such as systemic lupus, and impairment of function of those organs most stressed during pregnancy— the liver, heart, kidneys, and lungs. Unlike egg donation, a carrier cannot be anonymous. If she is married, her husband must be supportive, and her children need to understand what is happening. For that reason, there is a great deal of contact with the team psychologist, who first has to match the parties, and who then must make certain that the interactions at all levels are good ones. More than any other IVF ancillary service, carrier gestation places an enormous administrative and time burden on the team. The carrier is artificially cycled with the biologic mother while the latter goes through the process of stimulation and egg retrieval. Egg retrieval sometimes is difficult because of previous surgery and present anatomy. Therefore, a retrieval may be done via vaginal ultrasonic approach as usual, or ultrasonically through the bladder or abdominal wall, or laparoscopically. As is the case with an egg recipient, the carrier, who usually has had her own natural menstrual cycle suppressed, will be supplemented hormonally until the placenta comes on line.

You may have read the term "gestational surrogate". We have objected to this in our medical writing since this may tend to confuse the process with surrogate parenting. That is a process by which a woman agrees to insemination with the sperm from the husband of the infertile woman. Thus, the surrogate not only delivers the child, but also has a genetic contribution. This is in contradistinction to a gestational carrier, who is genetically inert from the pregnancy. Both of these solutions require pre-treatment consultation with a knowledgeable lawyer. Contracts must be drawn up and certain "what-if" scenarios explored. Among these are the issue of multiple gestation/embryo reduction, and genetic testing with its consequences, depending on the age of the biologic mother. For these and many other reasons, there are few programs which offer the service. Over the past decade, we have had 93 women in our program, and although the total amount of time and expertise spent is enormous, the emotional reward of helping a couple achieve their biologic pregnancy is worth it. As you might guess, it is far from easy to recruit gestational carriers. Most of the time, they are relatives or extremely close friends of the biologic parents. The birth certificate is a potentially sticky issue; check into the laws in your state, if a program is available. In Pennsylvania, where I practice, I sign an affidavit that the child is that of the biologic parents, and the birth certificate is signed in their favor; otherwise, they would have to adopt their child with added expense and time heaped on an already intricate process.

Table 18.10
Reasons for Gestational Carrier
Pregnancy

- **Congenital Uterine Absence**

  (Rokitansky Syndrome)

- **Surgical Removal**

DES	Cervical Incompetence
Myomas	Congenital Abnormality
Adenomyomas	Uterine Scar Tissue

- **Medical Condition**

Diabetes Mellitus	Heart Disease
Immunologic Disease	Kidney Disease
Liver Disorders	Pulmonary Insufficiency

19

A Summary: Algorithms of Care

An algorithm can be defined as a set of rules used to solve a problem in a finite number of steps. Put within an everyday working context rather than a dictionary framework, algorithms help us to deal with scenarios that start with "if this, then that". Algorithms are helpful guides in teaching situations and for elaboration of standard operating procedures. On the other hand, slavish devotion to algorithms dulls the thinking process, and funnels patients with unusual problems into pre-selected treatment patterns. With the thought in mind that we are dealing with a two edged sword, let us summarize some of the diagnosis-specific treatment protocols presented earlier in this book.

Figure 19.1 shows the general approach to infertility according to the age of the female partner. For women 35 or younger, the procedures within the box represent the initial approach to infertility of twelve months or more. Our philosophy is that women over 35 with at least six months of infertility should be screened with a clomiphene citrate challenge test. Treatment thereafter is mainly dependent on the results of that survey. Younger patients with any evidence of ovulatory disturbance or infertility of unknown etiology should be screened as well.

Figure 19.2 summarizes the approach when anovulation is suspected or when endocrine factors are at play. Thyroid dysfunction is common in women within the reproductive age group, but in actuality is a rare cause for infertility. Women with androgen excess are likely to have some form of polycystic ovarian syndrome. Today, the diagnosis is made more often

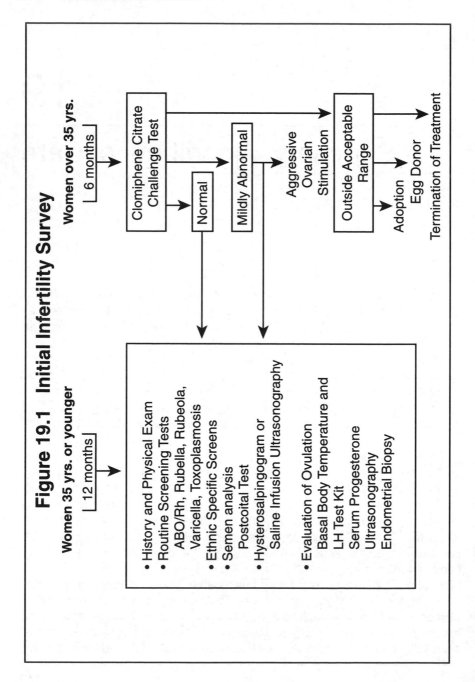

Figure 19.1   Initial Infertility Survey

Figure 19.2 Anovulation/Endocrine Factors

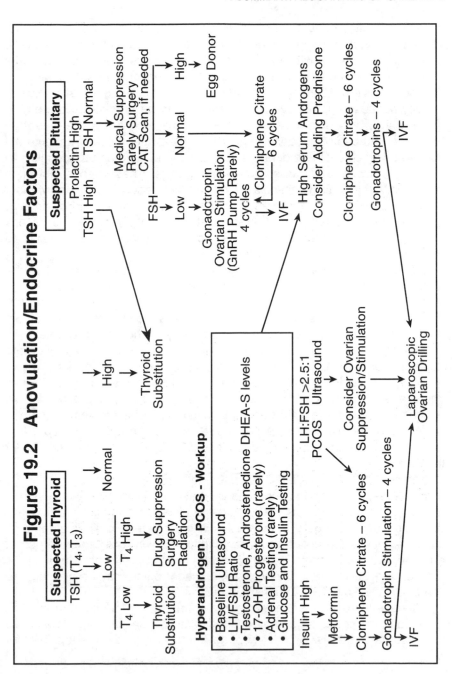

according to ultrasound criteria rather than by traditional endocrine testing. The insulin story is important, and I believe that testing for insulin levels, and treating patients with insulin sensitizing agents who show elevated peripheral resistance to insulin, is a great step forward in dealing with this common problem. Clomiphene citrate is almost always the first choice of therapy because it is relatively inexpensive, can be administered orally, is non-invasive, and is associated with a multiple pregnancy rate less than that seen with use of gonadotropins. Slightly less than 50% of patients will conceive with clomiphene citrate, and use beyond six months adds little to the pregnancy rate. Laparoscopic ovarian surgery has been a last ditch approach, but actually is associated with a high response rate, and without the risk of multiple pregnancy seen with use of gonadotropins. Considering the cost of those agents and the associated laboratory tests, laparoscopy as a primary approach in patients not conceiving or responding to clomiphene citrate is quite reasonable.

Figure 19.3 outlines how we deal with tubal factors. Blockage of the tube at the uterine junction can be treated with catheter techniques in the radiology department or in the operating room with the expectation of 30% or more pregnancy rate by one year. Distal disease, on the other hand, must be treated surgically, usually by laparoscopy. Although cure rates are excellent for minimal disease, most infertile patients present with moderate to severe tubal pathology, which gives poor pregnancy yield along with a relatively high ectopic pregnancy rate. As each year goes by, IVF rates improve, and today there's no question that medically speaking, IVF is superior to tubal surgery for dealing with infertility. The problem in the real world is that the insurance carriers have not yet learned this lesson, and they continue to fund hopeless repetitive tubal surgical procedures rather than IVF.

The algorithm for dealing with suspected endometriosis when infertility is the issue is really quite simple. As illustrated in figure 19.4, the keystone is a laparoscopic diagnosis and surgical eradication of implants with sharp dissection, electrosurgery, or laser all having equal results. The golden time for pregnancy is the first six to nine months following surgery, and use of any suppressive drug therapy such as Lupron or danazol is counterproductive during this interval. Gonadotropins may be helpful, and IVF or GIFT is saved as a final solution.

Although the uterus is the workhorse of pregnancy for nine months, it is not a common cause for infertility. Congenital anatomical variants such as the bicornate uterus or the septate uterus may be responsible for

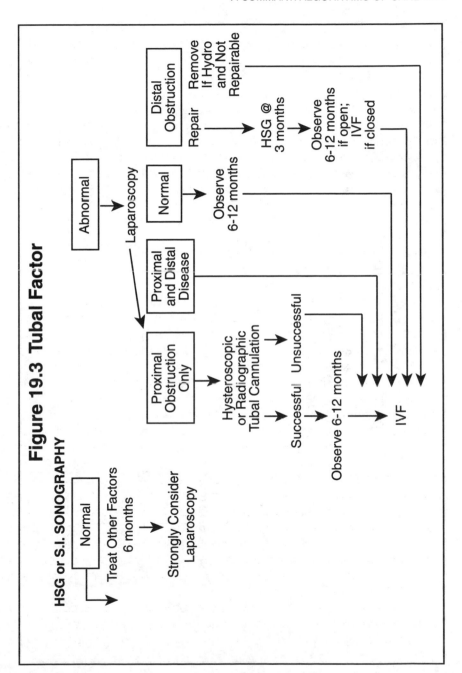

Figure 19.3 Tubal Factor

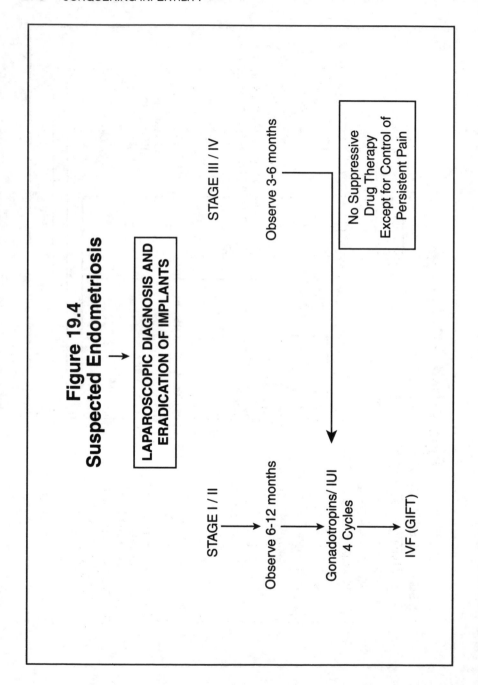

Figure 19.4
Suspected Endometriosis

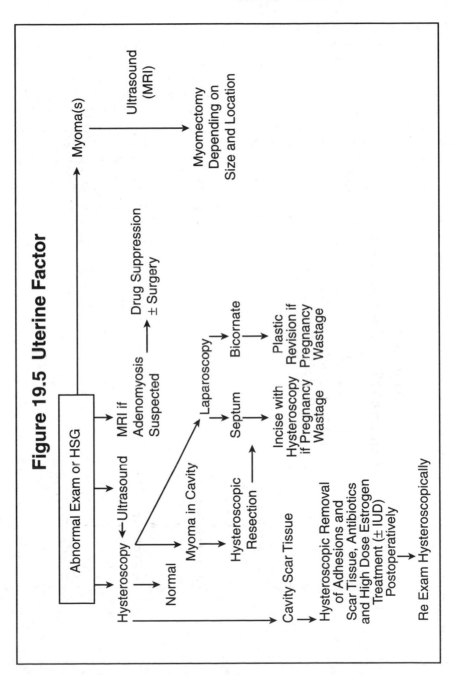

Figure 19.5 Uterine Factor

pregnancy loss but not infertility. Acquired problems such as myomas, or scar tissue, can usually be surgically corrected with good results (figure 19.5).

Perhaps nothing is more frustrating for the infertile couple than to be told that all the tests are normal, and that the reason for infertility remains unknown. Figure 19.6 deals with this issue. With a good work-up, less than 10% of couples should fall into this category. Even if this is the case, assisted reproductive technology, such as IVF or GIFT, may solve the issue without really knowing why the treatment worked. This may be intellectually less than totally acceptable, but the end result of pregnancy constitutes a quite satisfactory bottom-line.

Figure 19.7a deals primarily with male factor testing and figure 19.7b shows treatment pathways for various seminal problems. Remember that sperm count varies tremendously from day-to-day, and that any seemingly minor illness can depress the semen analysis for 70 days thereafter. While IVF with ICSI is a dramatic cure, not all patients need this extreme approach. Direct treatment of the male by a competent urologist with correction of infection or varicocele may be all that is necessary. Intrauterine insemination is yet another attractive treatment modality which is neither invasive nor overly expensive.

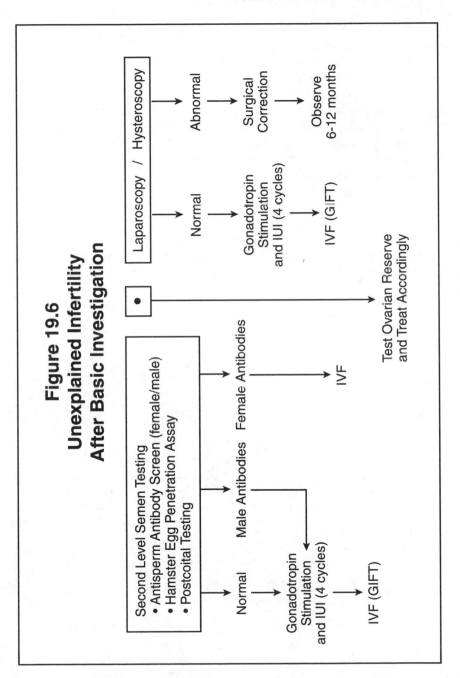

Figure 19.6
Unexplained Infertility
After Basic Investigation

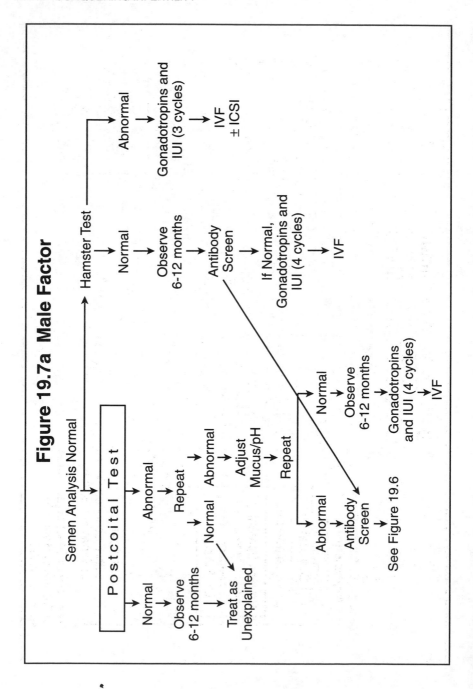

Figure 19.7a Male Factor

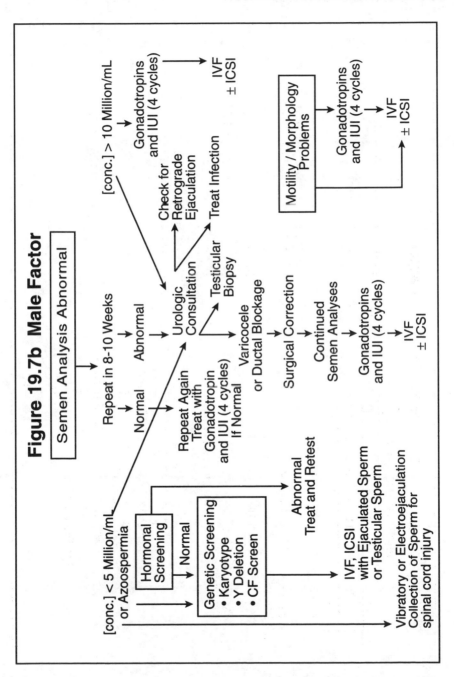

Figure 19.7b Male Factor

20

Resolution

The word "resolve" can be used to mean that a decision has been made for a particular course of action; it can also describe the determination with which we deal with adversity. An equally acceptable meaning is the ability to bring a situation to a conclusion. All in turn apply to the infertile couple. First, they resolve to conquer infertility by entering the treatment program. Resolve is needed to endure the stresses of protracted therapy. At some point resolution is needed, either with the birth of a child, or the realization that treatment has failed.

The advent of assisted reproduction has given couples choices never dreamed possible even a few years ago. Although sperm donation has a century of history, egg donors, gestational carriers and surrogate parenting are new entries. Embryo freezing, egg, and testicular tissue cryopreservation for subsequent use are now clinically possible. The science fiction of just a few years ago has become standard routine in the laboratory. Preimplantation evaluation with the possibility of genetic splicing to correct DNA coding errors is on the horizon. Following successes in large mammals, the prospect of human cloning looms on the horizon. It is a thorny issue that will not go away, and should be dealt with by society in general and not by legislative bodies. Whether these technologies are to become standard practice within the community is up to society rather than bureaucrats who may make a decision within a knowledge vacuum and who are subjected to pressure by a vocal minority. The population of infertile patients must take the lead in educating the general public in order to reach the conclusion that infertility is indeed a major disability with interruption of one of life's basic processes. Childless couples cry out for tolerance of procedures which might not be acceptable to their critics, but which are desperately needed for reproductive success.

Development of in vitro fertilization techniques with quite reasonable pregnancy yields should have been responsible for even a greater reduction in fallopian tube surgery than has been seen. Only the continued stubborn stand taken by the insurance industry is responsible for operations which are invasive, sometimes dangerous, and which offer little for success, but which are performed because they are covered by insurance and IVF is not.

Every fertility specialist has committed to memory hundreds of vignettes, each unique, and each involving intense emotions ranging from despair to elation. The thread common to all of these is an attitude of resolve, determination to endure temperature charts, scheduled intercourse, injections, and postoperative pain. Fortunately, more couples than ever before can now achieve a happy resolution. Innovative approaches to ovulation disorders can achieve pregnancy in a high percentage of cases. In vitro fertilization pregnancy rates for women less than 40 now approach 40% per cycle. Although the initial population served by this technique was that of tubal infertility, immunologic infertility and endometriosis also respond well to IVF. It is male fertility, however, which has had the biggest boost in recent years from special IVF techniques. When intrauterine insemination has failed or is unrealistic because of the severity of seminal impairment, ICSI comes to the rescue with pregnancy rates almost equal to those of regular IVF. We still need to do a lot of work in the area of improving egg quality and in embryo selection. This will allow us to reduce the number of embryos transferred to the uterus and thus reduce the multiple pregnancy rate associated with IVF, which we all agree is unacceptably high.

When you enter a treatment protocol, you should have more than a cursory idea of what tests are necessary, what treatments are to be employed, and the expected pregnancy rate per cycle of treatment. By all means, do some reading, ask many questions, and find a therapy team that is willing and able to communicate with you. A second opinion may be necessary; don't worry about bruising the ego of your present therapist. Often, a fresh eye may generate a different approach, or, reassure all involved that the present course is correct.

We remain quite limited in our ability to improve egg quality when this is the issue. Postponement of pregnancy in our society becomes more marked with each succeeding survey. Perhaps in the not so distant future, egg banks will be established as a safeguard against age-related infertility for the female. Until then, it is important that women understand that this reproductive hazard may have no symptoms. I do not think that it is radical to suggest that women have dynamic ovarian testing as part of the yearly gynecologic visit when they reach the middle 30s and wish to postpone their reproductive option.

Many patients state that they are determined to have "my own baby" or none at all. If you find yourself in this situation, be aware that this attitude need not be written in stone. Very often strong opinions about basic philosophies change during infertility treatment when choices become limited. We live in a society in which many people acquire instant families through re-marriage. Most have no trouble in learning to love their new children. Parenting is an art quite distinct from the ability to procreate. For some people, resolution means remaining childless and diverting energies to careers, humanitarian services, and other interests. Some choose to become foster parents and others will adopt. Sometimes marriages seem to grow stronger because of this adversity, but it is also true that some marriages are destroyed by this problem. In a world subject to overcrowding, the anguish of infertility is frequently ignored. The pain can be intense and of long duration. I hope this book has proven informative, and helpful to all who are attempting to conquer infertility.

Index